Chemical Warfare Toxicology

Volume 2: Management of Poisoning

Issues in Toxicology

Series Editors:
Professor Diana Anderson, *University of Bradford, UK*
Dr Michael D. Waters, *Michael Waters Consulting, N. Carolina, USA*
Dr Timothy C. Marrs, *Edentox Associates, Kent, UK*

Advisor to the Board:
Dr Alok Dhawan, *Ahmedabad University, India*

Titles in the Series:

1: Hair in Toxicology: An Important Bio-Monitor
2: Male-mediated Developmental Toxicity
3: Cytochrome P450: Role in the Metabolism and Toxicity of Drugs and other Xenobiotics
4: Bile Acids: Toxicology and Bioactivity
5: The Comet Assay in Toxicology
6: Silver in Healthcare
7: *In Silico* Toxicology: Principles and Applications
8: Environmental Cardiology
9: Biomarkers and Human Biomonitoring, Volume 1: Ongoing Programs and Exposures
10: Biomarkers and Human Biomonitoring, Volume 2: Selected Biomarkers of Current Interest
11: Hormone-Disruptive Chemical Contaminants in Food
12: Mammalian Toxicology of Insecticides
13: The Cellular Response to the Genotoxic Insult: The Question of Threshold for Genotoxic Carcinogens
14: Toxicological Effects of Veterinary Medicinal Products in Humans: Volume 1
15: Toxicological Effects of Veterinary Medicinal Products in Humans: Volume 2
16: Aging and Vulnerability to Environmental Chemicals: Age-related Disorders and their Origins in Environmental Exposures
17: Chemical Toxicity Prediction: Category Formation and Read-Across
18: The Carcinogenicity of Metals: Human Risk Through Occupational and Environmental Exposure
19: Reducing, Refining and Replacing the Use of Animals in Toxicity Testing
20: Advances in Dermatological Sciences
21: Metabolic Profiling: Disease and Xenobiotics
22: Manganese in Health and Disease
23: Toxicology, Survival and Health Hazards of Combustion Products

24: Masked Mycotoxins in Food: Formation, Occurrence and Toxicological Relevance
25: Aerobiology: The Toxicology of Airborne Pathogens and Toxins
26: Chemical Warfare Toxicology, Volume 1: Fundamental Aspects
27: Chemical Warfare Toxicology, Volume 2: Management of Poisoning

How to obtain future titles on publication:
A standing order plan is available for this series. A standing order will bring delivery of each new volume immediately on publication.

For further information please contact:
Book Sales Department, Royal Society of Chemistry, Thomas Graham House, Science Park, Milton Road, Cambridge, CB4 0WF, UK
Telephone: +44 (0)1223 420066, Fax: +44 (0)1223 420247
Email: booksales@rsc.org
Visit our website at www.rsc.org/books

Chemical Warfare Toxicology
Volume 2: Management of Poisoning

Edited by

Franz Worek
Bundeswehr Institute of Pharmacology and Toxicology, Munich, Germany
Email: franzworek@bundeswehr.org

John Jenner
Defence Science and Technology Laboratory, Porton Down, UK
E-mail: jjenner@dstl.gov.uk

Horst Thiermann
Bundeswehr Institute of Pharmacology and Toxicology, Munich, Germany
E-mail: horstthiermann@bundeswehr.org

ROYAL SOCIETY OF CHEMISTRY

Issues in Toxicology No. 27

Print ISBN: 978-1-78262-803-3
Two-volume set print ISBN: 978-1-78262-804-0
PDF eISBN: 978-1-78262-807-1
EPUB eISBN: 978-1-78262-808-8
ISSN: 1757-7179

A catalogue record for this book is available from the British Library

Published by The Royal Society of Chemistry,
Thomas Graham House, Science Park, Milton Road,
Cambridge CB4 0WF, UK

Registered Charity Number 207890

For further information see our web site at www.rsc.org

Printed in the United Kingdom by CPI Group (UK) Ltd, Croydon, CR0 4YY, UK

Preface

The international community has undertaken great efforts to abandon chemical weapons. This endeavour resulted in an agreement, the Chemical Weapons Convention, which entered into force on 29th April 1997 and has been ratified and implemented by, at present, 192 state parties. This convention bans the production, stockpiling and use of chemical weapons, and up to now more than 90% of the declared stockpiles have been destroyed.

Despite this great success, recent events have demonstrated the continuing threat of chemical warfare agents. The repeated homicidal use of the chemical warfare nerve agent sarin in Syria in 2013, the suspected perpetual use of chlorine in Syria and most recently supposed attacks with sulphur mustard in Syria and Iraq illustrate the capacity and intent to deploy chemical warfare agents against military units and civilians.

The decreasing likelihood of state use of chemical weapons and increasing interest of terrorist groups in using toxic chemicals as weapons will have a great impact on the spectrum of future threat agents, modes of dissemination and, consequently, preparation of countermeasures for military forces and the general population.

The intention of this book, *Chemical Warfare Toxicology* is to provide an overview of the toxicological properties of relevant chemical warfare agents including nerve, blistering and lung agents, and opioids. The main focus of this multi-author book is to give an update on recent findings for a broad range of topics related to chemical warfare agents. This includes chapters on new insight into the toxicology and pathophysiology of nerve, blistering and lung agents, established and experimental means for diagnosis and verification of exposure to chemical warfare agents, novel approaches for the treatment of nerve agent poisoning, and an update on the use of, and human exposure to, chemical warfare agents.

Issues in Toxicology No. 27
Chemical Warfare Toxicology, Volume 2: Management of Poisoning
Edited by Franz Worek, John Jenner, and Horst Thiermann

Published by the Royal Society of Chemistry, www.rsc.org

The chapters of this book are authored by experts covering the broad range of topics related to chemical warfare agents. The authors are regarded as authorities in the fields of toxicology and military medicine, presenting state of the art information for academic, clinical and governmental audiences.

The first volume, *Fundamental Aspects*, covers the fundamentals of the toxicology of nerve agents and vesicants whilst the second volume, *Management of Poisoning*, describes aspects of the treatment after exposure to these and other chemical warfare agents.

References to Material in The National Archives

Over the years, many of the reports produced as accounts of Government research have found their way into the public records of the originating nation. In the USA the military reports relating to Chemical Warfare Agents that are available for public review are indexed by the Defense Technical Information Center (DTIC) and can be accessed *via* the website http://www.dtic.mil. In the UK, similar reports are held in The National Archives and can be accessed through the website http://www.nationalarchives.gov.uk. In this book, the references to reports in The National Archives (UK) are referenced using the system used by the archive, so that each report can be searched for and located using its unique reference number. The number consists of a two letter code identifying the contributing department and a series number. The series number may consist of two numbers separated by a forward slash. A piece may be a single item or a collection of documents. If the reference is part of a collection, an additional item number may be added to identify the document within the piece. For example, WO 1234/56/7 would indicate item 7 of piece 1234/56 entered into the archive by the War Office.

Issues in Toxicology No. 27
Chemical Warfare Toxicology, Volume 2: Management of Poisoning
Edited by Franz Worek, John Jenner, and Horst Thiermann

Published by the Royal Society of Chemistry, www.rsc.org

Contents

Volume 1: Fundamental Aspects

Issues in Toxicology No. 27
Chemical Warfare Toxicology, Volume 2: Management of Poisoning
Edited by Franz Worek, John Jenner, and Horst Thiermann

Published by the Royal Society of Chemistry, www.rsc.org

Volume 2: Management of Poisoning

CHAPTER 1

Treatment of Nerve Agent Poisoning

HORST THIERMANN*[a], NADINE AURBEK[a], AND FRANZ WOREK[a]

[a]Bundeswehr Institute of Pharmacology and Toxicology, Neuherbergstraße 11, 80937 Munich, Germany
*E-mail: horstthiermann@bundeswehr.org

1.1 Introduction

Therapy of nerve agent poisoning is a challenge for clinical toxicologists, specialists in intensive care units, medical doctors and all other medical personnel. The reason for this is manifold. Generally, nerve agents belong to a larger group of organophosphorus (OP) compounds whose single members present a high variability in physicochemical, toxicodynamic and toxicokinetic properties. Moreover, different types of absorption, *e.g.* inhalation, percutaneous exposure and oral ingestion, may affect the kinetics of poisoning dramatically. Hence, the onset of signs and symptoms may vary substantially and valuable time for an initial treatment may be lost if no adequate triggers to treat are available. Therapeutic approaches, therefore, may be complicated by simultaneously ongoing reactions within the body, *e.g.* aging, which frequently reduce the size of the therapeutic window in a dramatic way.

On the other hand, handling of victims itself may be a challenging problem, as secondary contamination may pose a life threatening risk for personnel

Issues in Toxicology No. 27
Chemical Warfare Toxicology, Volume 2: Management of Poisoning
Edited by Franz Worek, John Jenner, and Horst Thiermann

Published by the Royal Society of Chemistry, www.rsc.org

and lead to contamination of medical facilities. This may also affect transport facilities, thereby preventing rapid transfer to the hospital.

Further uncertainties may arise from inadequate information about antidotal therapy as recommendations basing on a high level of evidence are not available. Thus, one has to rely on appropriate extrapolation from animal studies or poisoning with similar compounds, *e.g.* OP pesticides. Later, alternative therapeutic strategies used in intensive care units have been discussed and may be helpful for patient oriented treatment. All of these aspects will be discussed in the following chapter.

1.2 OP Compounds

1.2.1 General Remarks That Are Relevant for Therapy

The generic structure of OP compounds was first described by Schrader in 1937.[1,2] Among the huge variety of compounds, only some of them were identified as potentially useful military nerve agents. Today, they are listed in the Annex on Chemicals, Schedule 1 of the Chemical Weapons Convention (http://www.opcw.org/chemical-weapons-convention/). The G-series agents include GA (tabun), GB (sarin), GD (soman) and GF (cyclosarin). The V-series agents (VX, CVX and RVX) were developed after World War II. All of them are chiral compounds with at least one (two in the case of soman) optically active centers. The isomers of nerve agents show marked differences regarding their stability in biological systems and their human toxicity. Due to big differences in their chemical structures nerve agents differ widely in their physiochemical properties (for a comparison see Volume 1, Chapter 3). All nerve agents are liquids at room temperature with boiling points higher than water. Their different volatility and vapor pressure lead to their classification into volatile (G-series) and non-volatile (V-series) nerve agents.[3–5] Nevertheless, modification of a single substance is possible, *e.g.* thickened soman is persistent while aerosolized VX can pose a very serious inhalational threat. Thereby, the physicochemical properties are determinative for military use and for exposure scenarios. Sarin for example will persist in soil in convenient climates (sunshine, slight wind, 15 °C) for several hours only, while V-agents may persist for a longer period in the soil, *e.g.* at cold temperature (−10 °C) and dry climates for up to 4 months.[6]

The military intention to find OP compounds with enhanced human toxicity was in contrast to the civilian attempt to reduce human toxicity of highly effective OP pesticides. OP compounds are used increasingly as pest-control agents in the agricultural industry, especially in the developing world. Today, OP pesticides that are highly toxic to humans are widely banned in developed countries, but a high variety of OP pesticides are still available and causing human OP poisoning, especially in third world countries. Mainly in the context of suicide attempts, OP pesticides account for about 3 million intoxications per year, leading to death in up to 260 000 cases.[7,8] A high number of studies on pesticide poisoning are available. However, differences between compounds regarding toxicity, physicochemical properties, reactions with target enzymes and metabolism affect the clinical course. In addition, different exposure scenarios, *e.g.* most frequently suicidal attempts involving ingestion of multiple lethal dose, 50% (LD_{50})'s, result in mega-dose poisoning. Hence, findings from OP pesticide poisoning need careful assessment before being translated to nerve agent poisoning.

1.2.2 Toxicology of OP Compounds

1.2.2.1 Toxicokinetic Aspects Relevant for Therapy

Exposure to OP compounds may be by ingestion, percutaneous absorption, inhalation or injection. In military or terrorist scenarios, exposure to vapor, aerosol or droplets of nerve agents appear relevant. Thus, exposure may either occur after inhalational or percutaneous absorption. As details on the toxicokinetics are discussed in Volume 1, Chapter 3 and 8, only a few aspects directly relevant for therapy are mentioned here. For further information please also refer to John *et al.*[9]

First, absorption through mucous membranes and distribution of volatile G-type nerve agents, *e.g.* tabun, sarin and soman, is expected to be very fast, thus leading to a very rapid onset of cholinergic crisis. Hence, treatment has to be started immediately, at best at the time of exposure. To address this special requirement during the Cold War, military forces equipped their personnel with autoinjectors for self and buddy aid that were to be applied as soon as a soldier suffered from the first signs and symptoms of cholinergic crisis. This strategy, nowadays, has to be expanded to scenarios of unexpected use of nerve agents in asymmetric military conflicts and terrorist attacks. In such scenarios, the majority of victims reaching medical facilities[10] are expected to be exposed to doses of less than 5 LD_{50}'s of the respective agent. Accordingly, the rapid binding and hydrolysis of G-agents by endogenous mechanisms will result in a comparatively short residence time in the systemic circulation. In conclusion, very early administration of effective antidotes is important and lifesaving. Long term therapy will only be necessary in severely poisoned victims or in patients developing complications as a result of an initial cholinergic crisis.

In contrast, after percutaneous exposure as typically expected in V-agent poisoning, toxic blood levels will develop more slowly. Development of a subcutaneous depot has been hypothesized from which the agent may be distributed to other compartments for a prolonged time. Initially, ongoing absorption of the agent results in distribution in the systemic circulation and binding to various proteins. This is reflected by a slow decrease of acetylcholinesterase (AChE) and butyrylcholinesterase (BChE) activities, and delayed agent transfer into tissues. As a consequence, systemic signs of poisoning become obvious after a time lag, which may be several hours. Hence, early diagnosis of exposure is essential to initiate antidote therapy prior to onset of life threatening signs (see Chapter 5). Toxic agent concentrations may persist for hours or even days and require intensive treatment for several days. In these patients, careful therapeutic monitoring is of greatest importance in order to avoid too early discontinuation of antidotal administration.

1.2.2.2 Toxicodynamics of Nerve Agents

1.2.2.2.1 Reactions of Nerve Agents with AChE. OP compounds, *i.e.* nerve agents and pesticides, inhibit serine esterases such as AChE (E.C. 3.1.1.7), BChE (E.C. 3.1.1.8), carboxylesterases and neuropathy target esterase (NTE; E.C. 3.1.1.5) by covalently binding to a serine residue of the enzyme's catalytic center. Inhibition of AChE is regarded as the main mechanism for nerve agent toxicity. The velocity of AChE inhibition is dependent on the chemical properties of the individual nerve agent and can be described by the second order inhibition rate constant (k_i; Table 1.1). AChE–OP compound conjugates determine further compound specific reactions that affect toxicity and therapeutic options (Chapter 5, Figure 5.2). The first reaction, spontaneous hydrolysis, often denoted as spontaneous reactivation, appears of minor importance for nerve agents, but may contribute to several specific features in OP pesticide poisoning. The second, a dealkylation reaction, denoted as aging, results in a stable complex, which can no longer be reactivated by nucleophiles under physiological conditions. From a therapeutic point of view, the aging velocity is decisive for the therapeutic window in which OP residues can be cleaved from the inhibited AChE by nucleophiles. AChE is located in synapses in close vicinity to receptors in the central and peripheral nervous system (nicotine and muscarine receptors), sympathetic and parasympathetic ganglia (nicotine receptors), and parasympathetic nerve endings

Table 1.1 Inhibition rate constants of OP compounds derived from erythrocyte AChE from humans and various animal species.[a]

	Inhibition rate constant k_i (10^6 M^{-1} min^{-1})			
	Guinea pig	Swine	Cynomolgus monkey	Human
G-agents				
Cyclosarin	160	268	735	439
Soman	45.9	75.8	250	193
Sarin	12.9	16.6	40.7	39.8
Tabun	3.8	5.0	12.0	18.2
V-agents				
VR	159	188	396	458
VX	81.7	44.3	119	115
OP pesticides				
Paraoxon-methyl	0.19	0.84	0.53	1.1
Paraoxon-ethyl	0.45	1.1	4.6	3.3

[a]Data from Worek and Thiermann.[13]

(muscarine receptors), neuromuscular junctions (nicotine receptors), as well as on membranes of red blood cells. AChE hydrolyzes acetylcholine (ACh), which mediates chemical synaptic transmission at cholinergic synapses. AChE is one of the most effective enzymes known, hydrolyzing approximately 10 000 ACh molecules per second. Inhibition of this decisive enzyme results in disturbance of neurochemical transmission, thereby initiating the clinical picture of cholinergic crisis (see below). For assessment of the toxicological effects of OPs as well as the therapeutic effectiveness of antidotes it has to be considered that AChE is encoded by a single gene,[11] resulting in the same functional structure of its active center in all tissues.[12] However, there are species differences in AChE structure, which, in part, lead to markedly different kinetic properties. This finding needs adequate appreciation when assessing new therapeutic approaches as most of the results are derived from animal experiments.

These differences also impact therapeutic measures and will be mentioned later again when discussing effective plasma concentrations of oximes.

1.2.2.2.2 Binding of Nerve Agents to Other Targets. As highly reactive compounds, nerve agents are able to interact with a variety of proteins in the body. Such binding reactions affect the toxicity of nerve agents as binding may reduce the amount of free nerve agent (*e.g.* binding to BChE and carboxylesterases) and chemical modifications of other proteins may induce pathophysiological effects (*e.g.* binding to AChE and NTE). The inhibitory potency of nerve agents towards AChE and BChE is in the same order of magnitude.[14] Therefore, BChE may scavenge nerve agents in the systemic circulation, thereby preventing or delaying distribution to cholinergic synapses. Indeed, this effect is the subject of research efforts directed towards producing human BChE in various expression systems in larger quantities. Unfortunately, BChE is inhibited by nerve agents and can only react stoichiometrically. Hence, large amounts of this bioscavenger need to be administered to achieve a therapeutic effect.[14] Accordingly, this therapeutic approach appears only rational for treatment of poisoning with highly toxic nerve agents, but will have only a marginal effect in poisoning with OP pesticides, which show lower toxicity and much higher plasma levels. In a similar way, although there are comparably high amounts of albumin present in the plasma, due to the low affinity, scavenging of nerve agents by this protein does not substantially contribute to an antidotal effect. At best, in severe poisoning, nerve agent adducts at albumin residues can be used for biomedical verification.[9] Similarly, chemical modifications of other proteins and enzymes generally require higher concentrations than expected in nerve agent poisoning for substantial interactions.[9] On the other hand, research is directed towards enhancing the hydrolytic activity of human (*e.g.* paraoxonase[15]) or bacterial (*e.g.* phosphotriesterase[16]) enzymes in order to develop catalytic bioscavengers (see Chapter 2). A further approach consists of the development of small molecule scavengers that are able to bind to or hydrolyze nerve agents.[17] These approaches are far from clinical use at present and are therefore not discussed here in detail.

1.3 Protective Measures and Decontamination

As outlined in Volume 1 Chapter 3 (see also Table 3.4), nerve agents are characterized by high human toxicity (Table 1.2).

Due to this high toxicity, the general population and accordingly medical personnel are at risk when exposed to low concentrations of nerve agents. An estimate of toxic levels that are relevant for medical personnel can be derived from the Acute Exposure Guideline Levels (AEGLs) developed by the US Environmental Protection Agency (USEPA) (Table 1.3). These values represent threshold exposure limits for the general public and are applicable to various emergency scenarios. These threshold values allow protection of the general public, including sensitive sub-populations (*e.g.* infants and children), but not hypersensitive or hyper-susceptible individuals.

The high toxicity of nerve agents, reflected by the AEGL values, emphasizes the need for effective protection of first responders and medical personnel. In view of the difficulty in detecting such low levels of agent, an anticipated dissemination of nerve agents calls for full protective gear. Especially for rescue operations in highly contaminated areas and activities in wet environments, butyl rubber suits are recommended. For other activities, semi-permeable suits are considered adequate and have the advantage of lower physical burden but provide limited protection against aerosols. Full protective gear is needed for as long as the absence of nerve agents is not verified.

Protective gear can impair the handling of patients, making procedures such as oro-tracheal intubation and venous puncture very difficult, and requires additional training.[19,20]

Not only medical personnel performing pre-hospital treatment must be protected. It is of decisive importance to protect medical facilities, including hospital personnel and other patients. It was one of the most important lessons learned from the Tokyo sarin attack that toxicologically relevant nerve agent concentrations may arise when patients exposed to even comparably low doses enter medical facilities without being adequately decontaminated.[21]

Table 1.2 Human lethality of nerve agents after percutaneous and inhalation exposure.

	LD_{50}			
	Sarin	Soman	Tabun	VX
Percutaneous[b] (μg kg^{-1})	24–28 × 10^3	18 × 10^3 (LD_{low})[a]	14–21 × 10^3	86 (LD_{low})[a]
Inhalation[c] mg min m^{-3} (vapor)	100	50	400	10

[a]LD_{low}: minimal amount of a chemical that has been shown to be lethal.
[b]Data from John *et al.*[9]
[c]Data from Sidell.[18]

Table 1.3 Acute exposure guideline levels of nerve agents.[a,b]

	10 min	0.5 h	4 h
	AEGL-1 (mg m^{-3})		
Tabun	0.0069	0.0040	0.0014
Sarin	0.0069	0.0040	0.0014
Soman/GF	0.0035	0.0020	0.0007
VX	0.00057	0.00033	0.00010
	AEGL-2 (mg m^{-3})		
Tabun	0.087	0.050	0.017
Sarin	0.087	0.050	0.017
Soman/GF	0.044	0.025	0.0085
VX	0.0072	0.0042	0.0015
	AEGL-3 (mg m^{-3})		
Tabun	0.76	0.38	0.14
Sarin	0.38	0.19	0.070
Soman/GF	0.38	0.19	0.070
VX	0.029	0.015	0.0052

[a]Three AEGLs have been defined as follows: "AEGL-1 gives the airborne concentration of a nerve agent above which it is predicted that the general population, including susceptible individuals, could experience notable discomfort, irritation, or certain asymptomatic nonsensory effects. However, the effects are not disabling, transient and reversible upon cessation of exposure. AEGL-2 gives the airborne concentration of a nerve agent above which it is predicted that the general population, including susceptible individuals, could experience irreversible or other serious, long-lasting adverse health effects or an impaired ability to escape. AEGL-3 gives the airborne concentration of a nerve agent above which it is predicted that the general population, including susceptible individuals, could experience life-threatening health effects or death".

[b]Data from the US Environmental Protection Agency http://www.epa.gov./oppt/aegl/pubs/results31.htm; search performed July 2015.

Decontamination itself is defined as reduction or removal of chemical agents by physical means or by chemical neutralization or detoxification. Decontamination efficacy is time dependent and at least provisional decontamination should be performed immediately after contamination.[22] In most cases, one will not know if and at which part of the body a nerve agent contamination occurred, making undressing and whole body decontamination mandatory for effective removal of agents from the body surface.

Generally, liquid and contaminated soil/dust have to be removed by any means as fast as possible. Percutaneous absorption is dependent on the barrier qualities of the stratum corneum, which is determined by factors including location on the body, thickness, and the presence and number of hair follicles.[23] Hair follicles in particular appear critical for nerve agents to bypass the corneal barrier.[23]

Various decontamination products are available on the market. Corrosive decontaminants, *e.g.* sodium hypochlorite (bleach), are highly effective but due to their irritating and damaging effects on skin are not recommended for skin decontamination.

At present, Reactive Skin Decontamination Lotion (RSDL) appears to be an appropriate decontaminant for humans in order to perform spot decontamination. RSDL was introduced in several military forces as a skin decontamination product to remove or neutralize chemical warfare agents, T-2 toxin and many pesticide related chemicals from the skin. It received a license from the US Food and Drug Administration (FDA) and has received a European CE Mark and an Australian TGA license (http://www.rsdl.com/skin-decontamination/rsdl/). However, RSDL is not approved for use in the eyes or in wounds, as it may impair wound healing.[23]

In conclusion, a decontaminant for skin, eye, wound and mucous membrane decontamination is not available at present.

If eyes are suspected to be contaminated, extensive rinsing should be performed with, ideally, physiological solutions, *e.g.* 0.9% saline solution, but sterile or at least clean water could be used. However, care should be taken in order to prevent eye damage due to vigorous procedures.

Equally, wounds should be extensively rinsed with sterile physiological solutions. Here, however, a thorough balance may be necessary in order to prevent secondary damage due to exposure to great amounts of fluid in large wounds.

In conclusion, effective personnel decontamination combines an immediate spot decontamination, *e.g.* by RSDL, followed by undressing and whole body decontamination by showering with plenty of water or soapy water at ambient temperature.

1.4 Clinical Picture of Nerve Agent Poisoning

1.4.1 Acute Nerve Agent Poisoning

The failure of inhibited AChE to hydrolyze the neurotransmitter ACh results in endogenous ACh flooding followed by over-stimulation of muscarinic and nicotinic ACh receptors. In general, the severity of signs of poisoning is dependent on the level of synaptic AChE inhibition. The localization of muscarinic and nicotinic synapses in the nervous system allows the differentiation between nicotinic and muscarinic mediated symptoms of OP poisoning.[24]

1.4.1.1 Central Nervous System

Central manifestations of ACh accumulation are mediated by nicotinic and muscarinic receptor over-stimulation and result in headache, confusion, ataxia, tremor, psychosis, convulsions, coma and central respiratory depression.

1.4.1.2 Autonomic Nervous System

1.4.1.2.1 Sympathetic Nervous System. Nicotinic ACh receptors are located at paravertebral sympathetic ganglions. In response to the preganglionic stimulus, postganglionic neurons release noradrenaline, which activates adrenergic receptors on the peripheral target tissues. Accordingly, overstimulation of

ACh receptors of the sympathetic nervous system induces a short lasting initial adrenergic/noradrenergic stimulation, which leads to secretion of adrenaline from the adrenal medulla and may cause transient tachycardia and increased blood pressure in the initial stage of poisoning.[25] In this phase, a systemic administration of atropine may aggravate tachycardia.

1.4.1.2.2 Parasympathetic Nervous System. ACh is the primary neurotransmitter of the parasympathetic nervous system and neurotransmission occurs in two stages: when stimulated, the preganglionic neuron releases ACh into the synaptic cleft, which acts on nicotinic receptors of postganglionic neurons; the postganglionic neuron then releases ACh to stimulate the muscarinic receptors at the target organs. The axons of presynaptic parasympathetic neurons are usually long and the ganglions located in or near their target organ. Muscarinic effects of OP poisoning occur at cholinergic end-organs resulting in vagal over-stimulation and cholinergic crisis with hypersecretion of secretory glands (rhinorrhea and bronchorrhea), smooth muscle contraction (bronchoconstriction, miosis and abdominal cramps) and, subsequent to the initial stage of poisoning, effects on the cardiovascular system (hypotension, bradycardia and arrhythmia). Hence, the parasympathetic nervous system overrides sympathetic effects and dominates during the typical cholinergic crisis.[25]

1.4.1.3 Somatic Nervous System

Nicotinic ACh receptors are located at muscle endplates of skeletal muscles. Consequences of AChE inhibition at neuromuscular junctions are muscle fasciculations and hyperreflexia followed by muscle weakness and depolarization block with reduced tendinous reflexes. Paralysis of the respiratory muscles finally may result in death.

1.4.1.4 Conclusion

The development of signs and symptoms of nerve agent poisoning varies depending on the dose and the route of exposure of the nerve agent. Local signs and symptoms (*e.g.* miosis after vapor exposure to the eyes or fasciculations at the exposure site after liquid exposure) may precede systemic effects (Chapter 5, Figure 5.3).

Different receptor systems are involved in the development of cholinergic crisis. The cause of death in the acute phase of nerve agent poisoning is respiratory dysfunction due to a combination of effects on respiration:

- Muscarinic induced bronchorrhea and bronchoconstriction (muscarine receptors)
- Impaired respiratory central drive (muscarine and nicotine receptors)
- Nicotinic mediated progressive respiratory muscle paralysis (nicotine receptors)

1.4.2 Intermediate Syndrome

Wadia *et al.*[26] reported on neurological manifestations in OP insecticide poisoning. The group described a phenomenon arising later, during atropine therapy, characterized by proximal limb weakness, areflexia and cranial nerve paralysis.[26] Later, in 1987, Senanayake and Karalliedde[27] defined an intermediate syndrome occurring in about 20% of patients poisoned by OP pesticides.[28] This syndrome typically develops 2–4 days after exposure when the signs of acute cholinergic syndrome are no longer obvious. It is characterized by weakness of respiration (diaphragm, intercostal muscles and accessory muscles including neck muscles) and proximal limb muscles. Such a syndrome has not yet been reported in cases of nerve agent poisoning.[29] However, in 1981, Weger and Szinicz[30] found in dogs, 3 weeks after having recovered from soman poisoning, a weakness of neck muscles making them unable to lift their heads. This feature was accompanied by a decrease in cholinesterase activity. Hence, there are no conclusive data ruling out the development of an intermediate syndrome in nerve agent poisoning. One should be cautious in order to avoid overlooking such a life threatening complication.

1.4.3 Organophosphate Induced Delayed Neuropathy

Organophosphate induced delayed neuropathy (OPIDN) is characterized by a symmetrical sensorimotor axonopathy that tends to be most severe in long axons. It usually causes weakness of peripheral muscles in the hands and feet with a variable sensory impairment that generally occurs 7–14 days after exposure to several OP compounds.[29,31,32] OPIDN is initiated by a sufficiently strong and extensive inhibition of the NTE. It appears that even aging of the inhibited NTE is necessary to induce OPIDN.[32] However, much higher nerve agent concentrations are necessary to inhibit NTE than those occurring during nerve agent poisoning in humans. Thus it appears unlikely that nerve agents possess the capability to cause OPIDN in survivors of poisoning.[29]

1.5 Pretreatment

One knows that poisoning by several nerve agents, *e.g.* soman and tabun, cannot be treated sufficiently with atropine and oximes. To enable survival of soldiers during an attack with these agents, the concept of medical prophylaxis was developed and belongs to the NATO doctrine.[33] This approach is based on early animal experiments[34,35] showing that administration of a carbamate prior to the nerve agent analog DFP resulted in convincing protection rates.[36] Finally, this finding was translated to human use and pyridostigmine bromide was approved by the FDA on 5th February 2003 for prophylaxis against the nerve agent soman (http://www.fda.gov/Drugs/EmergencyPreparedness/BioterrorismandDrugPreparedness/ucm130342.htm). This concept aims to carbamylate synaptic AChE partially, thus preventing phosphylation by a nerve agent. After clearance of unbound nerve agent from the body, decarbamylation of AChE is expected to result in a small fraction of active AChE in the synaptic cleft, resulting in improved survival. It was estimated that carbamylation of 20–40% of AChE should be sufficient for a relevant protective effect. To this end, a daily oral dose of 3 × 30 mg pyridostigmine is required prior to nerve agent exposure.[33] Although a variety of side effects may occur under such treatment, fewer than 1% of the US troops had to discontinue pyridostigmine administration during the Gulf War Conflict.[22] Meanwhile, it was shown experimentally that after pyridostigmine prophylaxis, soman may not lead to a complete inhibition of AChE. It appears that a very small portion of AChE remains active under such conditions,[37] which might be decisive for survival. It is notable that the pretreatment approach only has relevance for military personnel and a few selected first responders.

1.6 Differences Between Nerve Agent and OP Compound Pesticide Poisoning

The acute toxicity of nerve agents and OP pesticides is induced by inhibition of AChE. Nevertheless, there are several decisive differences between nerve agent and pesticide poisoning that have to be considered when translating research results on the therapeutic effectiveness of oximes. Generally, only a few compounds fulfilled the requirements to be developed as nerve agents. Principally, they were selected as chemical warfare agents because of their higher toxicity towards humans. This is reflected by the low lethal doses, which are a result of their high inhibitory potency (the k_i of nerve agents is in the range of 10^{-7} to 10^{-8} *versus* 10^{-3} to 10^{-6} for pesticides). Accordingly, the toxic concentration of a nerve agent in the body is generally lower compared with pesticides. In addition, inhalation and percutaneous exposure are most likely with nerve agents while severe pesticide poisonings occur after suicide attempts with oral uptake of large doses. This leads to resorption of huge amounts of the poison, and results in high and persistent concentrations in the body. Moreover, in order to optimize the efficacy of pesticides, commercial products contain different solvents and stabilizers. These ingredients may induce additional toxic effects and may aggravate the toxicity of neat agents. As an example, a study by Eddleston *et al.* may be mentioned,[38] in which a possible contribution of solvents to the toxicity of dimethoate in minipigs was shown.

The aforementioned factors may effect therapeutic strategies and appear to influence dramatically the assessment of oxime effectiveness. Generally, in most clinical reports, cohorts of patients were formed who were poisoned by different pesticides. Although data on severity of intoxication are mostly presented, clear stratification is hampered due to different and often unknown pesticide doses, different times to first treatment and access to hospital care, and different strategies of treatment, *etc.* Moreover, most studies included only small numbers of patient, which almost prevents the formation of sub-groups with comparable parameters. Thus, it is no surprise that oxime effectiveness (see below) in OP pesticide poisoning is still a matter of debate. It is a challenge to extract the relevant results from current pesticide research and translate them to nerve agent poisoning.

A further important aspect is the number of poisonings. In general, single patients poisoned by OP pesticides need treatment, while the homicidal use of nerve agents may result in a mass casualty scenario. Accordingly, individual patient care in well equipped intensive care units cannot be expected in nerve agent exposure scenarios. Triage, artificial ventilation and drug administration are the major tasks to ensure survival of the maximum number of patients. The capacity for artificial ventilation will for sure be the limiting factor and requires the availability and early administration of effective antidotes to restore the respiratory drive, to reduce bronchoconstriction and bronchorrhea and to improve respiratory muscle function.

1.7 Therapeutic Regimen of Nerve Agent Poisoning

1.7.1 General Considerations

Signs of nerve agent induced cholinergic crisis are characteristic. They may develop rapidly, especially after inhalational exposure and may frequently lead to comatose and seizing patients with severe respiratory distress resulting in death within minutes.[10,18] Hence, even the suspicion of OP poisoning necessitates the immediate start of antidotal treatment. Aside from clinical signs, ongoing inhibition of AChE, especially from percutaneous nerve agent exposure, may be an appropriate trigger to treat (see Chapter 5) in cases with delayed onset. In general, the identity of the nerve agent will be unknown initially, requiring a standardized emergency therapy to counteract the cholinergic crisis. Individualized therapy based on the nerve agent and severity of poisoning may follow later on. The standard post exposure antidotal treatment of OP poisoning includes a muscarinic receptor antagonist, usually atropine, an oxime as a reactivator of OP inhibited AChE, usually pralidoxime or obidoxime, and an anticonvulsant, usually diazepam, in combination with further symptomatic treatment, *e.g.* artificial ventilation.

1.7.2 Atropine

Atropine represents the cornerstone in antidotal treatment of OP poisoning. Adequate administration facilitates effective suppression of life threatening muscarinic symptoms.

Atropine (racemic D-hyoscyamine/L-hyoscyamine) belongs to the family of tropane alkaloids that are biosynthesized in flowering plants of the Solanaceae family, *e.g.* *Atropa belladonna* (deadly nightshade), *Datura stramonium* (thorn apple) and *Hyoscyamus niger* (henbane).[39] Its pharmacological action results from competitive antagonism of ACh at muscarinic (M1–M5) receptors. Although atropine lacks selectivity for muscarinic receptors, there is a hierarchy of relative sensitivity, which is most probably determined by the degree of parasympathetic tuning of the single end organs as well as the contribution of intramural neurons and reflexes.[40] At low doses, salivary and bronchial secretion and sweating are depressed. Larger doses result in dilatation of pupils, inhibition of the lens to near vision and blocking of vagal effects on the heart leading to an increased heart rate. A further increase in dose results in inhibition of micturition and decrease of gut tone and motility.[40] Still higher dosing leads to inhibition of gastric motility and particular secretion.[40] A certain consideration of atropine's effects on the central nervous system is necessary. At doses used in clinical routine (0.5–1 mg), only mild vagal excitation due to stimulation of the medulla and higher cerebral centers is expected in adults. Higher doses, however, are associated with more prominent central nervous system effects, finally resulting, at the highest concentrations, in depression associated with circulatory collapse and respiratory failure.

Accordingly, atropine poisoned patients present with peripheral and central signs of poisoning that allow clinical diagnosis.[25] The peripheral anticholinergic syndrome is dominated by tachycardia, inability to sweat and dry mucosa. Frequently, the head is red, gastrointestinal tone is reduced with disturbances of defecation. Most striking is a nearly complete lack of sweat at the armpits and the typical mydriasis accompanied by loss of accommodation. Initially, patients may present tired with somnolence. This behavior will turn to agitation, restlessness, irritability, disorientation (time, location) and hallucination (optical) or delirium.[25] These symptoms may be followed by possibly repetitive epileptic seizures and deep coma. Spontaneous muscle twitching and choreoathetoid movements can be observed, occasionally. Children are more sensitive than adults and especially vulnerable for epileptic seizures accompanied by hypoxic residuals.[25]

Hence, atropine therapy requires a balance between beneficial and adverse effects. As the antidotal mechanism is based on competition, the atropine dose has to be carefully adjusted to clinical sings, thereby avoiding adverse side effects.

1.7.2.1 Self and Buddy Aid

Due to the threat of an attack with nerve agents during the Cold War, soldiers were equipped with atropine to be administered *via* autoinjectors for self and buddy aid. It was agreed that autoinjectors would be filled with 2 mg atropine sulfate, a dose that is still regarded as standard today. This decision was based on the finding that 2 mg appeared to be reasonably effective while higher doses are expected to produce embarrassing effects on troops with operational responsibilities.[18] At the dose of 2 mg, an increase in heart rate of about 35 beats per min, dry mouth, dry skin, mydriasis and disturbance of accommodation may be expected. These effects might last for 4–6 h with the exception of blurred vision, which may persist for about 24 h.[18] In particular, the signs of reduced sweating need careful consideration, as this may contribute substantially to disability during exhausting tasks on a military mission or during a complex mass casualty scenario. The administration of three autoinjectors (6 mg) may result in mild mental disorder (*e.g.* drowsiness or forgetfulness), together with other peripheral signs of poisoning, when administered in the absence of nerve agent poisoning.[18] Accordingly, many armed forces are equipped with autoinjectors containing about 2 mg of atropine sulfate. It depends on national doctrine whether the autoinjectors contain atropine alone, *e.g.* AtroPen, 2.0 mg atropine sulfate, or whether they are additionally filled with an oxime, *e.g.* pralidoxime [antidote treatment-nerve agent autoinjector (ATNAA), containing 600 mg pralidoxime and 2.1 mg atropine] or obidoxime (ATOX II, containing 220 mg obidoxime and 2 mg atropine sulfate), and also depends on how many autoinjectors are planned to be distributed to each soldier. In many countries, three autoinjectors containing a total of 6 mg atropine sulfate, frequently together with an oxime, are used. In general, it is recommended to use the first autoinjector when the initial signs appear. After 5–10 min, the second autoinjector should be administered if no improvement occurs, followed by the third after a further 5–10 min in the case of no improvement. In severe cases, all three autoinjectors should be administered at the same time. This medical strategy, however, presupposes training of the soldiers in handling of autoinjectors, awareness of the signs of poisoning and distribution of autoinjectors to the soldiers. In many countries, this distribution is dependent on an assessment of the military situation and, therefore, needs an adequate nerve agent threat level for delivery in time. In the civilian environment, autoinjectors will not be of relevance for self and buddy aid.

1.7.2.2 *Treatment by Medical Specialists*

In a mass casualty scenario with a nerve agent, a huge number of patients may arrive simultaneously in conditions that may be described as "poor", "moderate" or "mild", as well as patients who think that they have been poisoned but have not (worried well).[10] Thus, dosing of atropine needs adequate assessment and the first challenge would be to differentiate the worried well, to whom no atropine should be administered.

One lesson learned from the Tokyo sarin attack, when people were exposed to nerve agent vapor, is that most patients are expected to suffer from miosis and headache (about 99 and 83%[41]). Further eye effects may be eye pain, blurred vision, dim vision, conjunctival injection and tearing.[41] As the eye is a first path of entry and directly exposed to nerve agent vapors in unprotected individuals, these effects may be induced locally without prior distribution in the body. The headache mentioned above may also be in part related directly to the local spasm of eye muscles. In such cases, local application of atropine or homatropine should be considered.[18]

Independent from the route of exposure, systemic signs have to be treated systemically with atropine. The lessons learned from the Iran–Iraq war[10] and the Tokyo sarin attack[41] show that the velocity of adequate atropinization is decisive. This is underlined by studies on OP pesticide poisoning showing a clear benefit from rapid atropinization (for a review see ref. 42 and 43). At present, the regimen suggested by Eddleston and colleagues[44] appears appropriate. It consists of starting with 2 mg followed by an assessment after 5–10 min and consecutive doubling of the dose (4–8 to 16–32 mg) if there is no clinical improvement. The criteria for adequate atropinization could be (i) clear lung on auscultation, (ii) heart rate >80 beats per min, systolic blood pressure >80 mmHg, (iii) dry axilla, and (iv) pupils no longer pinpoint.[44] As there is an ongoing discussion on the appropriate dose, an alternative concept, basing on experiences from Iran, is presented. In this concept, it is suggested to start with 2 mg in mild, 2–10 mg in moderate and 10 mg in severe cases, maintaining a status of mild to moderate atropinization until the patient becomes asymptomatic.[45,46]

One important aspect when suggesting fast atropinization needs to be considered. In several textbooks, it is stated that hypoxic patients may be at risk of developing ventricular tachycardia or fibrillations when treated with atropine and, thus, atropine should be avoided if possible before resuscitation with oxygen or artificial ventilation.[47] In a recent review, however, it was convincingly shown that atropine induced life threatening dysrhythmias in OP pesticide poisoned patients are rather unlikely.[48]

In conclusion, fast and adequate atropinization is key for survival and should be initiated as soon as possible. In situations in which intramuscular (i.m.) or intravenous (i.v.) administration is not possible intraosseous administration should be considered.

After reaching adequate atropine levels, atropine should be administered *via* an i.v. line in severe cases. Experiences from patients with pesticide poisoning allow the conclusion that in the post acute phase, a dose of 0.5–1 mg h^{-1} should be sufficient,[25] although the dose should be adjusted to clinical conditions. Generally, however, it appears that patients with severe nerve agent poisoning tend to require lower doses of atropine than patients with severe OP pesticide poisoning.[46] In any case, the criteria mentioned above can be used even later on during a stay at the intensive care unit or a field hospital to ensure adequate atropinization. However, it should be considered that, especially during a later stage of cholinergic crisis, "over-atropinization" should be avoided. Foroutan[10] found that several patients may develop a "atropine immunization", resulting in the requirement of higher dosages of atropine each day; these patients occasionally went on to die.[10] A similar observation was also seen in OP pesticide poisoning treated in the toxicological intensive care unit in Munich in the 1980s and 1990s. Here, after stopping atropine, it appeared that patients re-developed cholinergic sings and even needed higher atropine doses for antagonism. As there was uncertainty, these high doses were not stopped until BChE activity increased substantially (personal communication, Prof. Zilker). Such high dosing most probably would not have been necessary if atropine weaning had been performed more resolutely.

However, atropine is not suitable to counteract symptoms mediated by overstimulation of nicotinic ACh receptors. Hence, nicotinic signs of OP poisoning are treated by restoration of AChE function by oximes. Thereby, the efficacy of oximes to reactivate OP inhibited AChE depends on the structure of the inhibiting agent and the oxime. As oxime and atropine are less effective to counteract convulsions, an anticonvulsant complements the pharmacological antidotal management of OP poisoning.

1.7.3 Oximes

1.7.3.1 General Background

As early as 1955, researchers in the USA[49] and UK[50] published independently that the pyridinium compound pralidoxime (*i.e.* 2-PAM iodide) efficiently reactivated phosphorylated cholinesterases. Only 3 years later, Namba and Hiraki came to the conclusion "Hithertoo, alkylphosphates poisoning has been treated mainly by atropine, but now atropine is replaced by pralidoxime".[51] Research programs on oximes were started in the 1950s and are still going on. Initially, the focus was on the identification of an oxime that is effective against soman. For more than two decades the main focus has been on the development of broad spectrum oximes covering the range of structurally different nerve agents. Unfortunately, no such compound has been identified so far.[52,53] At present, only pralidoxime, obidoxime, TMB-4 and HI-6 are in clinical use. Pralidoxime is most extensively used (*e.g.* in the USA, UK and Asian states) while obidoxime is in use in several European countries (*e.g.* Germany and The Netherlands).[54] TMB-4 is only used in autoinjectors in Israel.[55] HI-6 has already been tested in a few selected OP pesticide poisoned patients[56] and is stockpiled in autoinjectors by a few nations (*e.g.* Canada and Sweden). Unfortunately, HI-6 is not commercially available at present. Several programs are running in order to develop HI-6 as a licensed drug. It should be mentioned that pralidoxime and obidoxime are licensed in several countries (*e.g.* pralidoxime by the FDA in the USA and obidoxime by the BfArM in Germany) for civilian use. The huge number of other oximes developed during the last few decades are far away from clinical use and are therefore not considered in this chapter.

Oximes are pyridinium compounds that break the covalent bond between OP compounds and AChE by nucleophilic attack, thus restoring enzyme function to OP inhibited AChE (for review see ref. 57 and 58). This reaction takes place at the active center at the bottom of an approximately 20 Å deep and 4 Å wide gorge[59,60] that is lined with aromatic amino acids[61] that interact with inhibitors and reactivators. These spatial constraints and the structure of the most bulky oximes do not provide optimal geometry for fast reactivation.[57] Thus, until now, a clear structure–activity relationship could not be established for oximes and individual OP compounds.[52,62–64] Moreover, as mentioned above, there are remarkable species differences in susceptibility to inhibition, spontaneous reactivation and aging that also affect reactivation substantially.[65–68]

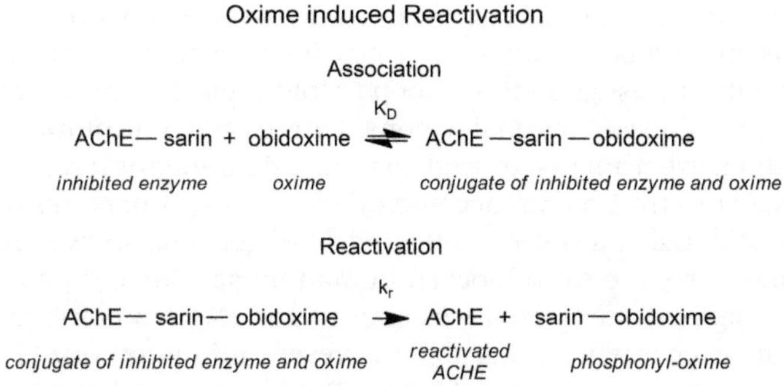

Figure 1.1 Reactivation process of inhibited AChE by oximes, exemplified by the nerve agent sarin and obidoxime.

The oxime induced reactivation consists of two steps (Figure 1.1).[57,69] First, there is a bimolecular reaction of the inhibited enzyme, *e.g.* sarin inhibited AChE, with an oxime, *e.g.* obidoxime, resulting in a conjugate of the inhibited enzyme and the oxime. The velocity of this reaction depends on the concentration of both reactants. As the concentration of AChE in the body is constant, an increase in the oxime concentration can lead to saturation, *i.e.* transformation of all inhibited enzymes into resulting Michaelis–Menten complexes. The oxime concentration necessary for saturation is dependent on the type of the inhibited enzyme as well as on the properties of the oxime, *e.g.* its affinity, which can be expressed by the dissociation constant K_D (*e.g.* 31 μM for obidoxime for sarin inhibited AChE[70]). In the second step, the reactivated enzyme is liberated. This reaction follows first-order kinetics and can be described by the reactivity constant k_r (*e.g.* 0.937 min^{-1} for reactivation of sarin inhibited AChE by obidoxime[70]), which can be translated easily into the reactivation half time. Notably, the velocity of this reaction, although dependent on the properties of the oxime (reactivity), is completely independent of the oxime concentration. The clinical relevance of this consideration is given by the fact that oxime concentrations resulting in about 50–70% saturation are sufficient. Higher concentrations only marginally enhance reactivation but may increase adverse events.[69] For assessment of the clinical effectiveness of a certain oxime, the reactivation half time of an oxime and the concentration necessary to achieve this half time have to be considered. It may be assumed that the shorter the reactivation half time at a tolerable oxime concentration, the more effective the oxime.

1.7.3.2 *Effectiveness of Oximes in Nerve Agent Poisoning*

From clinical experience of patients poisoned with parathion and treated with obidoxime, it is known that a reactivation half time of about 5 min is sufficient to achieve substantial reactivation if the poison load in the patient is not too high.[57,69,71–77] This reactivation half time can safely be achieved with ~10 μM obidoxime in parathion/paraoxon poisoned patients.[69,71,73,78] Moreover, it was clearly shown that substantial reactivation was associated with improvement of neuromuscular transmission, indicating clinical benefit.[78–81] For ethical reasons, comparable investigations are not possible in patients poisoned by nerve agents. Hence, it appears rational to consider results from complex organ tissues and animal experiments. Indeed, in mouse diaphragms it was shown that oxime induced reactivation was accompanied by recovery of paraoxon blocked muscle force.[82,83] Using a comparable model, Seeger *et al.* showed that 30 µM HI-6 was able to restore sarin blocked human muscle force.[84] Finally, in percutaneously exposed minipigs it was shown that HI-6, in combination with cooling of the exposure site, was able to prevent inhibition of AChE by VR[85] and VX.[86] In these animals, signs of VX or VR toxicity did not become visible if HI-6 was administered as soon as red blood cell AChE activity was inhibited to 30% of its baseline activity.[86,87]

The species differences mentioned above have to be taken into account when estimating effective oxime concentrations in humans (see Section 1.2.2.1). Kinetic *in vitro* studies showed almost identical kinetic properties of erythrocyte, brain and muscle AChE when inhibited by OP and reactivated by oximes within one species.[88–94] According to these and clinical data,[78–81] erythrocyte AChE is considered to be a suitable surrogate for synaptic AChE and was used for the determination of reactivation kinetics of a larger number of OP compounds and oximes.[95] These data were used for further calculations of the relationship between reactivation half time and oxime concentration (Figure 1.2).[57,69,77]

Figure 1.2 illustrates that at low oxime concentrations, the reactivation half times increase; however, at higher oxime concentration they show asymptotic behavior, indicating that an increase in oxime concentration above a certain level (saturation, see above) no longer results in a substantial reduction in the respective half time. Moreover, although the curves behave in a roughly similar manner, the respective oxime concentrations and half times are dependent on the OP compound as well as on the oxime. As concluded from the data above, reactivation half times should be below about 10 min (*e.g.* 5 min was found to be effective for reactivation of paraoxon inhibited AChE in humans, see above). This approach allows estimation of required oxime concentrations. However, the actual use of these oxime concentrations in humans is dependent on the tolerability, which is compound dependent. Limited human data indicate that maximum oxime concentrations of ≤50 µM can be achieved after administration of one autoinjector and that these concentrations are well tolerated (see Sections 1.7.3.6–1.7.3.8). According to the data shown in Figure 1.2 obidoxime, pralidoxime and HI-6 would meet the criteria for sarin and VX, HI-6 and obidoxime for VR, HI-6 for GF, and only obidoxime for diethyl-OP pesticides. AChE can hardly be reactivated by any oxime after tabun exposure and in the case of soman, sufficient reactivation is prevented by fast aging (aging half time in humans is about 2 min). In order to visualize this, the oxime concentrations necessary to achieve reactivation half times of 5, 10 and 50 min have been calculated (see Figure 1.2) and are given in Table 1.4, with the values fulfilling the criteria marked.

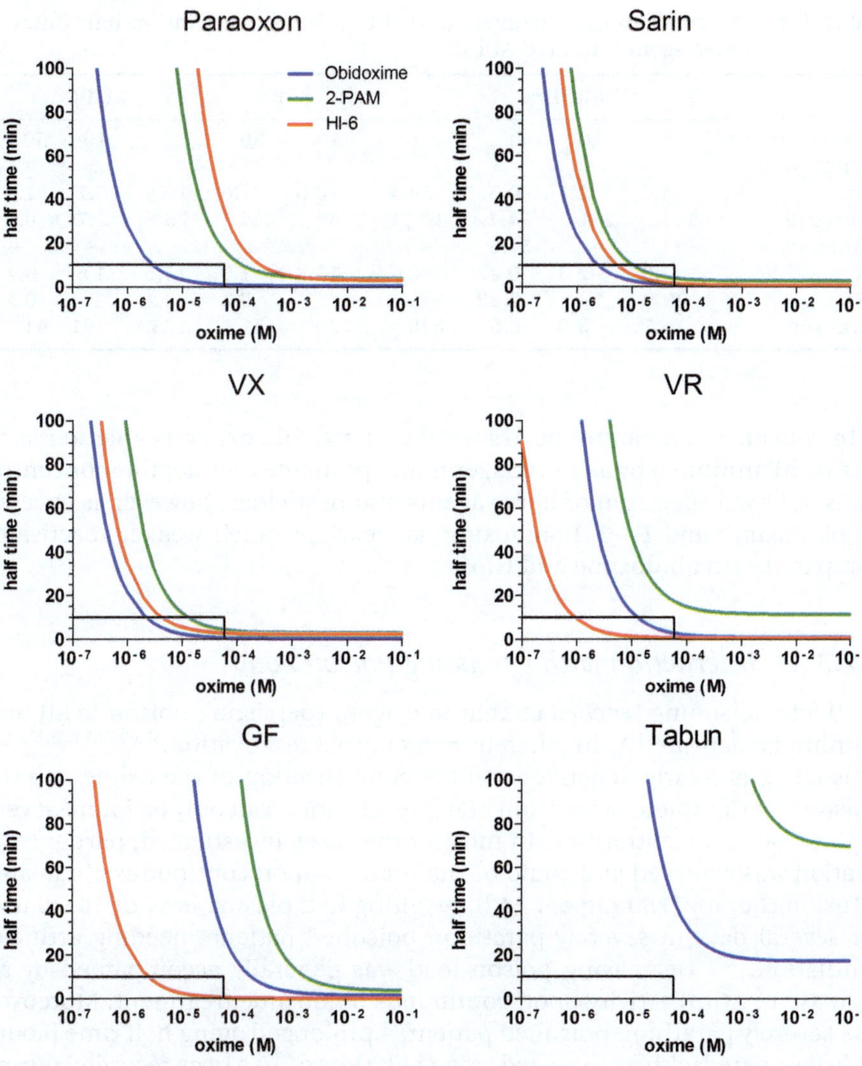

Figure 1.2 Relationship between reactivation half time and oxime concentration. Using the equation: half time = $\ln 2 \times (1 + K_D/[\text{oxime}])/k_r$, the relationship was calculated for the reactivation of red blood cell AChE under steady-state conditions with paraoxon, sarin, VX, VR and tabun, and obidoxime, 2-PAM and HI-6. The *x*-axes are plotted in log scale. The boxes highlight the clinically relevant data: oxime concentration ≤50 μM and reactivation half times ≤10 min.

Unfortunately, the kinetic constants for TMB-4 were not available and a respective calculation could not be performed. Generally, it appears that TMB-4 is a good reactivator;[96] however, its toxicity[96,97] prevents its general use. As, additionally, this oxime is not readily available on the general market, it is not considered in detail, here.

Table 1.4 Concentrations of oximes needed to achieve reactivation half times of nerve agent inhibited AChE.

	Obidoxime			Pralidoxime			HI-6		
Reactivation half time (min)	5	10	50	5	10	50	5	10	50
Sarin	5.4	2.5	0.5	34.4	10.6	1.6	12.9	5.7	1.0
Cylosarin	512	201	34.4	10097	1943	261	5.6	2.7	0.5
Tabun	—	—	51.6	—	—	—	—	—	—
VX	5.0	2.3	0.4	50.7	13.3	1.93	15.5	4.6	0.7
VR	29.9	13.1	2.28	—	—	9.2	2.2	1	0.2
Paraoxon	6.7	3.0	0.6	828	129	41	1239	291	41

In conclusion, it cannot be assumed that a single oxime is able to reactivate AChE inhibited by all nerve agents and pesticides at tolerable concentrations. A broad spectrum of nerve agents and pesticides, however, is covered by obidoxime and HI-6. Pralidoxime is clearly a much weaker reactivator compared with obidoxime and HI-6.

1.7.3.3 *Interaction with Persisting Poison Load*

Pesticide poisoning teaches us that free agent (persisting poison load) may re-inhibit reactivated AChE, thereby reducing net reactivation.[57,69,73,74,76,77,81,98] This effect is clearly dependent on the concentration of the oxime and the poison.[57,69] Complete prevention of net reactivation can only be found at very high poison concentrations. In most of the cases investigated, partial reactivation was achieved and could be maintained upon continuous obidoxime infusion therapy (750 mg per 24 h, resulting in a plasma level of 10–20 μM) for several days in severely parathion poisoned patients needing artificial ventilation.[73,98] Decreasing poison load was generally accompanied by an increase in AChE activity upon continuous obidoxime treatment. Moreover, in a severely parathion poisoned patient, a prolonged aging half time (about 66 h, compared with an expected aging half time of 30 h) was recorded during obidoxime infusion.[77] This remarkable finding indicates that oxime treatment may even prolong the therapeutic window for agents that undergo fast aging. On the other hand, a fast reactivation–re-inhibiton–reactivation cycle may contribute to accelerated degradation of the poison. Such an approach may be a therapeutic option when infusing erythrocytes, *i.e.* AChE, together with an effective oxime.

Due to the rather rapid elimination of G-type nerve agents, a high and persisting poison load is unlikely. In contrast, percutaneous exposure to V-agents will result in a slow increase of agent concentration followed by a plateau for hours, or possibly days. Hence, re-inhibition due to relevant poison load will be a problem, especially in patients with initially successful oxime treatment and inadequate continuation of oxime administration.

1.7.3.4 Oxime Dosing Strategies

Finally, the question on the dose of the oxime remains. When using autoinjectors (single bolus dose, *e.g.* 220 mg obidoxime, 600 mg pralidoxime or 500 mg HI-6), maximum concentrations of ~40 µM for obidoxime, and ~50 µM for pralidoxime and HI-6 can be expected,[71] with elimination half times of approximately an hour (1.4 h for obidoxime, 1.3 h for pralidoxime and 1.0 h for HI-6[71]). These doses should allow sufficient reactivation in sarin inhalation poisoning in military or terrorist scenarios as outlined above. In contrast, obidoxime and pralidoxime may be only marginally effective in GF poisoning and HI-6 would be better. Using three autoinjectors simultaneously would result in maximal concentrations of about 120 µM for obidoxime, 145 µM for pralidoxime or 155 µM for HI-6.[71] Under such conditions, in GF poisoning reactivation half times of 14 min for obidoxime and 85 min for pralidoxime at the maximal concentration can be estimated. Aside from the highly effective HI-6, at the most obidoxime could reactivate GF inhibited AChE under such conditions. Due to the expected short half time of G-agents under the conditions considered, one autoinjector filled with an effective oxime should be sufficient in most cases. In severe cases, repetitive doses may be appropriate; the necessity of an infusion therapy should be the exception. In tabun poisoning no effective reactivation may be expected and in soman poisoning fast aging will prevent reactivation under realistic conditions.

Reactivation of V-agents needs a different assessment. Generally, obidoxime, HI-6 and pralidoxime appear to be good reactivators for VX, while pralidoxime appears less efficient in VR poisoning. Slow and progressive inhibition of AChE was shown in percutaneous VX poisoning, which opens a therapeutic window for oxime administration prior to the onset of signs of poisoning. Indeed, in swine percutaneously exposed to VX and treated with repetitive HI-6 injections when red blood cell AChE activity had dropped to approximately 30% that of controls, severe signs of poisoning could be prevented until the end of the experiment (6 h).[99] These data emphasize the need to start oxime therapy as early as possible and to continue oxime administration, either by repetitive bolus injections or by continuous infusion, for as long as free agent is circulating in the body. Generally, it appears preferable to maintain an effective concentration by infusion[100] rather than having oscillating concentrations, thereby preventing concentrations from falling below the effective concentration for a certain time period.[101] A bolus dose of obidoxime, *e.g.* 220 mg (the amount in an autoinjector) or 250 mg (the amount in commercially available ampoules), should be followed by 750 mg per 24 h resulting in a plasma level of 10–20 µM. This dose regimen is licensed by the German authorities (BfArM). For pralidoxime, aside from autoinjectors (bolus doses of 600 mg pralidoxime per autoinjector), a bolus dose of 30 mg kg^{-1} followed by continuous infusion of 8–10 mg kg^{-1} h^{-1}[57,102] was recommended for OP pesticide poisoning, resulting in plasma concentrations of 80–100 µM.[57] No human safety data on HI-6 doses above 500 mg of the dichloride salt are available, making it difficult to recommend an infusion.

1.7.3.5 Monitoring of Oxime Therapy

These considerations allow definition of the following prerequisites for an effective oxime treatment:

- Reactivation of inhibited AChE with the oxime of choice is possible
- Aging does not prevent substantial reactivation
- Net reactivation is not prevented by re-inhibition due to a high poison load
- Oxime therapy is maintained for a sufficient period of time
- Oxime is administered at a dose that results in an effective concentration

To assess these prerequisites, the laboratory determination of cholinesterase status, described in Chapter 5 can be used. Activity of red blood cell AChE or plasma BChE are suitable parameters for laboratory confirmation of an exposure to OP compounds. Measurement of the reactivatability (incubation of a patient's blood dilution with a specified oxime concentration for a defined period of time followed by determination of AChE activity) allows assessment as to whether reactivation is possible at all or whether aging has occurred. Measurement of the inhibitory activity (incubation of a patient plasma sample with test AChE for a defined time period followed by determination of AChE activity) enables a rough estimation of the poison load in the patient. When reactivation is possible but the poison load is high, net reactivation is prevented and red blood cell activity remains inhibited.

These parameters enable a rough estimation of the period over which oximes should be administered. In conclusion, oxime therapy should be maintained for as long as reactivation is possible and as long as inhibitory activity is present in the patient's blood.

1.7.3.6 Obidoxime

Obidoxime was synthesized by Lüttringhaus and Hagedorn in 1964,[103] and many European countries have currently fielded obidoxime for military use as well as in the civilian sector.[54]

The recommended obidoxime plasma level for effective reactivation of nerve agent and OP pesticide inhibited AChE is 10–20 μM (see above).[57,104] This recommendation is based on experimental findings[95,98] and substantiated by clinical data from OP pesticide poisoning.[69,73,74,77–81,81,105] Using an autoinjector, *e.g.* ATOX II filled with 220 mg obidoxime, a maximum plasma concentration of about 40 μM may be estimated.[98] With an elimination half time of about 1.4 h, an appropriate concentration (above 10 μM) can be maintained for 2–3 h. If obidoxime is needed for a longer period, a repetitive bolus dose, or better, a continuous infusion can be used. The established therapeutic regime of an initial i.v. bolus of 250 mg obidoxime followed by continuous administration of 750 mg per 24 h obidoxime was derived based on pharmacokinetic data, assessed in healthy male volunteers.[57,101] Retrospective pharmacokinetic studies of poisoned patients confirm the achievement of the targeted obidoxime plasma level in this regimen.[106] Early recommendations or attempts to administer repetitive bolus doses up to 6 g per day can be regarded as obsolete (see above).

The use of obidoxime chloride was investigated in healthy volunteers in the 1960s and 1970s.[107–109] Generally, single doses up to 10 mg kg^{-1} were well tolerated. A peculiar side effect was reported by Sidell[107] as a generalized warmth that became localized in the skin around the mouth as well as inhibition of face muscles and a menthol like sensation within 15 min of a 250 mg obidoxime i.m. injection. Later, a menthol like sensation in the rhino-pharyngeal space during inspiration was experienced.[107,108] When the dose was increased (>10 mg kg^{-1}), in addition to dry mouth, a hot feeling in the throat, experiences of paresthesia, a transient mild to moderate increase of systolic and diastolic blood pressure (~11–17 mmHg), and increased heart rate (30 beats per min) occurred.[107] In a study targeting side effects on the liver after two injections of 250 mg obidoxime i.m., no hepatotoxic effect was recorded.[110] At higher doses, some authors associated hepatic dysfunction in terms of cholestatic icterus and elevation of liver enzymes with obidoxime administration in OP pesticide poisoning.[111–114] Indeed, after high dose obidoxime treatment, *e.g.* 7.7 g over 3 days (day 1: 16 × 250 mg, day 2: 9 × 250 mg, day 3: 6 × 250 mg) and 6.75 g over 3 days, in two patient with severe parathion poisoning, transient signs of cholestasis occurred, while in one patient treated with 750 mg no signs of hepatotoxicity were registered.[112] Von Gaisberg and Dieterle reported on a parathion poisoned patient who had been treated with 22 ampoules of obidoxime within a short time. The patient similarly developed signs of cholestasis that ameliorated during ongoing therapy.[113] In a retrospective study by Finkelstein and colleagues,[114] 5 (9.4%) out of 53 organophosphate poisoned patients receiving the highest cumulative doses of obidoxime (6 mg kg^{-1} every 4 h) suffered from impaired liver function that returned to normal within 3–5 weeks. Moreover, in this study, several patients developed cardiac arrhythmias. In these patients, frequency of cardiac arrhythmias correlated with the doses of both antidotes when the highest doses of atropine and obidoxime were administered. In patients receiving low obidoxime doses but high atropine doses, frequency of cardiac arrhythmias were correlated with the atropine dose. Finally, in patients developing prolongation of the Q-T interval, no correlation to the obidoxime dose could be found.[114] Prinz[115] reported on a parathion poisoned patient treated with 3 × 250 mg obidoxime and elevated liver parameters were recorded. Detailed investigation, however, revealed that these parameters were most probably due to recent viral hepatitis.[115] Finally, in a study using 250 mg obidoxime as bolus followed by 750 mg per day for a severely organophosphate poisoned patients no obvious hepatic toxicity was correlated with obidoxime. Here, elevations of serum transaminases were mild to moderate and transient, often subsiding during ongoing obidoxime therapy.[116] Thereby, hepatotoxicity was assessed thoroughly in patients who died in this study but no correlation to obidoxime treatment could be found.[116]

In conclusion, the administration of a bolus dose of 250 mg obidoxime as well as a dose regimen using 250 mg obidoxime, followed by 750 mg per day appears to be safe. Both dose regimens are covered by the license of BfArM.

1.7.3.7 Pralidoxime

Pralidoxime was developed in the 1950s by Wilson and colleagues.[49,117,118] Four salts of pralidoxime are in clinical use for antidotal treatment of OP poisoning, pralidoxime chloride (2-PAM, molecular weight 172.6 Da), pralidoxime iodide (molecular weight 264.1 Da), pralidoxime methanesulfonate (P2S, molecular weight 232.3 Da) and pralidoxime methylsulfate (Contrathion, molecular weight 248.3 Da). The chloride salt is used widely, whereas P2S and Contrathion are used only in a few countries such as France, Belgium and the UK.[96,119] It should be mentioned in particular that pralidoxime iodide may cause thyroid toxicity if given for a long period. The concentrations given above refer to pralidoxime chloride if not indicated otherwise.

Autoinjectors are available filled with, for example, 600 mg pralidoxime chloride, 500 mg pralidoxime methanesulfonate[120] or 350 mg of pralidoxime methyl sulphate.[121] Healthy young volunteers administered with doses of up to 10 mg kg^{-1} i.m. or i.v. experienced a slight and transient increase in heart rate (about 10 beats per min) that lasted for about half an hour.[122] Blood pressure was not affected significantly.[122] Mild and transient symptoms of dizziness, double and blurred vision, and diplopia were recorded.[122] When higher doses were administered (15–45 mg kg^{-1} i.v.), pralidoxime clearly showed cardiovascular activity. A period of marked increase in systolic and diastolic blood pressure was followed by a period of hypotension 3–4 h later. Heart rate was not changed significantly.[123] Dizziness, blurred vision, diplopia were also recorded when 15–30 mg kg^{-1} pralidoxime iodide[124] or pralidoxime methanesulfonate[125] was administered to healthy volunteers. Medicis and colleagues[126] compared administration of 16 mg kg^{-1} pralidoxime chloride i.v. over 30 min (traditional short infusion) with a regimen consisting of a loading dose of 4 mg kg^{-1} over 15 min followed by 3.2 mg kg^{-1} h^{-1} for 3.75 h (total dose 16 mg kg^{-1}). It turned out that the loading dose regime was clearly better tolerated. Dizziness and blurred vision occurred only in the traditional short infusion group. Apart from a significant increase in diastolic blood pressure in the traditional short infusion group when compared with the loading dose group, no further cardiovascular effects were reported.[126] Notably, a maximum concentration of 14 μg l^{-1} (80 μM) pralidoxime chloride was achieved with the level above approximately 60 μM for about an hour in the traditional group (data estimated from the graph shown in the manuscript[126]), while in the loading dose group, a permanent level of about 10–30 μM was maintained. Both rapid i.v. injection of pralidoxime [both iodide (0.6–1.0 g i.v.; 1–4 injections per day) and chloride (0.5–1.0 g i.m.; 1–4 injections)] and high doses (not specified) were associated with transient impairment of respiration[97] in OP pesticide poisoned patients. One severely coumaphos poisoned patient even experienced cardiac arrest (asystolia) after administration of 2 g pralidoxime iodide over 10 min.[127] It remains unclear whether a small amount of narcoleptics (self medication with tranquillizers) or hydrocarbons from the solvent contributed to this serious adverse event in the patient.[127] In a therapeutic accident, approximately 4–5 g of pralidoxime chloride was infused rapidly within 10–20 min to a patient who was just recovering from OP compound poisoning treated successfully with pralidoxime. He developed blurred vision, rigidity of extremities, neurological disorders, substantial increase in blood pressure (190/110 mmHg) and tachycardia (116 beats per min). Finally, the patient needed artificial ventilation and sedation. Nevertheless, he could be discharged from the hospital after an uneventful recovery.[128]

Substantially higher doses of pralidoxime are recommended in OP pesticide poisoning[57,101,129,130] since the previously proposed concentration of 4 µg ml^{-1} was considered inappropriate. Eddleston and colleagues administered a 2 g pralidoxime chloride loading dose over 20 min followed by constant infusion of 0.5 g h^{-1} for a maximum of 6 days[53] to OP pesticide poisoned patients and compared them to saline administered controls. The pralidoxime regimen resulted in a plasma level of about 100 µM. Although clear reactivation could be shown in patients poisoned by diethyl- and dimethyl-type OP pesticides, this finding was not correlated with a better survival rate. Regarding analysis of adverse events, a significant increase in blood pressure and tachycardia was reported in the pralidoxime group during the first 3 days. The reason for the failure of clinical benefit despite substantial reactivation was not analyzed in detail.[53] Goel and colleagues[131] showed clear regeneration of red blood cell AChE activity in eight OP pesticide poisoned patients following pralidoxime infusion over the first 24 h after exposure. However, probably due to the small number of patients, a better survival rate could not be shown in this study, either. In contrast, in other studies using either a high pralidoxime dosing regimen of 1 g pralidoxime infusion every hour (24 g per day), compared with 1 g every 4 h (6 g per day) after a 2 g loading dose,[132] or a dosage regimen tailored to the severity of poisoning and the level of BChE activity,[133] there was a clear benefit for morbidity and mortality. Accordingly, there is an ongoing debate on the effectiveness of oximes in OP pesticide poisoning and adequate studies are urgently needed (see above).

From the aspect of safety, autoinjector doses appear to be safe in adults. For children, a dose correction appears necessary. When using higher pralidoxime doses, *e.g.* according to the World Health Organization (WHO) recommended regimen (30 mg kg^{-1} pralidoxime chloride bolus followed by 8 mg kg^{-1} h^{-1} infusion) in severe nerve agent poisoning with persisting poison load as assumed in VX poisoning, adverse events may develop.

1.7.3.8 HI-6

Despite its experimentally proven antidotal efficacy in the treatment of nerve agent poisoning, HI-6 is not yet licensed for clinical use. One major problem appears to be the production of large quantities of good manufacturing practice grade HI-6. Another important limitation of HI-6 use is its poor stability in aqueous solutions[134,135] and the low solubility of the dichloride salt at low temperatures.[136,137] In particular, the latter feature requires relatively sophisticated dry–wet autoinjectors.[136–139] Nevertheless, HI-6 is available for military use in some countries such as the Czech Republic, Sweden and Canada.

Several studies have examined the safety of HI-6 administration. Single doses of up to 500 mg kg^{-1} HI-6 dichloride turned out to be well tolerated in humans. No adverse effects concerning the cardiovascular, respiratory, central nervous system, muscle or visual function have been reported after use of HI-6.[56,140,141] During treatment of OP poisoned patients i.m. administration of 500 mg HI-6 was conducted four times a day up to a cumulative dose of 14 g, no adverse effect occurred that could be related to the oxime.[56] These data indicate that HI-6 dichloride might be more tolerable than pralidoxime and obidoxime.

1.7.3.9 Benzodiazepines

One feature of nerve agent poisoning is the development of central over-excitation. Clinically, this feature is characterized by central seizures [identified by electroencephalography (EEG)] and convulsions (outward manifestations; for review see ref. 142). Extensive research was undertaken to improve therapy of nerve agent induced seizures (for review see ref. 142–144). Generally, this research is based on animal and *in vitro* experiments, mainly focused on poisoning with soman. It is assumed that the course of seizure development can be divided into three phases: (i) a short cholinergic phase; (ii) a transitional phase characterized by high cholinergic activity and increasing glutamatergic activity; and (iii) a predominate glutamatergic phase.[144] Therapeutic problems arise when initial therapy is delayed and anticholinergic drugs are no longer effective. In the past decades, a huge variety of established and experimental drugs were tested to counteract nerve agent induced seizures and convulsions. Unfortunately, all of these experiments were done *in vitro* or in animals, and it remains uncertain whether, or in which way, these results can be extrapolated to humans.

Clinical reports on convulsions in nerve agent poisoning are rare. Foroutan[10] reported that he used diazepam, which was the only anticonvulsant available in chemical emergency units during the Iran–Iraq war. Therefore, diazepam was not only used as classical anticonvulsant but also during the "spastic stage" that was seen during recovery from sarin poisoning. No EEG recordings were available for these incidents.

Later on, during the Japan (Matsumoto in 1994 and Tokyo in 1995) sarin attacks, diazepam was used successfully. Yanagisawa *et al.* reported that severely poisoned patients, who had survived the attack in Masumoto but suffered from loss of consciousness and generalized seizures, had been treated successfully with atropine, benzodiazepines, i.v. fluids and other systematic therapies.[145] In the patients treated at St Luke's International

Hospital, Tokyo, Japan, after the sarin attack, convulsions were rare events (three patients, 2.7%).[41] These patients were supplied with atropine, pralidoxime and diazepam. It appeared that pralidoxime and diazepam reduced the frequency and severity of convulsions and fasciculations, although it was difficult to distinguish between convulsions and fasciculations in unconscious patients.[41]

When looking at patients with OP pesticide poisoning there is a comparable pattern. There are no randomized clinical trials or cohort studies on benzodiazepines in the treatment of acute OP pesticide poisoning.[102] However, benzodiazepines, such as diazepam, lorazepam and midazolam, are recommended.[102] Based on observations of single patients in medically controlled scenarios, Zilker[25] even suggests to start early with low doses of diazepam in anxious patients with mild signs of OP pesticide poisoning. If adequate artificial ventilation is not possible due to severe spasm, relaxation (*e.g.* by pancuronium) may be necessary.[25] Midazolam and fentanyl are considered appropriate for prolonged sedation of artificially ventilated patients.[25] Inadequate responses of severely poisoned patients to benzodiazepines requires the use of barbiturates.

The US military field autoinjectors contain 10 mg of diazepam (labelled CANA) as an anticonvulsive antidote against nerve agents.[33] It is, however, assumed that higher doses, *e.g.* up to 30–40 mg could be necessary.[33] This recommendation is in accordance with the one given by Balali-Mood and Saber, *i.e.* 5–10 mg diazepam i.v. in the absence of convulsions and a bolus of 10–20 mg i.v. in the presence of convulsions.[46] Balali-Mood and Saber further suggest that the dose of diazepam recommended by WHO of 5–10 mg i.v. over 3 min can be repeated every 10–15 min in adult patients up to a maximum of 30 mg.[46]

McDonough and colleagues have shown in guinea pigs that midazolam is able to stop seizures fast and at a lower dose compared with other benzodiazepines (avizafone, clonazepam, diazepam and lorazepam).[146] Accordingly, midazolam appears to be an alternative to diazepam in nerve agent poisoning. However, midazolam may induce respiratory depression, which may limit its use in the field.

In conclusion, diazepam remains the recommended drug for the emergency treatment of organophosphate induced seizures and convulsions.

1.7.3.10 Magnesium

Magnesium (Mg), one of the most abundant cations in the body, is distributed up to 99% intracellularly, including in the skeleton.[147] Mg in bone belongs either to the mineral lattice or to an elutable surface limited mineral pool that may serve as a reservoir for the maintenance of constant plasma concentrations. The normal serum concentration of Mg^{+} amounts to 1.5–2.5 mEq l^{-1} (1.8–3.0 mg dl^{-1}), of which about a third to a half is bound to plasma proteins.[148] Its plasma concentration is tightly held within the normal range by the kidneys.[147] Mg has an elimination half time of about 4 h (product information: $MgSO_4$, 2015) and roughly 80% of an i.v. Mg load is excreted in the urine within 24 h after admission in healthy subjects.[147]

Mg has been proposed as an adjunct to conventional therapy in OP poisoning.[149,31] Pajoumand presented a study on OP pesticide poisoned patients treated, in addition to conventional therapy, with Mg ($MgSO_4{\cdot}7H_2O$, at a dose of 4 g per day i.v.). The mortality in 11 patients with OP poisoning was lower and the hospital stay shorter than in the group without Mg administration, but neither type nor dose of OPs ingested were provided and only a small amount of data on clinical course during therapy (*e.g.* markers for severity, complications, cause of death and time of death) could be found. In addition, 82% of the patients were treated with obidoxime in the $MgSO_4$ group but only 55% in the group without $MgSO_4$ therapy. Thus, a better rate of reactivation achieved by obidoxime when compared with pralidoxime could also be the reason for the different outcome.[149]

Moreover, a conclusive explanation for the potential beneficial effect of Mg is not established. Pajoumand and colleagues[149] refer to a study by Petroianu *et al.*[150] that showed, in artificially ventilated and anaesthetized minipigs, an excessive increase in blood pressure and heart rate as well as a drop of hematocrit could be prevented upon $MgSO_4$ infusion over 150 min in control animals as well as in animal poisoned by paraoxon (54 mg kg^{-1}). The dose of $MgSO_4$ and fluid used to achieve this effect, however, was significantly higher in the poisoned animals.[150] In conclusion, the study of Petrouianu cannot be used as an explanation for the beneficial effects in the Pajoumand study (no data on blood pressure, heart rate or hematocrit were provided). Moreover, in human poisoning, cardiovascular failure and respiratory depression appear to be life threatening for a long period (*e.g.* several days) after $MgSO_4$ administration.

Another possible explanation for a potential beneficial effect could be alleviation of seizures arising during OP poisoning. Administration of $MgSO_4$ in order to achieve a continuous plasma level of about 3.5–7 mEq l^{-1} (4.2–8.4 mg dl^{-1}) is recommended for the treatment of eclamptic convulsions.[148] The situation for pregnant woman and the different mechanism discussed in this special context (for review see ref. 148), however, cannot be transferred to human OP pesticide poisoning without detailed scientific assessment. Pajoumand *et al.* do not provide further data on possible seizures. Moreover, Katalan and colleagues[151] investigated the effect of Mg in sarin poisoned rats treated with atropine, TMB-4 and $MgSO_4$. They concluded that there is no advantage in using $MgSO_4$ as an anticonvulsant in antidotal treatment against warfare agents such as sarin.[151]

The effect of Mg on neuromuscular function has been known since the 1950s.[152] Since Mg is able to reduce the stimulating effect of ACh on muscles, it was obvious to investigate whether such an effect may be beneficial in OP poisoning. Singh and colleagues performed the decisive study,[153] investigating the effect of $MgSO_4$ (4 g i.v.; 20% $MgSO_4{\cdot}7H_2O$) in OP pesticide poisoned patients who were initially treated with appropriate atropine doses and pralidoxime. Although the group could detect a slight effect on the pattern of neuromuscular transmission, they clearly pointed out that they had not found any indication of improvement in any clinical parameters and concluded that it is unlikely that $MgSO_4$ is therapeutically beneficial in acute OP poisoning.

Finally, $MgSO_4$ (20% $MgSO_4 \cdot 7H_2O$) was administered to four dosing groups [4 mg i.v. (n = 16), 8 mg i.v. (n = 8), 12 mg i.v. (n = 8) or 16 mg i.v. (n = 8)] in OP poisoned patients.[154] In this study, no adverse events of $MgSO_4$ were observed. As this study assessed the safety of $MgSO_4$, no analysis of the beneficial effects of $MgSO_4$ was performed. For such an assessment, a higher number of patients would have been necessary.[154]

In conclusion, although Mg appears to be well tolerated in OP poisoned patients, a clear beneficial effect has not been demonstrated so far. Thus, the administration of $MgSO_4$ cannot be recommended in nerve agent poisoning at present. This assessment is in agreement with the analysis of Blain.[102]

1.7.3.11 *Alkalinization by Sodium Bicarbonate*

As early as 1983, Cordoba and colleagues investigated modifications of the acid–base equilibrium and use of sodium bicarbonate as an aid in the treatment of toxicity in dogs poisoned with a LD_{100} of DDVP (*O*–*O*-dimethyl 2-2 dichlororine vinylphosphate).[155] They reported that upon treatment with sodium bicarbonate, a recovery of the acid–base balance and survival of 84.4% of the dogs were achieved. Since then, the effect of sodium bicarbonate has been investigated in a few studies in rats also poisoned by DDVP.[156,157] In the investigation of Bajgar and Portman, also on DDVP in rats, the nerve agent sarin and pyridostigmine were included when the effects of sodium bicarbonate were assessed.[158] Moreover, some case series or clinical trials[156,159,160] have been published in which patients poisoned by various pesticides, in addition to conventional treatment (atropine/atropine in combination with an oxime), were administered sodium bicarbonate in order to achieve alkalinization.

All of the authors came to the conclusion that alkalinization by sodium bicarbonate has a beneficial effect in OP poisoning. However, the highest benefit was achieved when sodium bicarbonate was administered in combination with standard antidotes (*e.g.* atropine or atropine in combination with an oxime).

Although no clear mechanism has been established, several mechanisms have been suggested to explain the beneficial effect: enhanced clearance of the poison from the body; improved efficacy of oximes; a direct effect on neuromuscular function; volume expansion with improved tissue perfusion; and bicarbonate induced release of lactate into the circulation.[161]

Furthermore, increased enzymatic and chemical hydrolysis of OP compounds by sodium bicarbonate was proposed.[160] However, it is rather unlikely that a small pH shift from 7.36 to 7.48 would increase the hydrolysis of an agent to such an extent that a substantial reduction of the body load could be achieved. In particular, the chemically and biologically stable V-agents would need harsher conditions for detoxification.[162,163]

On the other hand, severe OP poisoning may result in acidic conditions,[160] which must be corrected by moderate alkalinization. In this respect, appropriate administration of sodium bicarbonate should have a therapeutic value without interfering with the OP compounds themselves.

In conclusion, there are inadequate scientific and clinical data to support alkalinization in nerve agent poisoning.

1.7.3.12 Supportive Treatment

The clinical picture of nerve agent poisoning is mainly dominated by cholinergic crisis. When the administration of atropine, an oxime and a benzodiazepine are not able to antagonize the clinical effect, further supportive measures have to be taken.

At first, it is crucial to maintain sufficient ventilation. On the spot, assisted or artificial ventilation has to be started as early as possible. Mouth-to-mouth ventilation has to be avoided. When the patients are transported to medical facilities, established ventilation protocols should be followed. Special care has to be taken of severe bronchospasm, marked bronchosecretion and pulmonary edema.[164] Similar protocols as used for OP pesticide poisoned patients could be used (see above).

Other complications, *e.g.* pneumonia and circulatory depression, have to be treated with standard emergency or intensive care protocols.

1.8 Summary and Outlook

Although the Chemical Weapon Convention came into force in 1997, the recent events in the Middle East clearly show that chemical warfare agents remain a threat. Thereby, possible scenarios are no longer mainly restricted to typical military confrontations but are now extended to asymmetric conflicts and terrorist attacks. In any case, if such an event occurs one has to expect a large number of patients calling for medical care. In particular, nerve agents are most dangerous due to their high toxicity.

To apply adequate treatment, medical personnel, equipment and facilities need protection. However, because especially volatile nerve agents lead very quickly to life threatening signs and symptoms, fast treatment will be necessary. Accordingly, diagnostic and therapeutic measures have to be provided while wearing protective clothing until the patients undergo decontamination.

The trigger to treat will be clinical diagnosis, based on the typical signs and symptoms of cholinergic crises. Inhibition of red blood cell AChE can be assessed on site and can confirm poisoning by anticholinergic compounds within several minutes. For treatment, atropine and an oxime are first line drugs. Atropine has to be applied rapidly and at a sufficient dose, *e.g.* starting with 2 mg and doubling the dose every 5–10 min until relief of cholinergic signs and symptoms. In severe cases, a continuous infusion may be necessary. Similarly, oximes, *e.g.* obidoxime, pralidoxime or HI-6, have to be injected as soon as possible. Oximes are used to resolve the nerve agent induced inhibition of AChE, thereby acting as causal antidotes. To achieve this goal, appropriate dosing is necessary as well as continuation for an adequate time period, which is dependent on the amount of poison absorbed as well as on the persistence of the poison in the body.

Unfortunately, under several circumstances, sufficient reactivation will not be possible, *e.g.* when the time to treatment is delayed (*e.g.* soman) or the nerve agent induced inhibition of AChE cannot be reactivated substantially by oximes (*e.g.* tabun). In such cases, supportive measures, *e.g.* artificial ventilation, will become decisive.

References

1. G. Schrader, *Die Entwicklung neuer insektizider Phosphorsäure-Ester*, Verlag Chemie, Weinheim, 1963.
2. G. Schrader, Organische Phosphorverbindungen als neuartige Insektizide, *Angew. Chem.*, 1950, **62**, 471–473.
3. H. P. Benschop, L. P. A. deJong and J. P. Langenberg, *Inhalation toxicokinetics of C (+/-) P (+/-)-soman and (+/-)-sarin in the guinea pig, Enzymes of the cholinsterase family*, ed. D. M. Ouinn, A. S. Balasubramanian, B. P. Doctor and P. Taylor, Plenum Press, New York, London, 1995, pp. 361–368.
4. O. Tenberken, J. Mikler, I. Hill, K. Weatherby, H. Thiermann, F. Worek and G. Reiter, Toxicokinetics of tabun enantiomers in anaesthetized swine after intravenous tabun administration, *Toxicol. Lett.*, 2010, **198**, 177–181.
5. O. Tenberken, H. Thiermann, F. Worek and G. Reiter, Chromatographic preparation and kinetic analysis of interactions between tabun enantiomers and acetylcholinesterase, *Toxicol. Lett.*, 2010, **195**, 142–146.
6. R. Trapp, The detoxification and natural degradation of chemical warfare agents, *Stockholm International Peace Research Institute (SIPRI)*, Taylor and Francis Ltd., London, Philadelphia, 1985.
7. M. Eddleston, S. Singh and N. Buckley, Acute organophosphorus poisoning, *Clin. Evid.*, 2003, 1542–1553.
8. D. Gunnell, M. Eddleston, M. R. Phillips and F. Konradsen, The global distribution of fatal pesticide self-poisoning: systematic review, *BMC Public Health*, 2007, 7(**357**), 357.
9. H. John, F. Balszuweit, K. Kehe, F. Worek and H. Thiermann, *Toxicokinetic aspects of nerve agents and vesicants, Handbook of toxicology of chemical warfare agents*, ed. R. C. Gupta, Academic Press, Amsterdam, Boston, Heidelberg, London, New York, Oxford, Paris, San Diego, San Franzisko, Singapore, Sydney, Tokyo, 2015, pp. 817–874.
10. J. Newmark, The birth of nerve agent warfare: lessons from Syed Abbas Foroutan, *Neurology*, 2004, **62**, 1590–1596.

11. J. Massoulie, L. Pezzementi, S. Bon, E. Krejci and F. M. Vallette, Molecular and cellular biology of cholinesterases, *Prog. Neurobiol.*, 1993, **41**, 31–91.
12. J. Massoulie, The origin of the molecular diversity and functional anchoring of cholinesterases, *Neurosignals*, 2002, **11**, 130–143.
13. F. Worek and H. Thiermann, The value of novel oximes for treatment of poisoning by organophosphorus compounds, *Pharmacol. Ther.*, 2013, **139**, 249–259.
14. N. Aurbek, H. Thiermann, F. Eyer, P. Eyer and F. Worek, Suitability of human butyrylcholinesterase as therapeutic marker and pseudo catalytic scavenger in organophosphate poisoning: a kinetic analysis, *Toxicology*, 2009, **259**, 133–139.
15. F. Nachon, X. Brazzolotto, M. Trovaslet and P. Masson, Progress in the development of enzyme-based nerve agent bioscavengers, *Chem. Biol. Interact.*, 2013, **206**, 536–544.
16. F. Worek, T. Seeger, G. Reiter, M. Goldsmith, Y. Ashani, H. Leader, J. L. Sussman, N. Aggarwal, H. Thiermann and D. S. Tawfik, Post-exposure treatment of VX poisoned guinea pigs with the engineered phosphotriesterase mutant C23: a proof-of-concept study, *Toxicol. Lett.*, 2014, **231**, 45–54.
17. F. Worek, T. Seeger, M. Zengerle, S. Kubik, H. Thiermann and T. Wille, Effectiveness of a substituted beta-cyclodextrin to prevent cyclosarin toxicity in vivo, *Toxicol. Lett.*, 2014, **226**, 222–227.
18. F. R. Sidell, Nerve agents, in *Medical aspects of chemical and biological warfare*, ed. F. R. Sidell, E. T. Takafuj and D. R. Franz, Office of The Surgeon General at TMM Publications, Washington, DC, 1997, pp. 129–179.
19. I. Hendler, O. Nahtomi, E. Segal, A. Perel, M. Wiener and J. Meyerovitch, The effect of full protective gear on intubation performance by hospital medical personnel, *Mil. Med.*, 2000, **165**, 272–274.
20. R. Ben-Abraham and A. A. Weinbroum, Laryngeal mask airway control *versus* endotracheal intubation by medical personnel wearing protective gear, *Am. J. Emerg. Med.*, 2004, **22**, 24–26.
21. A. T. Tu, *Chemical terrorism: horrors in tokyo subway and matsumoto city*, Alaken Inc., Fort Collins, 2002.
22. U.S. Army Medical Research Institute of Chemical Defense (USAMRICD), *Medical management of chemical causalties handbook*, Chemical Causualty Care Division, Aberdeen Proving Ground, 2000.
23. E. D. Clarkson and R. K. Gordon, Rapid decontamination of chemical warfare agent from the skin, in *Handbook of toxicology of chemical warfare agents*, ed. R. C. Gupta, Academic Press, Amsterdam, Boston, Heidelberg, London, New York, Oxford, Paris, San Diego, San Franzisko, Singapore, Sydney, Tokyo, 2015, pp. 1127–1139.
24. B. Ballantyne and C. T. Marrs, Overview of the biological and clinical aspects of organophosphates and carbamates, in *Organophospates and Carbamates*, ed. B. Ballantyne and C. T. Marrs, Butterworth-Heinemann Ltd., Oxford, 1992, pp. 3–14.

25. T. Zilker, *Klinische Toxikologie für die Notfall- und Intensivmedizin*, UNI-MED Verlag Ag, Bremen, 2008.
26. R. S. Wadia, C. Sadagopan, R. B. Amin and H. V. Sardesai, Neurological manifestations of organophosphorous insecticide poisoning, *J. Neurol., Neurosurg. Psychiatry*, 1974, **37**, 841–847.
27. N. Senanayake and L. Karalliedde, Neurotoxic effects of organophosphorus insecticides. An intermediate syndrome, *N. Engl. J. Med.*, 1987, **316**, 761–763.
28. L. Karalliedde, D. Baker and T. C. Marrs, Organophosphate-induced intermediate syndrome: aetiology and relationships with myopathy, *Toxicol. Rev.*, 2006, **25**, 1–14.
29. L. Karalliedde, H. Wheeler, R. Maclehose and V. Murray, Possible immediate and long-term health effects following exposure to chemical warfare agents, *Public Health*, 2000, **114**, 238–248.
30. N. Weger and L. Szinicz, Therapeutic effects of new oximes, benactyzine and atropine in Soman poisoning: part I. Effects of various oximes in Soman, Sarin, and Vx poisoning in dogs, *Fundam. Appl. Toxicol.*, 1981, **1**, 161–163.
31. M. Balali-Mood and K. Balali-Mood, Neurotoxic disorders of organophosphorus compounds and their managements, *Arch. Iran Med.*, 2008, **11**, 65–89.
32. M. Ehrich and B. S. Jortner, *Organophosphorus-induced delayed neuropathy, Handbook of Pesticide Toxicology*, ed. R. I. Krieger, Academic Press, San Diego, San Francisco, New York, Boston, London, Sydney, Tokyo, 2001, pp. 987–1006.
33. J. Newmark, Nerve agents, *Neurologist*, 2007, **13**, 20–32.
34. G. B. Koelle, Protection of cholinesterase against irreversible inactivation by di-isopropyl fluorophosphate in vitro, *J. Pharmacol. Exp. Ther.*, 1946, **88**, 232–237.
35. R. Koster, Synergisms and antagonisms between physostigmine and di-isopropyl fluorophosphate in cats, *J. Pharmacol. Exp. Ther.*, 1946, **88**, 39–46.
36. R. H. Inns and T. Marrs, *Prophylaxis against anticholinesterase poisoning, Clinical and experimantal toxicology of organophosphates and carbamates*, ed. B. Ballantyne and T. C. Marrs, Butterworth Heinenmann, Oxford, 1992, pp. 602–610.
37. N. M. Herkert, H. Thiermann and F. Worek, In vitro kinetic interactions of pyridostigmine, physostigmine and soman with erythrocyte and muscle acetylcholinesterase from different species, *Toxicol. Lett.*, 2011, **206**, 41–46.
38. M. Eddleston, J. M. Street, I. Self, A. Thompson, T. King, N. Williams, G. Naredo, K. Dissanayake, L. M. Yu, F. Worek, H. John, S. Smith, H. Thiermann, J. B. Harris and C. R. Eddie, A role for solvents in the toxicity of agricultural organophosphorus pesticides, *Toxicology*, 2012, **294**, 94–103.
39. H. John, T. Binder, H. Hochstetter and H. Thiermann, LC-ESI MS/MS quantification of atropine and six other antimuscarinic tropane alkaloids in plasma, *Anal. Bioanal. Chem.*, 2010, **396**, 751–763.

40. J. H. Brown and P. Taylor, Muscarinic receptor agonists and antagonists, in *Goodman and Gilman's the pharmacological basis of therapeutics*, ed. L. L. Brunton, J. S. Lazo and K. L. Parker, McGraw-Hill, New York, Chicago, San Franzisko, Lisbon, London, Madrid, Mexico City, Milan, New Delhi, San Juan, Seoul, Singapore, Sydney, Toronto, 2006, pp. 183–200.
41. T. Okumura, N. Takasu, S. Ishimatsu, S. Miyanoki, A. Mitsuhashi, K. Kumada, K. Tanaka and S. Hinohara, Report on 640 victims of the Tokyo subway sarin attack, *Ann. Emerg. Med.*, 1996, **28**, 129–135.
42. N. J. Connors, Z. H. Harnett and R. S. Hoffman, Comparison of current recommended regimens of atropinization in organophosphate poisoning, *J. Med. Toxicol.*, 2014, **10**, 143–147.
43. M. J. Abedin, A. A. Sayeed, A. Basher, R. J. Maude, G. Hoque and M. A. Faiz, Open-label randomized clinical trial of atropine bolus injection *versus* incremental boluses plus infusion for organophosphate poisoning in Bangladesh, *J. Med. Toxicol.*, 2012, **8**, 108–117.
44. M. Eddleston, N. A. Buckley, H. Checketts, L. Senarathna, F. Mohamed, M. H. Sheriff and A. Dawson, Speed of initial atropinisation in significant organophosphorus pesticide poisoning–a systematic comparison of recommended regimens, *J. Toxicol., Clin. Toxicol.*, 2004, **42**, 865–875.
45. M. Balali-Mood and K. Balali-Mood, Neurotoxic disorders of organophosphorus compounds and their managements, *Arch. Iran Med.*, 2008, **11**, 65–89.
46. M. Balali-Mood and H. Saber, Recent advances in the treatment of organophosphorous poisonings, *Iran J. Med. Sci.*, 2012, **37**, 74–91.
47. J. W. A. Heath and T. Meredith, *Atropine in the management of anticholinesterase poisoning, Clinical and Experimental Toxicology of Organophosphates Carbamates*, ed. B. Ballantyne, C. T. Marrs and W. N. Aldridge, Butterworth-Heinemann, Oxford, 1992, pp. 543–554.
48. L. A. Konickx, K. Bingham and M. Eddleston, Is oxygen required before atropine administration in organophosphorus or carbamate pesticide poisoning? – A cohort study, *Clin. Toxicol.*, 2014, **52**, 531–537.
49. I. B. Wilson and S. Ginsburg, A powerful reactivator of alkylphosphate-inhibited acetylcholinesterase, *Biochim. Biophys. Acta*, 1955, **18**, 168–170.
50. A. F. Childs, D. R. Davies, A. L. Green and J. P. Rutland, The reactivation by oximes and hydroxamic acids of cholinesterase inhibited by organo-phosphorus compounds, *Br. J. Pharmacol. Chemother.*, 1955, **10**, 462–465.
51. T. Namba and K. Hiraki, PAM (Pyridine-2-aldoxime methiodide) therapy for alkylphosphate poisoning, *J. Am. Med. Assoc.*, 1958, **166**, 1834–1839.
52. G. Horn, T. Wille, K. Musilek, K. Kuca, H. Thiermann and F. Worek, Reactivation kinetics of 31 structurally different bispyridinium oximes with organophosphate-inhibited human butyrylcholinesterase, *Arch. Toxicol.*, 2015, **89**, 405–414.
53. M. Eddleston, P. Eyer, F. Worek, E. Juszczak, N. Alder, F. Mohamed, L. Senarathna, A. Hittarage, S. Azher, K. Jeganathan, S. Jayamanne, M. L. von, A. H. Dawson, M. H. Sheriff and N. A. Buckley, Pralidoxime in acute organophosphorus insecticide poisoning–a randomised controlled trial, *PLoS Med.*, 2009, **6**, e1000104.

54. H. Thiermann, F. Worek and K. Kehe, Limitations and challenges in treatment of acute chemical warfare agent poisoning, *Chem. Biol. Interact.*, 2013, **206**, 435–443.
55. Y. Bentur, I. Layish, A. Krivoy, M. Berkovitch, E. Rotman, S. B. Haim, Y. Yehezkelli and E. Kozer, Civilian adult self injections of atropine-trimedoxime (TMB4) auto-injectors, *Clin. Toxicol.*, 2006, **44**, 301–306.
56. R. Kusic, D. Jovanovic, S. Randjelovic, D. Joksovic, V. Todorovic, B. Boskovic, M. Jokanovic and V. Vojvodic, HI-6 in man: efficacy of the oxime in poisoning by organophosphorus insecticides, *Hum. Exp. Toxicol.*, 1991, **10**, 113–118.
57. P. Eyer, The role of oximes in the management of organophosphorus pesticide poisoning, *Toxicol. Rev.*, 2003, **22**, 165–190.
58. J. L. Willems and F. M. Belpaire, *Anticholinesterase poisoning: an overview of pharmacotherapy, Clinical and Experimental Toxicology of Organophosphates and Carbamates*, ed. B. Ballantyne, C. T. Marrs and W. N. Aldridge, Butterworth-Heinemann, Oxford, 1992, pp. 536–542.
59. J. L. Sussman, M. Harel, F. Frolow, C. Oefner, A. Goldman, L. Toker and I. Silman, Atomic structure of acetylcholinesterase from Torpedo californica: a prototypic acetylcholine-binding protein, *Science*, 1991, **253**, 872–879.
60. Y. Bourne, P. Taylor, P. E. Bougis and P. Marchot, Crystal structure of mouse acetylcholinesterase. A peripheral site-occluding loop in a tetrameric assembly, *J. Biol. Chem.*, 1999, **274**, 2963–2970.
61. P. H. Axelsen, M. Harel, I. Silman and J. L. Sussman, Structure and dynamics of the active site gorge of acetylcholinesterase: synergistic use of molecular dynamics simulation and X-ray crystallography, *Protein Sci.*, 1994, **3**, 188–197.
62. T. Wille, F. Ekstrom, J. C. Lee, Y. P. Pang, H. Thiermann and F. Worek, Kinetic analysis of interactions between alkylene-linked bis-pyridiniumaldoximes and human acetylcholinesterases inhibited by various organophosphorus compounds, *Biochem. Pharmacol.*, 2010, **6**, 941–946.
63. M. Winter, T. Wille, K. Musilek, K. Kuca, H. Thiermann and F. Worek, Investigation of the reactivation kinetics of a large series of bispyridinium oximes with organophosphate-inhibited human acetylcholinesterase, *Toxicol. Lett.*, 2016, **244**, 136–142.
64. N. Aurbek, N. M. Herkert, M. Koller, H. Thiermann and F. Worek, Kinetic analysis of interactions of different sarin and tabun analogues with human acetylcholinesterase and oximes: is there a structure-activity relationship?, *Chem.-Biol. Interact.*, 2010, **187**, 215–219.
65. F. Worek, G. Reiter, P. Eyer and L. Szinicz, Reactivation kinetics of acetylcholinesterase from different species inhibited by highly toxic organophosphates, *Arch. Toxicol.*, 2002, **76**, 523–529.
66. F. Worek, P. Eyer, N. Aurbek, L. Szinicz and H. Thiermann, Recent advances in evaluation of oxime efficacy in nerve agent poisoning by in vitro analysis, *Toxicol. Appl. Pharmacol.*, 2007, **219**, 226–234.
67. F. Worek, T. Wille, N. Aurbek, P. Eyer and H. Thiermann, Reactivation of organophosphate-inhibited human, Cynomolgus monkey, swine and guinea pig acetylcholinesterase by MMB-4: a modified kinetic approach, *Toxicol. Appl. Pharmacol.*, 2010, **249**, 231–237.

68. F. Worek, N. Aurbek, J. Wetherell, P. Pearce, T. Mann and H. Thiermann, Inhibition, reactivation and aging kinetics of highly toxic organophosphorus compounds: pig *versus* minipig acetylcholinesterase, *Toxicology*, 2008, **244**, 35–41.
69. H. Thiermann, L. Szinicz, F. Eyer, F. Worek, P. Eyer, N. Felgenhauer and T. Zilker, Modern strategies in therapy of organophosphate poisoning, *Toxicol. Lett.*, 1999, **107**, 233–239.
70. F. Worek, H. Thiermann, L. Szinicz and P. Eyer, Kinetic analysis of interactions between human acetylcholinesterase, structurally different organophosphorus compounds and oximes, *Biochem. Pharmacol.*, 2004, **68**, 2237–2248.
71. F. Worek, L. Szinicz, P. Eyer and H. Thiermann, Evaluation of oxime efficacy in nerve agent poisoning: development of a kinetic-based dynamic model, *Toxicol. Appl. Pharmacol.*, 2005, **209**, 193–202.
72. F. Eyer and P. Eyer, Enzyme-based assay for quantification of paraoxon in blood of parathion poisoned patients, *Hum. Exp. Toxicol.*, 1998, **17**, 645–651.
73. F. Eyer, F. Worek, P. Eyer, N. Felgenhauer, M. Haberkorn, T. Zilker and H. Thiermann, Obidoxime in acute organophosphate poisoning: 1-clinical effectiveness, *Clin. Toxicol.*, 2009, **47**, 798–806.
74. F. Eyer, V. Meischner, D. Kiderlen, H. Thiermann, F. Worek, M. Haberkorn, N. Felgenhauer, T. Zilker and P. Eyer, Human parathion poisoning. A toxicokinetic analysis, *Toxicol. Rev.*, 2003, **22**, 143–163.
75. P. Eyer, F. Worek, H. Thiermann and M. Eddleston, Paradox findings may challenge orthodox reasoning in acute organophosphate poisoning, *Chem.Biol. Interact.*, 2010, **187**, 270–278.
76. H. Thiermann, F. Eyer, N. Felgenhauer, R. Pfab, T. Zilker, P. Eyer and F. Worek, Pharmacokinetics of obidoxime in patients poisoned with organophosphorus compounds, *Toxicol. Lett.*, 2010, **197**, 236–242.
77. H. Thiermann, U. Mast, R. Klimmek, P. Eyer, A. Hibler, R. Pfab, N. Felgenhauer and T. Zilker, Cholinesterase status, pharmacokinetics and laboratory findings during obidoxime therapy in organophosphate poisoned patients, *Hum. Exp. Toxicol.*, 1997, **16**, 473–480.
78. H. Thiermann, F. Worek, P. Eyer, F. Eyer, N. Felgenhauer and T. Zilker, Obidoxime in acute organophosphate poisoning: 2-PK/PD relationships, *Clin. Toxicol.*, 2009, **47**, 807–813.
79. H. Thiermann, L. Szinicz, P. Eyer, T. Zilker and F. Worek, Correlation between red blood cell acetylcholinesterase activity and neuromuscular transmission in organophosphate poisoning, *Chem.-Biol. Interact.*, 2005, **157–158**, 345–347.
80. H. Thiermann, T. Zilker, F. Eyer, N. Felgenhauer, P. Eyer and F. Worek, Monitoring of neuromuscular transmission in organophosphate pesticide-poisoned patients, *Toxicol. Lett.*, 2009, **191**, 297–304.
81. H. Thiermann, L. Szinicz, P. Eyer, N. Felgenhauer, T. Zilker and F. Worek, Lessons to be learnt from organophosphorus pesticide poisoning for the treatment of nerve agent poisoning, *Toxicology*, 2007, **233**, 145–154.

82. H. Thiermann, P. Eyer, F. Worek and L. Szinicz, Effects of oximes on muscle force and acetylcholinesterase activity in isolated mouse hemidiaphragms exposed to paraoxon, *Toxicology*, 2005, **214**, 190–197.
83. H. Thiermann, P. Eyer and F. Worek, Muscle force and acetylcholinesterase activity in mouse hemidiaphragms exposed to paraoxon and treated by oximes in vitro, *Toxicology*, 2010, **272**, 46–51.
84. T. Seeger, K. V. Niessen, P. Langer, J. Gerhardus, F. Worek, H. Friess, R. Bumm, A. L. Mihaljevic and H. Thiermann, Restoration of nerve agent inhibited muscle force production in human intercostal muscle strips with HI 6, *Toxicol. Lett.*, 2011, **206**, 72–76.
85. J. Mikler, C. Tenn, F. Worek, G. Reiter, H. Thiermann, M. Garrett, S. Bohnert and T. W. Sawyer, Immobilization of Russian VX skin depots by localized cooling: implications for decontamination and medical countermeasures, *Toxicol. Lett.*, 2011, **206**, 47–53.
86. T. W. Sawyer, J. Mikler, F. Worek, G. Reiter, H. Thiermann, C. Tenn, K. Weatherby and S. Bohnert, The therapeutic use of localized cooling in the treatment of VX poisoning, *Toxicol. Lett.*, 2011, **204**, 52–56.
87. J. Mikler, C. Tenn, F. Worek, G. Reiter, H. Thiermann, M. Garrett, S. Bohnert and T. W. Sawyer, Immobilization of Russian VX skin depots by localized cooling: implications for decontamination and medical countermeasures, *Toxicol. Lett.*, 2011, **206**, 47–53.
88. S. Eckert, P. Eyer, H. Muckter and F. Worek, Kinetic analysis of the protection afforded by reversible inhibitors against irreversible inhibition of acetylcholinesterase by highly toxic organophosphorus compounds, *Biochem. Pharmacol.*, 2006, **72**, 344–357.
89. S. Eckert, P. Eyer, N. Herkert, R. Bumm, G. Weber, H. Thiermann and F. Worek, Comparison of the oxime-induced reactivation of erythrocyte and muscle acetylcholinesterase following inhibition by sarin or paraoxon, using a perfusion model for the real-time determination of membrane-bound acetylcholinesterase activity, *Biochem. Pharmacol.*, 2008, **75**, 698–703.
90. N. M. Herkert, G. Lallement, D. Clarencon, H. Thiermann and F. Worek, Comparison of the oxime-induced reactivation of rhesus monkey, swine and guinea pig erythrocyte acetylcholinesterase following inhibition by sarin or paraoxon, using a perfusion model for the real-time determination of membrane-bound acetylcholinesterase activity, *Toxicology*, 2009, **258**, 79–83.
91. N. M. Herkert, N. Aurbek, P. Eyer, H. Thiermann and F. Worek, Comparative study of oxime-induced reactivation of erythrocyte and muscle AChE from different animal species following inhibition by sarin or paraoxon, *Toxicol. Lett.*, 2010, **194**, 94–101.
92. N. M. Herkert, G. Freude, U. Kunz, H. Thiermann and F. Worek, Comparative kinetics of organophosphates and oximes with erythrocyte, muscle and brain acetylcholinesterase, *Toxicol. Lett.*, 2012, **209**, 173–178.

93. N. M. Herkert, G. Lallement, D. Clarencon, H. Thiermann and F. Worek, Comparison of the oxime-induced reactivation of rhesus monkey, swine and guinea pig erythrocyte acetylcholinesterase following inhibition by sarin or paraoxon, using a perfusion model for the real-time determination of membrane-bound acetylcholinesterase activity, *Toxicology*, 2009, **258**, 79–83.
94. N. M. Herkert, S. Eckert, P. Eyer, R. Bumm, G. Weber, H. Thiermann and F. Worek, Identical kinetics of human erythrocyte and muscle acetylcholinesterase with respect to carbamate pre-treatment, residual activity upon soman challenge and spontaneous reactivation after withdrawal of the inhibitors, *Toxicology*, 2008, **246**, 188–192.
95. F. Worek, H. Thiermann, L. Szinicz and P. Eyer, Kinetic analysis of interactions between human acetylcholinesterase, structurally different organophosphorus compounds and oximes, *Biochem. Pharmacol.*, 2004, **68**, 2237–2248.
96. C. Bismuth, R. H. Inns and T. C. Marrs, *Efficacy, toxicity and clinical use of oximes in anticholinesterase poisoning, Clinical and experimental toxicology of organophosphates and carbamates*, ed. B. Ballyntyne and T. C. Marrs, Butterworth-Heinemann Ltd., Oxford, 2015, pp. 555–577.
97. S. Z. Xue, X. J. Ding and Y. Ding, Clinical observation and comparison of the effectiveness of several oxime cholinesterase reactivators, *Scand. J. Work, Environ. Health*, 1985, **11**(**suppl. 4**), 46–48.
98. F. Worek, L. Szinicz, P. Eyer and H. Thiermann, Evaluation of oxime efficacy in nerve agent poisoning: development of a kinetic-based dynamic model, *Toxicol. Appl. Pharmacol.*, 2005, **209**, 193–202.
99. D. Steinritz, F. Worek, J. Mikler and H. Thiermann, On-site therapy monitoring of nerve agent poisoning, *Clin. Toxicol.*, 2012, **50**(**4**), 335.
100. J. Willems, *Pralidoxime methylsulphate in the treatment of organophosphours poisoning, Role of Oximes in the Treatment of Anticholinesterase Agent Poisoning*, ed. L. Szinicz, P. Eyer and R. Klimmek, Spektrum Akademischer Verlag, Heidelberg, Berlin, Oxford, 1996, pp. 69–73.
101. P. Eyer, *Optimal oxime dosage regimen, a pharmacokinetic approach, Role of Oximes in the Treatment of Anticholinesterase Agent Poisoning*, ed. L. Szinicz, P. Eyer and R. Klimmek, Spektrum Akademischer Verlag, Heidelberg, Berlin, Oxford, 1996, pp. 33–51.
102. P. G. Blain, Organophosphorus poisoning (acute), *BMJ Clin. Evid.*, 2011, **2011**(5), 2102.
103. A. Lüttringhaus and I. Hagedorn, Quartäre Hydroxyiminomethylpyridiniumsalze. Das Dichlorid des Bis-[4-hydroxyiminomethylpyridinium-(1)-methyl]äthers ("LüH6"), ein neuer Reaktivator der durch organische Phosphorsäureester gehemmten Acetylcholin-Esterase, *Arzneimittelforschung*, 1964, **14**, 1–5.
104. P. Eyer, Use of obidoxime in OP poisoning, *Hum. Exp. Toxicol.*, 1996, **15**, 78.
105. H. Thiermann, T. Seeger, S. Gonder, N. Herkert, B. Antkowiak, T. Zilker, F. Eyer and F. Worek, Assessment of neuromuscular dysfunction during poisoning by organophosphorus compounds, *Chem.Biol. Interact.*, 2010, **187**, 256–269.

106. H. Thiermann, F. Eyer, N. Felgenhauer, R. Pfab, T. Zilker, P. Eyer and F. Worek, Pharmacokinetics of obidoxime in patients poisoned with organophosphorus compounds, *Toxicol. Lett.*, 2010, **197**, 236–242.
107. F. R. Sidell and W. A. Groff, Toxogonin: blood levels and side effects after intramuscular administration in man, *J. Pharm. Sci.*, 1970, **59**, 793–797.
108. W. D. Erdmann, I. Bosse and P. Franke, Zur Resorption und Ausscheidung von Toxogonin nach intramuskulärer Injektion am Menschen, *Dtsch. Med. Wochenschr.*, 1965, **33**, 1436–1438.
109. G. A. Simon, M. S. Tirosh and H. Edery, Administration of obidoxime tablets to man. Plasma levels and side reactions, *Arch. Toxicol.*, 1976, **36**, 83–88.
110. G. Boelcke, W. Creutzfeldt, W. D. Erdmann, J. W. Gaaz and G. Jacob, Studies on liver toxicity of obidoxim (Toxogonin) in humans, *Dtsch. Med. Wochenschr.*, 1970, **95**, 1175–1178.
111. H. J. Prinz, Therapie akuter Alkylphosphat-Vergiftungen, *Dtsch. Ärzteblatt*, 1967, **36**, 1845–1849.
112. D. Barckow, G. Neuhaus and W. D. Erdmann, Treatment of parathion (E 605) poisoning with the cholinesterase-reactivating substance obidoxime (Toxogonin), *Arch. Toxikol.*, 1969, **24**, 133–146.
113. U. von Gaisberg and K. Dieterle, Organ-Parenchymschäden nach E-605-Vergiftung bzw. hochdosierter Toxogoninbehandlung, *Dtsch. Ärzteblatt*, 1967, **35**, 1791–1796.
114. Y. Finkelstein, A. Kushnir, B. Raikhlin-Eisenkraft and U. Taitelman, Antidotal therapy of severe acute organophosphate poisoning: a multihospital study, *Neurotoxicol. Teratol.*, 1989, **11**, 593–596.
115. H. J. Prinz, [Severe percutaneous poisoning with parathion (E 605)] Eine schwere percutane Vergiftung mit Parathion (E 605), *Arch. Toxicol.*, 1969, **25**, 318–328.
116. F. Eyer, F. Worek, P. Eyer, N. Felgenhauer, M. Haberkorn, T. Zilker and H. Thiermann, Obidoxime in acute organophosphate poisoning: 1-clinical effectiveness, *Clin. Toxicol.*, 2009, **47**, 798–806.
117. R. D. Birtley, J. B. Roberts, B. H. Thomas and A. Wilson, Excretion and metabolism of [14C]-pyridostigmine in the rat, *Br. J. Pharmacol.*, 1966, **26**, 393–402.
118. I. B. Wilson and S. Ginsburg, Reactivation of acetylcholinesterase inhibited by alkylphosphates, *Arch. Biochem.*, 1955, **54**, 569–571.
119. N. A. Buckley, M. Eddleston and L. Szinicz, Oximes for acute organophosphate pesticide poisoning, *Cochrane. Database. Syst. Rev.*, 2005, CD005085.
120. R. M. Dawson, Review of oximes available for treatment of nerve agent poisoning, *J. Appl. Toxicol.*, 1994, **14**, 317–331.
121. C. Abbara, J. Rousseau, A. Turcant, G. Lallement, E. Comets, I. Bardot, P. Clair and B. Diquet, Bioavailability of diazepam after intramuscular injection of its water-soluble prodrug alone or with atropine-pralidoxime in healthy volunteers, *Br. J. Pharmacol.*, 2009, **157**, 1390–1397.
122. F. R. Sidell and W. A. Groff, Toxogonin: oral administration to man, *J. Pharm. Sci.*, 1971, **60**, 860–863.

123. B. Calesnick, J. A. Christensen and M. Richter, Human toxicity of various oximes. 2-Pyridine aldoxime methyl chloride, its methane sulfonate salt, and 1,1′-trimethylenebis-(4-formylpyridinium chloride), *Arch. Environ. Health*, 1967, **15**, 599–608.
124. B. V. Jager and G. N. Stagg, Toxicity of diacetyl monoxime and of pyridine-2-aldoxime methiodide in man, *Bull. Johns. Hopkins. Hosp.*, 1958, **102**, 203–211.
125. A. Sundwall, Plasma concentration curves of N-methylpyridinium-2-aldoxime methane sulfonate (P2S) after intraveneous, intramuscular and oral administration in man, *Biochem. Pharmacol.*, 1960, **5**(**3**), 225–230.
126. J. J. Medicis, C. M. Stork, M. A. Howland, R. S. Hoffman and L. R. Goldfrank, Pharmacokinetics following a loading plus a continuous infusion of pralidoxime compared with the traditional short infusion regimen in human volunteers, *J. Toxicol., Clin. Toxicol.*, 1996, **34**, 289–295.
127. B. Scott, Toxicity and Clinical Use of Prilocaine, *Proc. R. Soc. Med.*, 1965, **58**, 420–422.
128. T. O. Jeong, J. B. Lee, Y. H. Jin and J. C. Yoon, Respiratory arrest caused by accidental rapid pralidoxime infusion, *Clin. Toxicol.*, 2015, **53**, 412.
129. M. K. Johnson, D. Jacobsen, T. J. Meredith, P. Eyer, A. J. Heath, D. A. Ligtenstein, T. C. Marrs, L. Szinicz, J. A. Vale and J. A. Haines, Evalution of antidotes for poisoning by organophosphorus pesticides, *Emerg. Med.*, 2000, **12**, 22–37.
130. M. K. Johnson, J. A. Vale, T. C. Marrs and T. J. Meredith, Pralidoxime for organophosphorus poisoning, *Lancet*, 1992, **340**, 64.
131. A. Goel, P. Aggarwal, S. Bhoi and V. Gupta, High-dose pralidoxime for organophosphorus poisoning, *Lancet*, 2007, **369**, 1425.
132. K. S. Pawar, R. R. Bhoite, C. P. Pillay, S. C. Chavan, D. S. Malshikare and S. G. Garad, Continuous pralidoxime infusion *versus* repeated bolus injection to treat organophosphorus pesticide poisoning: a randomised controlled trial, *Lancet*, 2006, **368**, 2136–2141.
133. P. Due, Effectiveness of high dose pralidoxime for treatment of organophosphate poisoning, *Asia Pac. J. Med. Toxicol.*, 2015, **3**, 97–103.
134. P. Eyer, I. Hagedorn and B. Ladstetter, Study on the stability of the oxime HI 6 in aqueous solution, *Arch. Toxicol.*, 1988, **62**, 224–226.
135. P. Eyer, B. Ladstetter, W. Schafer and J. Sonnenbichler, Studies on the stability and decomposition of the Hagedorn-oxime HLo 7 in aqueous solution, *Arch. Toxicol.*, 1989, **63**, 59–67.
136. H. Thiermann, R. Schreiner and P. Eyer, Dissolution kinetics of unstable drugs in two-compartment autoinjectors: analysis of the individual shaking behaviour and influence of various shaking parameters on the dissolution rate of HI 6 in an automated system, *Int. J. Pharm.*, 1998, **170**, 23–32.
137. H. Thiermann, S. Seidl and P. Eyer, HI 6 dimethanesulfonate has better dissolution properties than HI6 dichloride for application in dry/wet autoinjectors., *Int. J. Pharm.*, 1996, **137**, 167–176.

138. U. Spohrer, H. Thiermann, R. Klimmek and P. Eyer, Pharmacokinetics of the oximes HI 6 and HLo 7 in dogs after i.m. injection with newly developed dry/wet autoinjectors, *Arch. Toxicol.*, 1994, **68**, 480–489.
139. A. Goransson-Nyberg, G. Cassel, T. Jeneskog, L. Karlsson, R. Larsson, M. Lundstrom and S. A. Persson, Treatment of organophosphate poisoning in pigs: antidote administration by a new binary autoinjector, *Arch. Toxicol.*, 1995, **70**, 20–27.
140. R. Kusic, B. Boskovic, V. Vojvodic and D. Jovanovic, HI-6 in man: blood levels, urinary excretion, and tolerance after intramuscular administration of the oxime to healthy volunteers, *Fundam. Appl. Toxicol.*, 1985, **5**, S89–S97.
141. J. G. Clement, D. G. Bailey, H. D. Madill, L. T. Tran and J. D. Spence, The acetylcholinesterase oxime reactivator HI-6 in man: pharmacokinetics and tolerability in combination with atropine, *Biopharm. Drug Dispos.*, 1995, **16**, 415–425.
142. J. Tattersall, Seizure activity post organophosphate exposure, *Front. Biosci., Landmark Ed.*, 2009, **14**, 3688–3711.
143. T. Myhrer and P. Aas, Choice of approaches in developing novel medical countermeasures for nerve agent poisoning, *Neurotoxicology*, 2014, **44**, 27–38.
144. J. H. McDonough, Jr. and T. M. Shih, Neuropharmacological mechanisms of nerve agent-induced seizure and neuropathology, *Neurosci. Biobehav. Rev.*, 1997, **21**, 559–579.
145. N. Yanagisawa, H. Morita and T. Nakajima, Sarin experiences in Japan: acute toxicity and long-term effects, *J. Neurol. Sci.*, 2006, **249**, 76–85.
146. J. H. McDonough, Jr., J. McMonagle, T. Copeland, D. Zoeffel and T. M. Shih, Comparative evaluation of benzodiazepines for control of soman-induced seizures, *Arch. Toxicol.*, 1999, **73**, 473–478.
147. R. K. Rude and F. R. Singer, Magnesium deficiency and excess, *Annu. Rev. Med.*, 1981, **32**, 245–259.
148. A. G. Euser and M. J. Cipolla, Magnesium sulfate for the treatment of eclampsia: a brief review, *Stroke*, 2009, **40**, 1169–1175.
149. A. Pajoumand, S. Shadnia, A. Rezaie, M. Abdi and M. Abdollahi, Benefits of magnesium sulfate in the management of acute human poisoning by organophosphorus insecticides, *Hum. Exp. Toxicol.*, 2004, **23**, 565–569.
150. G. Petroianu, L. M. Toomes, A. Petroianu, W. Bergler and R. Rufer, Control of blood pressure, heart rate and haematocrit during high-dose intravenous paraoxon exposure in mini pigs, *J. Appl. Toxicol.*, 1998, **18**, 293–298.
151. S. Katalan, S. Lazar, R. Brandeis, I. Rabinovitz, I. Egoz, E. Grauer, E. Bloch-Shilderman and L. Raveh, Magnesium sulfate treatment against sarin poisoning: dissociation between overt convulsions and recorded cortical seizure activity, *Arch. Toxicol.*, 2013, **87**, 347–360.
152. C. J. Del and L. Engbaek, The nature of the neuromuscular block produced by magnesium, *J. Physiol.*, 1954, **124**, 370–384.

153. G. Singh, G. Avasthi, D. Khurana, J. Whig and R. Mahajan, Neurophysiological monitoring of pharmacological manipulation in acute organophosphate (OP) poisoning. The effects of pralidoxime, magnesium sulphate and pancuronium, *Electroencephalogr. Clin. Neurophysiol.*, 1998, **107**, 140–148.
154. A. Basher, S. H. Rahman, A. Ghose, S. M. Arif, M. A. Faiz and A. H. Dawson, Phase II study of magnesium sulfate in acute organophosphate pesticide poisoning, *Clin. Toxicol.*, 2013, **51**, 35–40.
155. D. Cordoba, S. Cadavid, D. Angulo and I. Ramos, Organophosphate poisoning: modifications in acid base equilibrium and use of sodium bicarbonate as an aid in the treatment of toxicity in dogs, *Vet. Hum. Toxicol.*, 1983, **25**, 1–3.
156. A. Wong and T. M. Santos, Use of sodium bicarbonate in organophosphate poisoning, *Hum. Exp. Toxicol.*, 1996, **15**, 79.
157. A. Wong, C. A. Sandron, A. S. Magalhaes and L. C. S. Rocha, Comaprative efficacy of pralidoxime vs. sodium bicarbonate in rats and humans severely poisoned with O-P-persticides, *J. Toxicol., Clin. Toxicol.*, 2000, **38**(**5**), 554.
158. J. Bajgar and R. Portmann, *The treatment of intoxication with selected organophosphates and a carbamate: comparison of different therapeutic approaches*, 2001, pp. 180–184.
159. M. Balali-Mood, M. H. Ayati and H. Ali-Akbarian, Effects of high doses of sodium bicarbonate in acute organophosphate pesticide poisoning, *J. Toxicol., Clin. Toxicol.*, 2003, **41**(**4**), 383.
160. M. Balali-Mood, M. H. Ayati and H. li-Akbarian, Effect of high doses of sodium bicarbonate in acute organophosphorous pesticide poisoning, *Clin. Toxicol.*, 2005, **43**, 571–574.
161. D. Roberts and N. A. Buckley, Alkalinisation for organophosphorus pesticide poisoning, *Cochrane. Database. Syst. Rev.*, 2005, CD004897.
162. G. Becker, A. Kawan and L. Szinicz, Direct reaction of oximes with sarin, soman, or tabun in vitro, *Arch. Toxicol.*, 1997, **71**, 714–718.
163. G. Becker, A. Kawan, D. Gutzeit, F. Worek and L. Szinicz, Direct reaction of oximes with crotylsarin, cyclosarin, or VX in vitro, *Arch. Toxicol.*, 2007, **81**, 415–420.
164. A. P. Volans, Sarin: guidelines on the management of victims of a nerve gas attack, *J. Accid. Emerg. Med.*, 1996, **13**, 202–206.

CHAPTER 2

Nerve Agents: Catalytic Scavengers as an Alternative Approach for Medical Countermeasures

PATRICK MASSON[a]

[a]Kazan Federal University, Neuropharmacology Laboratory, 18 Kremlevskaya St. Kazan 420008, Russia
*E-mail: pym.masson@free.fr

2.1 Introduction

Organophosphorus agents (OPs) are pesticides (*e.g.* parathion, malathion, chlorpyrifos and dichlorvos); drugs and pro-drugs (*e.g.* echothiophate, métrifonate and cyclophosphamide); flame retardants and anti-wear agents [*e.g.* tricresyl phosphate (TCP)]; and chemical warfare nerve agents (CWNAs). CWNAs include G-agents: tabun, sarin, soman, cyclohexyl-sarin (cyclosarin); V-agents: VX, VR (RVX), CVX; and "Novichoks": A-230, A-232, A-234.[1,2] OP pesticides and all other toxic OPs, excluding classical CWNAs, can be considered as "non-traditional nerve agents" (NTAs). NTAs are potential CWNAs and terrorist threat agents. Highly toxic OPs may result from cytochrome P_{450} mediated metabolic oxidation of parent thiono-phosphoesters, *e.g.* paraoxon from parathion,[3] or 2-(*o*-cresyl)-4*H*-1,3,2-benzodioxaphosphoran-2-one

Issues in Toxicology No. 27
Chemical Warfare Toxicology, Volume 2: Management of Poisoning
Edited by Franz Worek, John Jenner, and Horst Thiermann

Published by the Royal Society of Chemistry, www.rsc.org

[CBDP; or cresyl-saligenin phosphate (CSP)] by cyclization of tri-*ortho*-cresyl phosphate (TOCP), a tri-cresyl phosphate (TCP) isomer.[4] TCP is a flame retardant and anti-wear agent present in jet engine oils and hydraulic fluids. High temperature pyrolysis of jet fighter engine oils may also lead to toxic OPs such as trimethylolpropane phosphate (TMPP).[5] Most OPs are potent irreversible inhibitors of cholinesterases (ChEs) and of many other serine hydrolases. However, TMPP is not an inhibitor of ChEs; it is a GABA antagonist, so toxic that it has been called "the poor man's nerve agent", and is also considered as a potential threat.[6]

Acetylcholinesterase (AChE; EC 3.1.1.7) plays a major role in the cholinergic system, terminating the action of acetylcholine. Inhibition of AChE causes blockade of cholinergic transmissions in the peripheral and central nervous systems (Figure 2.1). It is the main cause of the acute toxicity of OPs.[7] Covalent modification of proteins and irreversible inhibition of other enzymes (non-cholinergic targets), including various serine hydrolases, plays a role in the sub-acute toxicity, delayed toxicity and non-cholinergic toxicity of OPs.[8,9] Although the sister enzyme butyrylcholinesterase (BChE; EC.3.1.1.8) has no known physiological function, its inhibition by OPs exerts a protection of the cholinergic system by stoichiometric scavenging of low doses of OPs. The concentration of BChE in human plasma is 50 nM.[10]

Emergency treatments of acute OP poisoning by pesticides and nerve agents (NAs), and management of casualties have significantly improved in the past 25 years.[11–15] However, classical pharmacological approaches are reaching their optimum limit. Attacks in Syria, where sarin was employed, revealed the limitations of current medical treatments.[16,17] Moreover, due to the possible storage of OP in depot sites and subsequent slow release in the blood stream, blood and tissue ChEs may remain inhibited for long periods of time post-exposure (Figure 2.1). Therefore, persistence of certain OPs in the body after exposure implies the need for prolonged treatments. This complication is particularly well documented for severe intoxications by parathion.[18]

The toxicity of OPs can be countered by reducing skin absorption, and lowering the OP concentration, [OP], in the blood compartment, thus preventing the transfer of OP molecules to cholinergic synapses and other physiological non-cholinergic targets. Neutralization of toxic molecules can be achieved by using stoichiometric traps or catalysts acting on exposed surfaces [*e.g.* active topical skin protectants (TSPs) and reactive skin decontamination lotions], or administered scavengers, acting in the bloodstream (Figure 2.1). There are several recent reviews about the use of (bio)scavengers for prophylaxis (pre-treatment) and post-exposure treatment of OP poisoning.[10,14,19]

2.2 The Scavenger Concept

Scavengers are chemicals or biomolecules that sequestrate and inactivate highly toxic chemicals before they reach biological targets. Scavengers can react stoichiometrically with toxic molecules or with a turnover as catalysts. Endogenous scavengers play a role in natural defenses against toxicants and

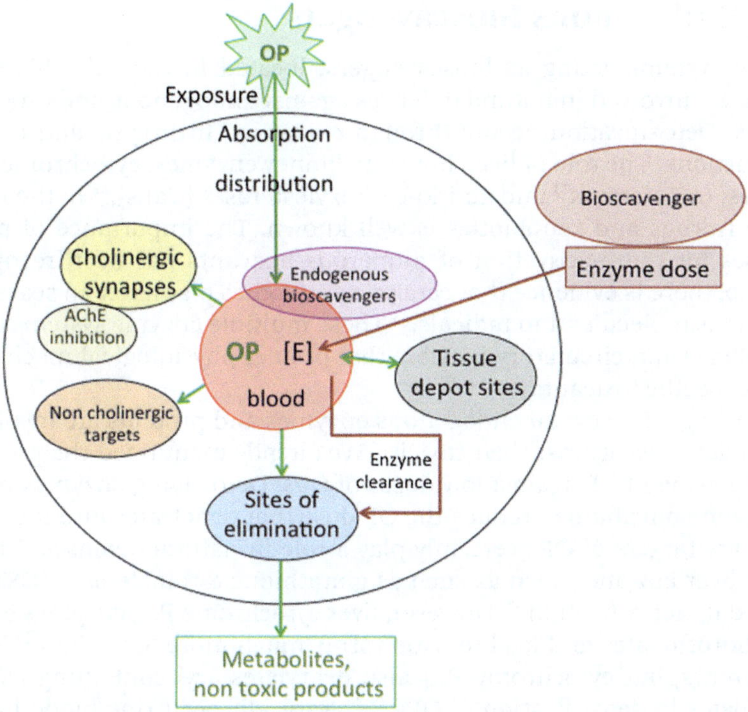

Figure 2.1 Biological fate and kinetic control of OPs in mammals. Routes of penetration of OPs are absorption through the skin, eyes and/or respiratory tract (nerve agents, pesticides and flame retardants), or ingestion (accidental or intentional self-poisoning). OP molecules distribute from the blood compartment into tissues, including depot sites, biophase (physiological targets, *i.e.* peripheral and central cholinergic synapses and secondary targets) and sites of elimination (liver and kidney). AChE is the main physiological target. Irreversible inhibition of AChE is responsible for acute toxicity. Reaction with secondary targets (CaEs, serine amidases, neuropathy target esterase, serine peptidases and other serine hydrolases, and various proteins) may be responsible for the non-cholinergic sub-lethal effects of OPs, delayed toxicity (neuropathies) and chronic toxicity from low dose exposure. Targets include endogenous bioscavengers. BChE is present in numerous tissues where it acts as an endogenous stoichiometric bioscavenger. In particular, its concentration in human plasma is about 50 nM. Therapeutic enzymes (exogenous stoichiometric/catalytic bioscavengers)—administered by injection, inhalation and any other delivery routes—act in the blood compartment (E) after absorption and distribution.

deleterious chemicals, *e.g.* free radicals. Exogenous scavengers are (bio)pharmaceuticals intended to be used for the protection of the body against ionizing radiation, reactive chemicals and poisonous xenobiotics, and deleterious side effects of drugs; they can be used for soft decontamination of the skin, mucosa, eyes and wounds, as well as for pre-treatment and post-exposure treatments.

2.3 Endogenous Bioscavengers

Enzyme systems acting as bioscavengers, located in the skin, blood and organs, are involved in natural defenses against endogenous and exogenous poisons. Detoxification occurs through oxidation, hydrolysis and conjugation reactions. The role of liver, lung and kidney enzymes, cytochrome P_{450},[20] oxidases, transferases[21] and amido-carboxylesterases (CaEs),[22] in the metabolism of drugs and xenobiotics is well known. The importance of plasma esterases for the inactivation of numerous toxicants has been recognized too. Also, there is evidence that catalytic antibodies play a role in scavenging deleterious molecules and radicals.[23] These multiple enzyme systems constitute cellular and circulatory barriers that protect physiological machineries against specific toxicants.

Regarding OPs, several endogenous enzymes and proteins are involved in natural defenses against their toxicity. We already mentioned the protective role of plasma BChE against low doses of OPs. Detoxifying enzymes present in the skin contribute to reduce the OP dose that penetrates into the body.[24] Secondary targets of OPs certainly play a role in natural defenses.[25] In particular, liver enzymes such as such as glutathione *S*-transferases (GSTs) are involved in detoxification.[26] However, liver cytochrome P_{450} enzymes activate phosphorothioates and lead to oxon forms much more toxic than their thiono parents, but cytochrome P_{450} also dearylates aryl containing OPs and participates in detoxification of OPs.[27,28] Naturally occurring blood bioscavengers significantly contribute to reduce the concentration of OP molecules reaching physiological targets. It has been shown that animal species with a high concentration of paraoxonase-1 (PON-1; EC 3.1.8.1) or CaE (EC 3.1.1.1) are relatively resistant to OPs.[29] Conversely, *knockout* mice for PON-1 are more sensitive to OPs.[30] Albumin slowly reacts with carbamoyl- and phosphoryl-esters. The albumin concentration in the blood and lymph system is so high (≈0.6 mM) that it may play a role in the neutralization of certain OPs[31,32] and carbamates at toxicologically relevant concentrations.[33]

The functional capacity of endogenous bioscavengers can be enhanced by increasing the expression of these macromolecules. An increase in the concentration of endogenous human BChE and AChE could be achieved by administration of proline rich polypeptides derived from ChE collagenic tail peptides [ColQ proline rich attachment domain (PRAD)] or peptides derived from the transmembrane anchor (PRIMA). This should promote folding, tetrameric assembly of enzymes, and thus increase their export from cells.[34] Endogenous expression of PON-1 and its plasma concentration can be positively modulated using hypolipemic drugs and polyphenols.[35,36]

2.4 Stoichiometric Scavengers

The first (bio)molecules that were studied for the purpose of making stoichiometric scavengers against OPs were cyclodextrins,[37] neutralizing antibodies,[38] activated charcoal and human plasma. Only hemodialysis on charcoal and transfusion of human plasma (plasmapheresis) have been used as adjuncts in the treatment of OP poisoning so far. Hemodialysis on a charcoal cartridge was successfully used on a Tokyo casualty who was resistant to the classical treatment of sarin poisoning.[39] The effects of fresh frozen plasma on ChE levels and outcomes in OP poisoned patients have been evaluated.[40,41] A recent *in vitro* study suggested that plasma therapy may be an effective adjunct to treatment of G-agent poisoning.[42] Plasma BChE and other OP scavenging proteins in plasma (*e.g.* albumin and PON-1) may have contributed to these results. At this point, it must be noted that human plasma does not contain CaEs.[43]

The interest in bioscavengers progressively emerged in the 1980s.[44] At the end of the 1980s, research on stoichiometric bioscavengers mostly focused on enzymes that specifically react with OPs: ChEs[45] and CaEs.[46–48] Then, after some 15 years of investigation, human BChE proved to be a safe and effective stoichiometric bioscavenger for pre- and post-exposure treatment of NA and OP pesticide poisoning.[49–53] Human plasma derived BChE was granted Investigational New Drug status by the US Food and Drug Administration in 2006 for protection against NAs.[50] Clinical trials on volunteers were accomplished a few years ago. However, results have not been released. The main problem with BChE, and any stoichiometric bioscavenger, is that enzymatic stoichiometric neutralization of several OP lethal dose, 50% (LD_{50})s requires administration of huge doses of enzyme; about 3 mg kg^{-1} of highly purified plasma BChE,[54] *i.e.* 200–300 mg for humans against 2 LD_{50}s of soman.

Therefore, large scale production of human BChE under good manufacturing practice (GMP) conditions has been the subject of intense research in the past 10 years. Several industrial processes have been proposed for production of the natural plasma enzyme or the recombinant one. The first process is purification of the natural BChE from a side product (Cohn fraction IV) of human plasma fractionation. However, although thousands of tons of outdated human plasma are available for preparing the enzyme, 1 l of human plasma provides less than 1 mg of GMP BChE. The purity of the enzyme has to be close to 100%, because any impurity, *e.g.* bacterial endotoxin or coagulation factors, could induce fatal iatrogenic effects. Thus, the cost of production is very high. Purification of the natural human plasma BChE has been developed by Saxena *et al.*,[55] Lockridge *et al.* (unpublished), and Baxter Healthcare Corporation (http://www.baxter.com), starting from the Cohn fraction IV. A new affinity chromatography method, using huprine derivatives[56] as immobilized ligands instead of procainamide, is expected to lower the cost of production of the plasma derived enzyme. The second process uses recombinant human BChE produced in the milk of transgenic goats. It has been developed by Nexia (http://www.nexiabiotech.com). Several grams of recombinant enzyme can be secreted in 1 l of milk. This enzyme has been named Protexia™. Since 2005, Pharmatheme (http://www.pharmathene.com) developed Protexia™ polyethylene glycol (PEG)ylated BChE conjugates[57] and fusion proteins.[58] However, production of recombinant human BChE in the milk of transgenic mammals has been discontinued due to the high cost and pharmacokinetic problems. Therefore, several companies are setting up large scale production of recombinant human BChE in Chinese hamster ovary (CHO) cells[59] and other cells. Thus, production of human BChE in transgenic tobacco has been made possible.[60–62] PlantForm in Canada (http://www.plantformcorp.com) has been engaged in the development of recombinant human BChE in tobacco that mimics the stability and pharmacokinetics of the plasma derived enzyme. In Russia, a program for the production of recombinant human BChE in *Agrobacterium* infected potatoes has been undertaken (Aliev *et al.*, unpublished).

As stated previously, secondary targets of OPs are potential bioscavengers. In particular, human serum albumin covalently binds OP molecules.[63] Thus, it may be hypothesized that the reactivity of reactive residues (tyrosine and serine) could be enhanced by genetic engineering and/or chemical modification. Engineered albumins might lead to new stoichiometric bioscavengers. However, the first attempt at direct tyrosine nitration (to lower the pK_a of tyrosine) did not improve its reactivity, possibly because of steric hindrance (Masson *et al.*, unpublished). Otherwise, conversion of human albumin into a catalytic bioscavenger is unrealistic because it would need to increase its OP hydrolase activity by several orders of magnitude.[31]

Small size stoichiometric scavengers could be an economic alternative to enzyme based stoichiometric bioscavengers. For instance, serine and tyrosine containing peptides capable of reacting with a sarin analog were selected from a random library of hexapeptides.[64,65] However, no data are available about the bimolecular rate constants of these reactions.

2.5 Pseudo-Catalytic Scavengers

Since the main limitation of the stoichiometric bioscavenger approach is the "pharaonic" cost of the enzyme dose needed for challenging OP molecules, a way to circumvent this problem is to reactivate *in vivo* the administered enzyme, converting the stoichiometric bioscavenger into a pseudo-catalytic bioscavenger. This concept could also be applied to small size OP reacting chemical scavengers by co-administering specific reactivators. Certain ChE mutants sensitive to OPs do not "age" after phosphylation, they are fully reactivatable. For instance, the human AChE mutant Y337A/F338A,[66] when associated with oximes, acts as a pseudo-catalyst in displacing the OP adduct. Enzyme reactivator coupled systems could lead to pseudo-catalytic bioscavengers.[67,68] This requires synthesis of new oximes displaying higher affinity for phosphylated ChEs and higher reactivation constants than current oximes, and a long residence time in the bloodstream. A study with wild-type human BChE showed that orientation of the oxime group toward the phosphorus atom of the adduct is crucial for fast reactivation of the enzyme. Several libraries of positively charged and uncharged molecules have been made by *in silico* design or click chemistry, and tested with success *in vitro* against tabun and soman inhibited human BChE,[69,70] and sarin, cyclosarin and VX inhibited human BChE.[71]

2.6 Catalytic Scavengers

Catalytic scavengers are either biomolecules, *i.e.* enzymes and catalytic antibodies, or artificial catalysts capable of trapping and degrading OPs with a turnover. These catalysts detoxify OPs either by hydrolyzing the phosphoester [organophosphorus acid anhydride hydrolase (OAAH)] activity, also called phosphotriesterase (PTE) activity, OP hydrolase (OPH; OPase) activity or by oxidizing their alkyl/aryl chains, thus leading to less toxic compounds.

The use of catalytic scavengers is based on the concept of fast and continuous degradation of OP molecules in the bloodstream. Thus, catalytic scavengers can be used for pre-treatment and/or post-exposure treatment. Prophylactic injection of catalytic scavengers capable of degrading OP quickly (alone or in association with current prophylactic countermeasures, *i.e.* pyridostigmine bromide, other carbamates and reversible ChE inhibitors, and anticholinergic drugs[14]) would allow first responders, firemen, explosive ordnance disposal technicians and medical personnel to operate safely in contaminated environments on contaminated casualties. Early studies established that intravenous or intramuscular administration of bioscavengers to chemical casualties should greatly improve the efficacy of current pharmacological countermeasures.[72,73]

Catalytic scavengers could also be used for protection of the skin, and decontamination of the skin, mucosa and open wounds.[74,75] Chemical catalysts and genetically engineered bacteria producing OP hydrolases could be introduced into water effluents of decontamination units and be used to purify contaminated water before recycling or washing up in the environment.[76]

2.7 Requirements for Operational Catalytic Scavengers

The general requirements for the use of catalytic (bio)scavengers as medical countermeasures against OP poisoning are as follows: (1) these catalysts must have a large activity spectra, and ideally, enantioselectivity for toxic stereoisomers; (2) their mass production under GMP conditions must be realizable at a reasonable cost; (3) long term storage without activity loss (in solution, lyophilized or adsorbed/bound on a matrix) must be possible under field conditions. Conformational stability of enzymes and other biopharmaceuticals can be optimized by chemical modification or addition of stabilizers. Otherwise, thermostable PTEs from hyperthermophilic bacteria[77,78] or mutated/evolved highly stable enzymes from mesophilic bacteria are promising alternatives to chemical modifications.

Other conditions depend on the administration route, delivery system or galenic formulation of (bio)scavengers. Enzymes can be injected intravenously or intramuscularly. Other routes have been considered such as the intranasal route against aerosolized or gaseous NAs. For instance, pre-treatment with aerosolized forms of BChE have been shown to protect against aerosolized paraoxon.[52] For parenteral administration, the toxicant concentration in the bloodstream has to be taken into account. However, the OP concentration, [OP], is always very low, even in the most severe cases of poisoning. For example, the sarin concentrations in serum of casualties after Matsumoto and Tokyo attacks were estimated between 1.5 and 30 nM, 14 h post-exposure.[79] Therefore, [OP] is well below the Michaelis constant (K_m) of enzymes for OP substrates. This determines first-order kinetics ([OP] $\ll K_m$) for hydrolysis of OP in the blood[80,81] as described by eqn (2.1):

$$v = \frac{k_{cat}}{K_m} \times [E] \times [OP] \tag{2.1}$$

In eqn (2.1), the product of the bimolecular rate constant (k_{cat}/K_m) and the enzyme active site concentration ([E]) is the first order rate constant (in min^{-1}). The enzyme dose to be injected for complete degradation of toxic molecules in a very short time depends on the enzyme's catalytic efficiency, *i.e.* k_{cat}/K_m. The higher the catalytic efficiency, the lower the enzyme dose to be administered. The actual [E] needed to drop the [OP] to a non-toxic concentration in time t is:

$$[E] = \frac{X}{k_{cat}/K_m \times t} \tag{2.2}$$

where X is the factor by which [OP] is reduced ($X = \ln[OP]_0/[OP]_t$).[81] In eqn (2.2), it is assumed that the biological stability and pharmacokinetics of the administered enzyme have been optimized, and that the enzyme concentration, [E], does not decrease significantly during the time course (t) of the detoxification process. Thus, the enzyme clearance has to be negligible (*cf.* Figure 2.1). Enzyme efficiency and stereospecificity can be increased by several orders of magnitude either by site directed mutagenesis, directed evolution or chemical engineering.[82,83]

The second constraint is, thus, to maintain the concentration, [E], in the bloodstream as high as possible for a long time. [E] is controlled by pharmacokinetics/pharmacodynamics and/or the frequency of repeated administrations of the enzyme. Fast clearance of glycoproteins is often due to glycosylation defects or the micro-heterogeneity of glycans. Fast clearance of non-glycosylated enzyme may result from their too small size.[84] The enzyme size can be increased by polymerization, fusion to other proteins (*e.g.* human albumin[58]) or conjugation to PEG, dextrans and other macromolecules. Non-covalent interactions of recombinant human BChE with co-expressed PRAD[85] or with added 15-mer to 50-mer polyproline peptides[86] promote assembly of monomers into enzyme tetramers. The residence time of the BChE tetramer is much longer than that of the monomeric enzyme. Glycosylation defects and micro-heterogeneity can be corrected by chemical modifications ("capping") of purified enzymes, *e.g.* PEGylation[87,88] or polysialylation,[85] or by selection of an appropriate expression system,[89] including over-expression of an additional glycosylation enzyme that increases the sialylation content of the expressed glycoprotein[62] or transient co-expression of a multigene vector carrying genes involved in the mammalian sialylation pathway.[90] All of these modifications reduce renal clearance and increase the biological half-life ($t_{1/2}$) or mean residence time (MRT) of the bioscavenger in the bloodstream.

Injection of homologous enzymes does not induce an immunologic response following a second injection.[91] Otherwise, immuno-tolerance of heterologous enzymes is a major issue. Bacterial enzymes and non-human eukaryotic enzymes are not suitable for use in humans, but conjugation to dextran, PEGylation or inclusion in nano-containers may reduce antigenicity and slow down clearance after multiple injections.[92–94] Another way to prevent immune response to heterologous enzymes is extracorporeal blood dialysis on immobilized enzyme medical devices. First, extracorporeal dialysis was successfully implemented in a patient for blood decontamination after the Tokyo subway attack.[39] Thus, incorporation of OP degrading enzymes in a plasmapheresis system coupled to a dialysis unit could greatly enhance the efficiency of dialysis. Enzymes can be easily immobilized on dialysis cartridges[95] or hollow fibers. Accessibility of OP molecules to the enzyme's active center must not be altered by the immobilization method or by matrix effects. The enzyme concentration per surface unit has to be maximized to reduce diffusion constraints. First-order kinetics take place under the conditions of immobilized enzymes in a continuous flow system. Thus, the reactive surface of the matrix and k_{cat}/K_m would have to be as high as possible and the flow rate reduced to increase the reactor efficiency.

Last, *in situ* transient production of enzymes will be possible in the future. Promising results of gene therapy attempts have been reported, using short induction gene vectors (adenoviral systems) for human PON-1,[96–101] human AChE,[102] human BChE,[103,104] mutated human BChE that displays high cocaine esterase[105] and human prolidase (PROL).[106]

Enzymes incorporated into skin lotions and eye drops, immobilized in foams and on tissues for skin and eye decontamination,[107] or in TSPs[108] act under conditions where local OP concentrations can be very high. Under such conditions, the enzyme reaction order in [OP] tends to zero, so that the reaction rate (v) is close to the maximum velocity ($v \rightarrow V_{max} = k_{cat} \times [E]$). Thus, the enzyme's efficiency depends on its concentration [E] and its catalytic constant k_{cat}. Thus, for external use, highly catalytically active enzyme preparations would have to be highly concentrated. Again, the bioscavenger cost is a serious operative limitation to this approach. Chemical catalytic scavengers such as functionalized cyclodextrins appear to be an alternative to enzymes for this purpose. Co-immobilization of different catalysts, enzymes or chemicals is a way to extend the spectra of agents to be degraded. This should allow simultaneous detoxification of G- and V-agents, as well as other CWNAs, OP pesticides and NTAs, and even the mysterious "fourth generation NAs". Indeed, exposure to multiple agents has to be considered. In this view, it should be remembered that during the war between Iran and Iraq, tabun and other OPs were combined with mustard gas in some attacks. We also must keep in mind that industrial chemicals contain numerous impurities and synthesis side-products that may be more toxic than the referenced agent. In asymmetric conflicts, eschatological and mafia like terrorism, the most extreme scenarios have to be anticipated.

2.8 Potential Enzymes

2.8.1 Phosphotriesterases

2.8.1.1 Bacterial PTEs

Bacterial PTEs (EC 3.1.8.1) detoxify OPs, including NAs.[109,110] These enzymes, which have been isolated from numerous strains, belong to a superfamily of amidohydrolases.[111,112] Four enzyme families showing different folds or topologies can be described: TIM-barrel fold, β-lactamase fold, pita bread fold and β-propeller fold.[112] They are encoded by the organophosphate degradation (*opd*) gene found in species of *Brevundimonas diminuta* (formerly *Pseudomonas diminuta*), *Flavobacterium* sp., *Agrobacterium radiobacter*[113] and *Pseudomonas pseudoalcaligenes*,[114] and genes similar to *opd* were also located in archaea.[77] PTEs are primarily lactonases, thus they are now called PTE like lactonases (PLL). The lactonase activity plays a role in bacterial communication as a *quorum* quencher. Indeed, virulence and formation of biofilms are regulated by the lactone concentration in the medium. The PTE activity is a promiscuous activity resulting from evolution of the lactonase activity. It is thought that evolution occurred within the last few decades.[78,115–117]

Brevundimonas diminuta PTE is a 72 kDa dimeric bimetallic (Zn^{2+}) enzyme. Its 3D structure has been solved.[118] However, its catalytic mechanism is still debated and the functional roles of divalent metal cations and amino acids in the active center are not yet fully understood.[112,119–123] Whereas the catalytic efficiency of *Brevundimonas diminuta* PTE for hydrolysis of paraoxon, the best substrate identified so far, is approaching the diffusion controlled limit ($k_{cat}/K_m = 2 \times 10^{-9}$ M^{-1} min^{-1}),[124] it is slow against NAs.[125–127] Meanwhile, early work on directed evolution of *Brevundimonas diminuta* PTE showed that only three amino acid changes dramatically enhanced the catalytic efficiency for a soman analog by approximately three orders of magnitude.[128] Further studies combining rational design, docking simulations based on mutant models or directed evolution led to randomized libraries of mutants and selection of variants with greatly improved catalytic activity against S_p enantiomers of NA chromogenic analogs, including VX, RVX and CVX analogs, and racemic real NAs.[83,129–131,240] For example, after five rounds of optimization, the mutant, called C23, is able to hydrolyze the toxic S_p isomers of the three V-agents with k_{cat}/K_m values of up to 5×10^6 M^{-1} min^{-1}.[130]

There have been numerous studies highlighting the potential of *Brevundimonas diminuta* PTE for decontamination or skin protection in addition to OP detection.[74,75,109,132,133] Administration of PTE before or after OP exposure was shown to improve pre-treatment and current treatment of OP intoxication.[49]

A recent study showed that the engineered mutant of this enzyme (C23),[130] administered in post-exposure treatment, can prevent the systemic toxicity of 2 LD_{50}s of P(−) VX in the guinea pig.[134] Although the $t_{1/2}$ of this enzyme in the bloodstream is short, ≈2.5 h, this is the first enzyme capable of challenging a V-agent, and in particular its most toxic enantiomer. However, in order to prevent abnormally fast pharmacokinetics and/or immunological responses due to injection of a bacterial enzyme, PTE could be PEGylated[135] or encapsulated. First attempts at using PTE encapsulated within sterically stabilized liposomes were promising, providing protection of rats from multiple LD_{50}s of OP pesticides.[136] An alternative route could be the detoxification of the blood by extracorporeal circulation through a hollow fiber cartridge containing immobilized PTEs (Masson *et al.*, unpublished results). PTEs possibly could also be used for skin protection as active components of TSPs or covalently coupled to the cornified layer of the epidermis.[137]

Brevundimonas diminuta PTE was also entrapped in additives for latex coatings of biodefensive surfaces. Such PTE based additives for paints and coatings were shown to retain the catalytic parameters and stability of the enzyme.[138] For decontamination of OPs in the environment and remediation of soils, an alternative approach, phytodegradation by transgenic plants expressing a bacterial PTE, has been considered as a potentially low cost, effective and environmentally friendly method.[139] A His-tagged PTE[140] was reported to degrade NAs, including VX, at a high rate. Since the enzyme was not genetically modified, it has been suggested that the presence of the His tag may play a role in this amazing property. Although neither 3D structure nor molecular dynamics studies are available for this enzyme, it was hypothesized that the His tag may increase the PTE flexibility, which in turn may increase the enzyme's capability to accommodate different OP molecules, and enhance its catalytic activity. However, without further studies supporting this hypothesis, the Occam's razor principle has to be applied.

Highly stable promiscuous lactonases/PTEs from hyperthermophilic archaea (*Sulfolobus solfataricus*, *Sulfolobus acidocaldarius*, *Sulfolobus islandicus* and *Vulcanisaeta moutnovskia*) have been isolated in hot springs and the volcano Solfatara. Stable PTE can also be created by mutagenesis of mesophilic lactonase/PTEs.[117] Owing to the high stability of these enzymes, long term storage at room temperature, field uses for decontamination, and pre- and post-exposure treatments have been considered. Other extremophile PTEs have been isolated from radio-resistant bacteria, *Deinococcus radiodurans* and *Agrobacterium radiobacter*. The 3D structures of several of them were determined.[78,114,115,141–145] These enzymes were expressed in *Escherichia coli* and mutated. Different mutagenesis strategies have been implemented: site directed mutagenesis; random mutagenesis; combinational active site mutagenesis; directed evolution; and rational design. The catalytic properties have been greatly improved against both OP pesticides and NA analogs.[115,142,146–150] For example, the k_{cat}/K_m of *Agrobacterium radiodurans* PTE for malathion was increased by more than three orders of magnitude ($1.9 \times 10^6\ M^{-1}\ min^{-1}$) by engineering through combinational active site saturation testing.[150]

2.8.1.2 Human Paraoxonase

The human PON-1 is a 45 kDa calcium dependent enzyme bound to high density lipoproteins (HDLs) with other apolipoproteins, such as the human phosphate binding protein (HPBP).[151] PON-1 and HPPB are tightly associated. HPBP binds inorganic phosphate in the blood. This non-glycosylated apolipoprotein was serendipitously discovered, and its 3D structure and complete amino acid sequence were determined.[152,153] HPBP belongs to the family of DING proteins.[154] The fact that HPBP stabilizes active human PON-1 suggests that it could be a functional chaperone.[151,155] The HPBP gene was synthesized and expressed in *Escherichia coli*.[153] However, co-crystallization of the human PON-1–HPBP complex has failed so far. Yet, this step is mandatory for the design of stable human PON-1 mutants with enhanced catalytic efficiency against toxic stereoisomers of G- and V-type NAs.

Although the primary activity of PON-1 is lactonase,[156,157] PON-1 displays two promiscuous activities, PTE and arylesterase. PON-1 shows a genetic polymorphism; the Q192 and R192 allozymes display small differences in activity against OPs and arylesters.[158]

A considerable body of biochemical, biological and toxicological data has been collected in the past two decades about the activities of human PON-1 and its relationship with lipoproteins and possible physiological functions,[159] but attempts at solving its 3D structure have failed. Certain amino acid residues essential for PON-1 activity were identified *via* chemical modification and site directed mutagenesis studies.[160] Later, molecular modeling[161,162] and the crystal structure of a hybrid rPON-1 (a synthetic construct created by shuffling rabbit, mouse, rat and human PON-1 genes expressed in *Escherichia coli*)[163] showed that human PON-1 is a six bladed β-propeller protein very similar in structure to *Loligo vulgaris* DFPase.[164] A catalytic mechanism for this eukaryotic Ca^{++} dependent PTE was then proposed.[165] This mechanism involves a calcium coordinated aspartate residue (D229) as the nucleophile that attacks the OP phosphorus atom to form a phosphoacyl intermediate that is subsequently attacked by a water molecule. A recent quantum mechanics/molecular mechanics simulation study suggests that D229 could activate water for nucleophilic attack on phosphorus rather than attacking the phosphorus atom directly.[166] Another mechanism was proposed; it involves the activation of another water molecule bound to Ca^{++} into a hydroxide ion that attacks the phosphorus center (Elias *et al.*, 2013). This mechanism is consistent with the common mechanism proposed for PTEs and PON-1.[119,157] Again, we must emphasize that knowledge of the molecular mechanism of NA hydrolysis is of the utmost importance for engineering PON-1 or DFPase based efficient catalytic bioscavengers.

As a naturally occurring enzyme present in human plasma, PON-1 is the most promising catalytic bioscavenger for pre- and post-treatment of OP poisoning.[167,168] The enzyme has been the subject of intensive research to improve its efficacy and functionalization. As regards its efficacy, the specific catalytic activity (k_{cat}/K_m) of PON-1 against OPs is 10^4 to10^6 M^{-1} min^{-1}.[80,158,169]

It has to be enhanced by one or two orders of magnitude to become effective for fast detoxification. However, its stereoselectivity also has to be optimized. Chimeric PON-1 mutants obtained by directed evolution exhibit enhanced PTE activity against the toxic enantiomers of NAs *in vitro* and *in vivo*.[168,170,171] These results show that this goal will be reached soon. However, the instability of PON-1 mutants could impinge on their biotechnological development. Indeed, as a HDL bound protein, PON-1 requires association to apolipoprotein partners in a hydrophobic environment (HDL or similar macromolecular complexes) to retain its stable active conformation[172–174] and long residence time in the bloodstream.[175]

Site directed mutagenesis of human PON-1 based on molecular modeling has led to double mutants capable of hydrolyzing G- and V-type NAs.[176] However, the catalytic efficiency of these mutants is modest and enantioselectivity is not changed compared with the wild-type enzyme. The directed evolution strategy has been more successful in producing chimeric PON-1 capable of degrading toxic isomers of coumarinyl NA analogs as well as real NAs of G-type. In particular, the enantioselectivity of evolved PON-1 was completely reversed. For instance, the activity against S_p cyclosarin was enhanced by 10^5 fold.[171,177,178] The most active evolved PON-1 mutant, IIG1, displays a k_{cat}/K_m of 10^6 to 10^8 M^{-1} min^{-1} against G-agents. This enzyme, administered at a dose of 1 mg kg^{-1}, was shown to prevent systemic toxicity after 2 LD_{50}s of cyclosarin in the guinea pig.[168] It was also shown to detoxify most G-type NAs at a high rate under first order conditions, but was ineffective against VX even under second order conditions ($k_{cat}/K_m = 1.4 \times 10^2$ M^{-1} min^{-1}).[168]

Gene therapy could also be considered to challenge NAs by using mutated/evolved paraoxonase genes coding for enzymes with high PTE activity against toxic enantiomers. As mentioned before, several preliminary works with different gene delivery vectors in mice showed increased PON-1 serum levels that reduced or even prevented the entry of OP into the brain, and reduced atherosclerosis signs.[96–98,100,101,179] Local delivery of the *PON-1* gene using the Sendai virus vector inhibited neonatal hyperplasia after arterial balloon injury in rabbits fed a high fat diet.[99] However, the catalytic efficiency of wild-type human PON-1 against NAs was too slow to provide *in vivo* protection against 2 LD_{50}s of G-agents. However, evolved PON-1 mutants are expected to be effective for gene therapy of OP poisoning. Indeed, a recent study showed that adenovirus expressed evolved PON-1 mutants challenged a cumulative 6.3 LD_{50} dose of paraoxon in mice, allowing asymptomatic prophylactic protection against this agent.[180]

2.8.1.3 Other Mammalian PTEs

Other known enzymes that display a PTE activity are involved in the degradation of OPs; these are PROLs, senescence marker protein (SMP) and platelet activating factor acetylhydrolase (PAF-AH).

PROLs (EC 3.4.13.9), first isolated from halophilic bacteria (*Alteromonas haloplanktis* and *Alteromonas* sp. JD6.5), are OPAA metallo-enzymes with a "pita bread" structure (Vyas *et al.*, 2010). This enzyme displays high activity against soman, sarin and cyclosarin ($k_{cat}/K_m \approx 5 \times 10^6$ to 10^7 M^{-1} min^{-1}), but is inactive against VX.[181] Thermostable PROLs have been isolated from hyperthermophilic archaea *Pyrococcus furiosus*[182] and *Pyrococcus horikoshii*;[183] they hydrolyze P–F and P–O bonds in NAs. Evolved mutants of these enzymes capable of degrading OPs over wide temperature ranges are of great interest for decontamination under mild conditions. Homologous PROLs were also isolated from human liver, kidney, erythrocytes and skin and expressed in *Escherichia coli*.[184–186] The recombinant human liver PROL displays a high catalytic activity against P(+) and P(−) isomers of sarin, soman and cylcosarin ($k_{cat}/K_m \approx 10^5$ M^{-1} min^{-1}).[184,187] However, it is inactive against VX and tabun.

Gene delivered human liver PROL using adenovirus produced high levels of active enzyme. However, this protects mice only against 1 LD_{50} of DFP,[106] and does not protect animals challenged with sarin, soman or cyclosarin.[187]

SMP-30 was first isolated from rat liver.[188] It is a six bladed-β-propeller metallo-lactonase structurally close to PON-1 and DFPase with promiscuous PTE activity.[189] The human and mouse enzymes display modest PTE activity against G-agents.[184,190] Engineering of this enzyme is still in the early stages.

PAF-AH is a group of 45 kDa lipoprotein (HDL and low density lipoprotein) associated phospholipases A2. These enzymes are structurally related to NTEs and are present both in human plasma and the brain. PAF-AH reacts with numerous OPs.[191–194] However, no site directed mutagenesis or directed evolution studies of human plasma PAF-AH for the creation of an OP hydrolase for the purpose of NA detoxification have been reported so far.

2.8.2 Engineered ChEs and CaEs

When ChEs and CaEs react with carboxyl-ester substrates, the acyl–enzyme intermediate is transient, the acyl group being rapidly displaced by a water molecule. On the contrary, in the case of phosphyl-esters (OPs), the stereochemistry of the phosphyl–enzyme intermediate restricts the accessibility of water to the phosphorus atom. In addition, water is a weak nucleophile. Thus, in most cases, hydrolysis of a phosphylated intermediate is very slow, and the enzymes remain inhibited. Therefore, OPs may be regarded as pseudo-substrates. It was postulated that introduction of a second nucleophile pole in the active center could activate a water molecule. This water molecule could subsequently attack the phosphorus atom on the back face, leading to breakage of the P–serine bond.[195]

X-ray determination of the 3D structure of the *Torpedo californica* AChE monomer[196] opened the way for the rational re-design of ChEs. Then, the possibility to convert a ChE into an OP hydrolase was demonstrated.[197] Human BChE was chosen as the model enzyme because its active center gorge is larger (500 Å^3) and less stereospecific than AChE's active center gorge (300 Å^3). Molecular modeling based on the structure of the *Torpedo californica* AChE model was used for making the first mutants of human BChE. The second nucleophilic pole was created in the oxyanion hole of the active center; a glycine residue was replaced by a histidine. The first mutant, G117H, was capable of slowly hydrolyzing paraoxon, sarin, echothiophate and VX, *e.g.* $k_{cat}/K_m = 1.5 \times 10^3\ M^{-1}\ min^{-1}$ for hydrolysis of VX and $1.6 \times 10^2\ M^{-1}\ min^{-1}$ for sarin.[197,198] However, this mutant was irreversibly inhibited by soman because serine adduct dealkylation ("aging") was faster than dephosphonylation. The dealkylation reaction involves a carbocationic transient that is stabilized by active site residues E197 and W82, and water molecules (for a recent review on "aging" see ref. 199). Mutation of E197 into D, Q or G considerably reduced the rate of "aging". As expected, the double mutant G117H/E197Q was capable of hydrolyzing soman.[200] However, the catalytic activity of this mutant was too slow to be of interest.

Construction of transgenic mice *knockout* for AChE and carrying the G117H mutant of human BChE were found to be less sensitive to OPs than wild-type animals.[201] Although transgenic mice expressed the G117H mutant in all organs, unlike the resistance of the blowfly, resistance to OPs cannot be explained by OP hydrolysis, which was too slow, but rather by G117H catalyzed hydrolysis of acetylcholine in cholinergic synapses.

More than 60 double or triple G117H based mutants were made.[202] The last mutants were designed using the X-ray structure of human BChE.[203] Unfortunately, none of them were more active than the G117H mutant.[81] At the same time, mutants of human AChE and *Bungarus fasciatus* AChE were made, using the same site directed mutagenesis approach.[204] Although these mutants were active against paraoxon, echothiophate and DFP, their activity was worse than that of the G117H BChE mutant. Actually, there is kinetic evidence that mutations at position G117 reduce the functionality of the oxyanion hole.[205] Thus, other mutations are needed to compensate for the structural and catalytic effects of the G117H mutation. However, the choice of proper mutations was not possible without knowledge of the structure, dynamics and catalytic mechanism of the simple G117H mutant.

The crystal structure of the G117H mutant conjugated to echothiophate and VX was solved.[206] Works are in progress to understand the mechanism of dephosphylation of this mutant.[206–210] Computational design of new G117H based mutants of BChE capable of hydrolyzing OPs is conceivable.[208] This new approach, called "intelligent" directed mutagenesis design, is based on simulation of transition states. Molecular dynamics simulation of the activation transition state of deacylation already has been successfully applied to the design of mutants of human BChE that hydrolyze (−)-cocaine at a high rate.[211,212] This approach was applied to the dephosphylation transition states of a G117H based mutant of human BChE with the intention of optimizing interactions favoring productive crossing of the energetic barrier for dephosphylation (Grigorenko *et al.*, unpublished). This will lead to a new generation of BChE mutants capable of hydrolyzing OPs at a high rate. Directed evolution of ChEs could be an alternative to computer based methods. Functional expression of ChEs is difficult in yeast and has failed both in bacteria and acellular systems to date, making the directed evolution approach difficult. However, a new adenoviral cloning method was used to construct human

BChE mutant libraries. This directed molecular evolution method in a mammalian cell based functional screen produced novel human BChE mutants that resist inhibition by OPs.[213] Thus, novel BChE mutants that hydrolyze OPs could be identified using this method. An alternative method is the creation of OP hydrolase activity in bacterial hydrolases that show sequence and fold homologies to human BChE. For this purpose, the *p*-nitrobenzyl esterase (pNBE) from *Bacillus subtilis* was re-designed.[210] Although the OP hydrolase activity of screened active variants of this enzyme was only modestly enhanced and kinetic complications were observed compared with the wild-type enzyme, this work demonstrated that pNBE is a valuable scaffold for re-engineering ChEs and other α/β-serine hydrolases into OP hydrolases.

Bioavailability and biological stability of mutated ChEs for i.v or i.m injection are important issues for therapeutic use of wild-type and mutant ChEs. The very first pharmacokinetic studies of highly purified human BChE injected to the rat showed that the $t_{1/2}$ or MRT of the enzyme in the bloodstream depends on sialylation of glycan chains.[44] Indeed, it is well documented that rapid elimination of asialoglycoproteins from the bloodstream is due to their capture by receptors located on the surface of hepatocytes. These receptors are specific to galactose, the sugar that precedes sialic acid at the terminus of complex glycan chains. Studies with other natural and recombinant ChEs confirmed the importance of sialic acid residues ending glycans.[214–217] It was found that the $t_{1/2}$ is inversely proportional to the number of unoccupied attachment sites of sialic acid.[218] To increase the $t_{1/2}$ of administered recombinant ChEs, all galactosyl residues have to be sialylated. Full sialylation of recombinant enzymes can be achieved using an expression system capable of synthesizing glycans similar to natural human glycoprotein glycans and adding sialidase inhibitors into the cell culture medium. Co-expression of human AChE and sialyltransferase in HEK 293 cells was found to lead to a fully sialylated recombinant enzyme.[218] Complete sialylation of recombinant human BChE produced in *Nicotiana benthamiana* was also achieved by co-expression of BChE with a gene stacking vector carrying six genes involved in sialylation of mammalian glycoproteins.[62] Alternatively, *in vitro* sialylation of purified enzymes can be performed using sialyltransferase or chemical methods.[219] Capping of BChE is possible by crosslinking polysialic acid chains.[85] PEGylation is also an effective chemical modification for increasing the $t_{1/2}$ of administered recombinant ChE.[57,216,217] Finally, pharmacokinetics can also be improved by increasing the protein size. For instance, the $t_{1/2}$ of a recombinant fusion protein human albumin–human BChE administered to juvenile pigs was ≈32 h compared with ≈3 h for recombinant BChE composed of 70% tetrameric enzyme.[58]

Engineering of CaE to make enzymes capable of hydrolyzing NAs has made recent progress. In fact, the discovery of a blowfly (*Lucilia cuprina*) resistant to OPs because it carries a mutated CaE (LcαE7)—in the oxyanion hole at G137 (G137D), a position homologous to G117 in human BChE—stimulated research on G117H based mutants of BChE. Although the OP hydrolase activity of the G137D is low, it is balanced by the abundance of the enzyme in the insect's organs.[220] The 3D structure of LcαE7 was solved.[221] Knowledge of this structure is a good starting point for engineering mutants with improved OP hydrolase activity. The human CaE1 is also of interest. The 3D structure of human CaE1–NA conjugates (with soman, tabun, sarin and cyclosarin) has been solved.[47,222] The enzyme was shown to reactivate spontaneously after phosphonylation by the most toxic P_s stereoisomer of sarin.[48] Computer design of CaE1 mutants for OP hydrolase activity was then undertaken. The first designed mutants are active against soman and cyclosarin, and display an enhanced rate of spontaneous dephosphonylation following sarin inhibition.[222] Thus, CaEs can be regarded as novel catalytic bioscavenger candidates.

2.8.3 Oxidases

2.8.3.1 Glutathione S*-Transferases*

GSTs (EC 2.5.1.18) are intracellular enzymes that catalyze glutathione conjugation to electrophilic substrates. They are involved in detoxification processes of endogenous compounds and xenobiotics, and their role in resistance to insecticides in insects is well established. There is evidence that GSTs contribute to OP detoxification in humans.[223] However, engineering of these enzymes has not been developed so far.

2.8.3.2 Laccases

Laccases (EC 1.10.3.2) are fungal phenol oxidoreductases that have been used for detoxification of numerous xenobiotics, including dyes and pesticides. The laccases from *Pleurotus ostreatus* and *Chaetomium thermophilium* were found to rapidly degrade VX and VR in the presence of 2,2′-azinobis(3-ethylbenzthiazoline-6-sulfonate) (ABTS) as a mediator.[224] Laccases from *Trametes versicolor* and *Coriolopsis polyzona* with ABTS display similar properties against the V-agents.[225] Oxidative cleavage of the P–S bond by laccases is of great interest because phosphorothiolates are almost resistant to wild-type PTEs/PLLs.

The heme-containing chloroperoxidase (EC 1.11.1.X) from *Caldariomyces fumago*, with peroxide as a co-substrate, is another efficient VX degrading enzyme.[226] Thus, oxidases and peroxidases are of interest for destruction of chemical weapons stockpiles, soil remediation, and decontamination of materials, protective equipment and water polluted by pesticides and NAs.[227] These enzymes could be used with other OP degrading enzymes for skin decontamination or incorporated into topical skin protection formulations. Although no work has been done on the combined action of oxidases and hydrolases, oxidation of P-bonded alkyl/aryl chains by oxidases is expected to alter the enantioselectivity of PTEs for parent OPs. Therefore, biopharmaceutical formulations of combined oxidases and PTEs may improve the efficiency of PTE based catalytic bioscavengers.

2.9 Catalytic Antibodies

Research on catalytic antibodies is like looking for the Holy Grail. Yet, some progress has been made.[228,229] However, the turnover rate of catalytic antibodies remains extremely slow, and their specificity is too narrow for practical interest as medical countermeasures. Resolution of the 3D structure of a "reactibody" fragment with an OP[230] has opened some hope for rational design and re-engineering of more active catalytic antibodies against OPs.[231,232]

2.10 Artificial Enzymes

Artificial enzymes based on macrocycles, dendritic polymers and supramolecular scaffolds represent an alternative to biomolecules. Only β-cyclodextrin based catalysts against OPs have been developed so far. β-Cyclodextrin derivatives bearing a nucleophilic group such as iodozobenzoic acid or a pyridinium oxime have been introduced on one glucosyl unit of the cyclodextrin ring.[234–237] These compounds display effective catalytic properties against certain NAs, in particular cyclosarin (second order detoxification constant $\approx 10^4\ M^{-1}\ min^{-1}$).[237,238] Prophylactic intravenous injection of one of these derivatives protected brain AChE and prevented systemic toxicity of 2 LD_{50}s of cyclosarin in guinea pigs.[239] This first *in vivo* test of a functionalized cyclodextrin clearly demonstrates the potential of artificial catalysts as catalytic scavengers for medical countermeasures of NA poisoning.

2.11 Future Directions

Enzymes and chemicals that degrade NAs with a turnover are the most promising alternative to current decontamination means and treatments of OP poisoning. In the near future, catalytic (bio)scavengers will be part of the arsenal of medical countermeasures for pre- and post-exposure treatments of OP poisoning, protective means (*e.g.* active TSPs and protective clothing suits) and decontamination tools.[233] Because of the narrow specificity and stereoselectivity of catalysts, multiple enzyme associations or reactive chemicals will be used to extend the activity spectrum of these catalysts.

Optimized OP degrading enzymes will be derived from naturally occurring human enzymes and from other organisms, including extremophile bacteria and archaea. Recombinant mutated, evolved and computer designed enzymes will be produced under GMP conditions, using prokaryotic expression systems (*Escherichia coli*), eukaryotic expression systems (yeast, insect and mammalian cell cultures), transgenic animals (worm, rabbit and goat) or transgenic plants (tomato, potato and tobacco). Although acellular biosynthetic systems have not been used yet for this purpose, their implementation could greatly reduce the costs of production of these enzymes. The goal of current research is to improve mass production of stable, highly active (high k_{cat}/K_m) and stereoselective engineered enzymes at low cost. Efforts concentrate primarily on bacterial PTEs and PON-1, but also on human BChE. Recent successes justify this approach.[178,213,241] In addition, improvements are focused on thermodynamic stability (storage stability at ambient temperature in solution or lyophilized) and *in vivo* operational stability, immuno-tolerance, and bioavailability. Recent implementation of the Rosetta based design and chemical modification led to mesophilic PTE mutants with improved heat stability.[241]

New potential enzymes have to be researched:

(1) Research of new natural enzymes, in particular in collections of bacterial strains[242] and in extreme biotopes,[243] or identification of such enzymes from genomic sequences of extremophiles, followed by expression of the synthetic gene in a mesophilic bacterial host, characterization of catalytic properties, X-ray structure determination and engineering.[143] Potential extremozymes, PLL and PROL, have been discovered in halophilic, hyperthermophilic, piezophilic, radioresistant bacteria and archaea;
(2) Identification of enzymes responsible for insect resistance to OP pesticides;
(3) Identification of secondary OP targets in humans.

Different strategies of enzyme engineering will continue to be implemented, *i.e.* site directed mutagenesis and directed evolution approaches. However, computational re-design of enzymes by combining molecular modeling/docking techniques, quantum chemical/molecular mechanics calculations and transition state simulations will be more and more successful.[244] In addition, chemical modifications and medium manipulations will improve stability and immuno-compatibility.

Re-design of known enzymes is another promising strategy that has already been successfully implemented. For instance, the active site of mouse adenosine deaminase, a zinc enzyme, was re-designed for hydrolysis of OPs. After maturation using directed evolution, the novel enzyme displayed k_{cat}/K_m activity greater than 10^7 fold the activity of the wild-type enzyme against R_p OPs.[245] Also, as mentioned, combination of rational design and directed evolution of *Bacillus subtilis* *p*-nitrobenzyl hydrolase led to libraries of variants with enhanced OP hydrolase activity.[210] Regarding artificial enzymes, research and screening of chemical libraries will benefit from computational chemistry methods.

In the future, gene therapy, which is still in its infancy, will offer the possibility of transitory production of human or humanized bioscavengers in the body. Further long term efforts are needed to engineer safe vectors that do not produce toxic viral proteins and/or induce an immune response. Recent studies give us reason to be optimistic.[246]

References

1. J. B. Tucker, *War of nerves: chemical warfare from World War I to al-Qaeda*, Pantheon Books, New York, 2006, xi+479 pages.
2. M. Balali-Mood and M. Abdollahi, *Basic and clinical toxicology of organophosphorus compounds*, Springer, London, 2014, xii+257 pages.
3. R. J. Foxenberg, B. P. McGarrigle, J. B. Knaak, P. J. Kostyniak and J. R. Olson, Human hepatic cytochrome P450-specific metabolism of parathion and chlorpyrifos, *Drug Metab. Dispos.*, 2007, **35**, 189–193.
4. M. Eto, J. E. Casida and T. Eto, Hydroxylation and cyclization reactions involved in the metabolism of tri-o-cresyl phosphate, *Biochem. Pharmacol.*, 1962, **11**, 337–352.
5. P. Masson, L. Schopfer, A. Saxena, J. Mikler and O. Lockridge, Endogenous human plasma catalytic bioscavengers for organophosphorus compounds do not protect against the toxicity of chemicals implicated in aerotoxic syndrome: an in vitro study, *J. Biol. Phys. Chem*, 2012, **12**, 89–97.
6. N. Antonov, *Khimicheskoe oruzhie na rubezhe dvikh stoletii (chemical weapons at the turn of the century)*, Progress, Moscow, 1994, 175 pages.
7. D. Maxwell, K. Brecht, I. Koplovitz and R. Sweeney, Acetylcholinesterase inhibition: does it explain the toxicity of organophosphorus compounds?, *Arch. Toxicol.*, 2006, **80**, 756–760.
8. J. E. Casida and G. B. Quistad, Organophosphate toxicology: Safety aspects of nonacetylcholinesterase secondary targets, *Chem. Res. Toxicol.*, 2004, **17**, 983–998.
9. J. E. Casida and G. B. Quistad, Serine hydrolase targets of organophosphorus toxicants, *Chem.-Biol. Interact.*, 2005, **157–158**, 277–283.
10. P. Masson and O. Lockridge, Butyrylcholinesterase for protection from organophosphorus poisons: catalytic complexities and hysteretic behavior, *Arch. Biochem. Biophys.*, 2010, **494**, 107–120.
11. J. Wetherell, M. Price, H. Mumford, S. Armstrong and L. Scott, Development of next generation medical countermeasures to nerve agent poisoning, *Toxicology*, 2007, **233**, 120–127.
12. H. Thiermann, L. Szinicz, P. Eyer, N. Felgenhauer, T. Zilker and F. Worek, Lessons to be learnt from organophosphorus pesticide poisoning for the treatment of nerve agent poisoning, *Toxicology*, 2007, **233**, 145–154.
13. M. Eddleston, N. A. Buckley, P. Eyer and A. H. Dawson, Management of acute organophosphorus pesticide poisoning, *Lancet*, 2008, **371**, 597–607.
14. P. Masson, Evolution of and perspectives on therapeutic approaches to nerve agent poisoning, *Toxicol. Lett.*, 2011, **206**, 5–13.
15. M. Moshiri, E. Darchini-Maragheh and M. Balali-Mood, Advances in toxicology and medical treatment of chemical warfare nerve agents, *Daru, J. Pharm. Sci.*, 2012, **20**, 81.
16. E. Dolgin, Syrian gas attack reinforces need for better anti-sarin drugs, *Nat. Med.*, 2013, **19**, 1194–1195.

17. Y. Rosman, A. Eisenkraft, N. Milk, A. Shiyovich, N. Ophir, S. Shrot, Y. Kreiss and M. Kassirer, Lessons learned from the syrian sarin attack: evaluation of a clinical syndrome through social medialessons learned from the syrian sarin attack, *Ann. Intern. Med.*, 2014, **160**, 644–648.
18. J. L. Willems, H. C. De Bisschop, A. G. Verstraete, C. Declerck, Y. Christiaens, P. Vanscheeuwyck, W. A. Buylaert, D. Vogelaers and F. Colardyn, Cholinesterase reactivation in organophosphorus poisoned patients depends on the plasma concentrations of the oxime pralidoxime methylsulphate and of the organophosphate, *Arch. Toxicol.*, 1993, **67**, 79–84.
19. F. Nachon, X. Brazzolotto, M. Trovaslet and P. Masson, Progress in the development of enzyme-based nerve agent bioscavengers, *Chem.-Biol. Interact.*, 2013, **206**, 536–544.
20. C. M. Brown, B. Reisfeld and A. N. Mayeno, Cytochromes P450: a structure-based summary of biotransformations using representative substrates, *Drug Metab. Rev.*, 2008, **40**, 1–100.
21. J. O. Miners, K. M. Knights, J. B. Houston and P. I. Mackenzie, In vitro–in vivo correlation for drugs and other compounds eliminated by glucuronidation in humans: pitfalls and promises, *Biochem. Pharmacol.*, 2006, **71**, 1531–1539.
22. T. Satoh and M. Hosokawa, Structure, function and regulation of carboxylesterases, *Chem.-Biol. Interact.*, 2006, **162**, 195–211.
23. A. Belogurov, A. Kozyr, N. Ponomarenko and A. Gabibov, Catalytic antibodies: balancing between Dr. Jekyll and Mr. Hyde, *BioEssays*, 2009, **31**, 1161–1171.
24. K. U. Schallreuter, N. C. J. Gibbons, S. M. Elwary, S. M. Parkin and J. M. Wood, Calcium-activated butyrylcholinesterase in human skin protects acetylcholinesterase against suicide inhibition by neurotoxic organophosphates, *Biochem. Biophys. Res. Commun.*, 2007, **355**, 1069–1074.
25. D. K. Nomura, K. Fujioka, R. S. Issa, A. M. Ward, B. F. Cravatt and J. E. Casida, Dual roles of brain serine hydrolase KIAA1363 in ether lipid metabolism and organophosphate detoxification, *Toxicol. Appl. Pharmacol.*, 2008, **228**, 42–48.
26. J. E. Casida and K. A. Durkin, Anticholinesterase insecticide retrospective, *Chem.-Biol. Interact.*, 2013, **203**, 221–225.
27. C. E. Furlong, Genetic variability in the cytochrome P450–paraoxonase 1 (PON1) pathway for detoxication of organophosphorus compounds, *J. Biochem. Mol. Toxicol.*, 2007, **21**, 197–205.
28. C. A. Ellison, Y. Tian, J. B. Knaak, P. J. Kostyniak and J. R. Olson, Human hepatic cytochrome P450-specific metabolism of the organophosphorus pesticides methyl parathion and diazinon, *Drug Metab. Dispos.*, 2012, **40**, 1–5.
29. E. Kaliste-Korhonen, K. Tuovinen and O. Hänninen, Interspecies differences in enzymes reacting with organophosphates and their inhibition by paraoxon in vitro, *Hum. Exp. Toxicol.*, 1996, **15**, 972–978.

30. D. M. Shih, L. Gu, Y.-R. Xia, M. Navab, W.-F. Li, S. Hama, L. W. Castellani, C. E. Furlong, L. G. Costa, A. M. Fogelman and A. J. Lusis, Mice lacking serum paraoxonase are susceptible to organophosphate toxicity and atherosclerosis, *Nature*, 1998, **394**, 284–287.
31. B. Li, F. Nachon, M.-T. Froment, L. Verdier, J.-C. Debouzy, B. Brasme, E. Gillon, L. M. Schopfer, O. Lockridge and P. Masson, Binding and hydrolysis of soman by human serum albumin, *Chem. Res. Toxicol.*, 2007, **21**, 421–431.
32. M. H. Tarhoni, W. G. Carter and D. E. Ray, Plasma albumin binding is a sensitive indicator of exposure to some, but not all organophosphorus pesticides, *Toxicology*, 2007, **240**, 173.
33. M. Sogorb, C. Álvarez-Escalante, V. Carrera and E. Vilanova, An in vitro approach for demonstrating the critical role of serum albumin in the detoxication of the carbamate carbaryl at in vivo toxicologically relevant concentrations, *Arch. Toxicol.*, 2007, **81**, 113–119.
34. R. L. Rotundo, Peptides that enhance acetylcholinesterase expression, US Patent No. 2011/0183922 A1, 2011.
35. C. Gouédard, R. Barouki and Y. Morel, Induction of the paraoxonase-1 gene expression by resveratrol, *Arterioscler., Thromb., Vasc. Biol.*, 2004, **24**, 2378–2383.
36. L. G. Costa, G. Giordano and C. E. Furlong, Pharmacological and dietary modulators of paraoxonase 1 (PON1) activity and expression: the hunt goes on, *Biochem. Pharmacol.*, 2011, **81**, 337–344.
37. B. Desire and S. Saint-Andre, Interaction of soman with beta-cyclodextrin, *Fundam. Appl. Toxicol.*, 1986, **7**, 646–657.
38. M. Glikson, R. Arad-Yellin, M. Ghozi, L. Raveh, B. S. Green and Z. Eshhar, Characterization of soman-binding antibodies raised against soman analogs, *Mol. Immunol.*, 1992, **29**, 903–910.
39. K. Yokoyama, Y. Ogura, M. Kishimoto, F. Hinoshita, S. Hara, A. Yamada, N. Mimura, A. Seki and O. Sakai, Blood purification for severe sarin poisoning after the tokyo subway attack, *JAMA, J. Am. Med. Assoc.*, 1995, **274**, 379.
40. M. Güven, M. Sungur, B. Eser, İ. Sarı and F. Altuntaş, The effects of fresh frozen plasma on cholinesterase levels and outcomes in patients with organophosphate poisoning, *Clin. Toxicol.*, 2004, **42**, 617–623.
41. H.-M. Qiu, S.-C. Zheng, W.-G. Wan and H.-J. Zou, [Meta-analysis of the effectiveness of plasma exchange in treatment of severe and acute organophosphate poisoning]. [Article in Chinese], *Zhonghua Lao Dong Wei Sheng Zhi Ye Bing Za Zhi*, 2011, **29**, 779–781.
42. T. Wille, H. Thiermann and F. Worek, In vitro kinetics of nerve agent degradation by fresh frozen plasma (FFP), *Arch. Toxicol.*, 2014, **88**, 301–307.
43. B. Li, M. Sedlacek, I. Manoharan, R. Boopathy, E. G. Duysen, P. Masson and O. Lockridge, Butyrylcholinesterase, paraoxonase, and albumin esterase, but not carboxylesterase, are present in human plasma, *Biochem. Pharmacol.*, 2005, **70**, 1673–1684.

44. J.-C. Douchet, P. Masson and P. Morélis, Elimination de la cholinestérase plasmatique humaine purifiée injectée au rat, *Trav. Sci. Serv. Santé Armées*, 1982, **3**, 342–347.
45. A. D. Wolfe, R. S. Rush, B. P. Doctor, I. Koplovitz and D. Jones, Acetylcholinesterase prophylaxis against organophosphate toxicity, *Fundam. Appl. Toxicol.*, 1987, **9**, 266–270.
46. M. R. Redinbo and P. M. Potter, Keynote review: mammalian carboxylesterases: from drug targets to protein therapeutics, *Drug Discovery Today*, 2005, **10**, 313–325.
47. C. D. Fleming, C. C. Edwards, S. D. Kirby, D. M. Maxwell, P. M. Potter, D. M. Cerasoli and M. R. Redinbo, Crystal structures of human carboxylesterase 1 in covalent complexes with the chemical warfare agents soman and tabun, *Biochemistry*, 2007, **46**, 5063–5071.
48. A. C. Hemmert, T. C. Otto, M. Wierdl, C. C. Edwards, C. D. Fleming, M. MacDonald, J. R. Cashman, P. M. Potter, D. M. Cerasoli and M. R. Redinbo, Human carboxylesterase 1 stereoselectively binds the nerve agent cyclosarin and spontaneously hydrolyzes the nerve agent sarin, *Mol. Pharmacol.*, 2010, **77**, 508–516.
49. B. P. Doctor and A. Saxena, Bioscavengers for the protection of humans against organophosphate toxicity, *Chem.-Biol. Interact.*, 2005, **157–158**, 167–171.
50. D. E. Lenz, C. A. Broomfield, D. T. Yeung, P. Masson, D. M. Maxwell and D. M. Cerasoli, Nerve agent bioscavengers: progress in development of a new mode of protection against organophosphorus exposure, in *Chemical Warfare Agents: Chemistry, Pharmacology, Toxicology and Therapeutics*, ed. J. A. Romano, B. J. Luckey and H. Salem, CRC Press, Boca Raton, Fl, 2007, pp. 175–202.
51. H. Mumford, C. J. Docx, M. E. Price, A. C. Green, J. E. H. Tattersall and S. J. Armstrong, Human plasma-derived BuChE as a stoichiometric bioscavenger for treatment of nerve agent poisoning, *Chem.-Biol. Interact.*, 2013, **203**, 160–166.
52. Y. J. Rosenberg, B. Laube, L. Mao, X. Jiang, S. Hernandez-Abanto, K. D. Lee and R. Adams, Pulmonary delivery of an aerosolized recombinant human butyrylcholinesterase pretreatment protects against aerosolized paraoxon in macaques, *Chem.-Biol. Interact.*, 2013, **203**, 167–171.
53. Y. J. Rosenberg, J. Gearhart, L. Mao, X. Jiang and S. Hernandez-Abanto, Protection against paraoxon toxicity by an intravenous pretreatment with polyethylene-glycol-conjugated recombinant butyrylcholinesterase in macaques, *Chem.-Biol. Interact.*, 2014, **210**, 20–25.
54. Y. Ashani and S. Pistinner, Estimation of the upper limit of human butyrylcholinesterase dose required for protection against organophosphates toxicity: a mathematically based toxicokinetic model, *Toxicol. Sci.*, 2004, **77**, 358–367.
55. A. Saxena, C. Luo and B. P. Doctor, Developing procedures for the large-scale purification of human serum butyrylcholinesterase, *Protein Expression Purif.*, 2008, **61**, 191–196.

56. X. Brazzolotto, M. Wandhammer, C. Ronco, M. Trovaslet, L. Jean, O. Lockridge, P.-Y. Renard and F. Nachon, Human butyrylcholinesterase produced in insect cells: huprine-based affinity purification and crystal structure, *FEBS J.*, 2012, **279**, 2905–2916.
57. Y.-J. Huang, Y. Huang, H. Baldassarre, B. Wang, A. Lazaris, M. Leduc, A. S. Bilodeau, A. Bellemare, M. Côté, P. Herskovits, M. Touati, C. Turcotte, L. Valeanu, N. Lemée, H. Wilgus, I. Bégin, B. Bhatia, K. Rao, N. Neveu, E. Brochu, J. Pierson, D. K. Hockley, D. M. Cerasoli, D. E. Lenz, C. N. Karatzas and S. Langermann, Recombinant human butyrylcholinesterase from milk of transgenic animals to protect against organophosphate poisoning, *Proc. Natl. Acad. Sci. U. S. A.*, 2007, **104**, 13603–13608.
58. Y.-J. Huang, P. Lundy, A. Lazaris, Y. Huang, H. Baldassarre, B. Wang, C. Turcotte, M. Cote, A. Bellemare, A. Bilodeau, S. Brouillard, M. Touati, P. Herskovits, I. Begin, N. Neveu, E. Brochu, J. Pierson, D. Hockley, D. Cerasoli, D. Lenz, H. Wilgus, C. Karatzas and S. Langermann, Substantially improved pharmacokinetics of recombinant human butyrylcholinesterase by fusion to human serum albumin, *BMC Biotechnol.*, 2008, **8**, 50.
59. Y. J. Rosenberg, A. Saxena, W. Sun, X. Jiang, N. Chilukuri, C. Luo, B. P. Doctor and K. D. Lee, Demonstration of in vivo stability and lack of immunogenicity of a polyethyleneglycol-conjugated recombinant CHO-derived butyrylcholinesterase bioscavenger using a homologous macaque model, *Chem.-Biol. Interact.*, 2010, **187**, 279–286.
60. B. C. Geyer, L. Kannan, P.-E. Garnaud, C. A. Broomfield, C. L. Cadieux, I. Cherni, S. M. Hodgins, S. A. Kasten, K. Kelley, J. Kilbourne, Z. P. Oliver, T. C. Otto, I. Puffenberger, T. E. Reeves, N. Robbins, R. R. Woods, H. Soreq, D. E. Lenz, D. M. Cerasoli and T. S. Mor, Plant-derived human butyrylcholinesterase, but not an organophosphorous-compound hydrolyzing variant thereof, protects rodents against nerve agents, *Proc. Natl. Acad. Sci. U. S. A.*, 2010, **107**, 20251–20256.
61. K. E. Larrimore, M. Barcus, L. Kannan, Y. Gao, C.-G. Zhan, S. Brimijoin and T. Mor, Plants as a source of butyrylcholinesterase variants designed for enhanced cocaine hydrolase activity, *Chem.-Biol. Interact.*, 2013, **203**, 217–220.
62. J. D. Schneider, A. Castilho, L. Neumann, F. Altmann, A. Loos, L. Kannan, T. S. Mor and H. Steinkellner, Expression of human butyrylcholinesterase with an engineered glycosylation profile resembling the plasma-derived orthologue, *Biotechnol. J.*, 2014, **9**, 501–510.
63. S.-J. Ding, J. Carr, J. E. Carlson, L. Tong, W. Xue, Y. Li, L. M. Schopfer, B. Li, F. Nachon, O. Asojo, C. M. Thompson, S. H. Hinrichs, P. Masson and O. Lockridge, Five tyrosines and two serines in human albumin are labeled by the organophosphorus agent FP-biotin, *Chem. Res. Toxicol.*, 2008, **21**, 1787–1794.
64. D. W. Landry and S. X. Deng, Peptides and methods for deactivation of organophosphorus-based nerve agents and insecticides, US Patent No. 07348403 B2, 2008.

65. Z. Zhu, S. X. Deng, J. Macdonald, M. Vinogradov and D. W. Landry, *Autophosphorylating peptides as the scavengers of nerve gas agents, 235th Am. Chem. Soc. National Meeting*, New Orleans, USA, 6–8 April, 2008, conference poster.
66. R. Cochran, J. Kalisiak, T. Kucukkilinc, Z. Radić, E. Garcia, L. Zhang, K.-Y. Ho, G. Amitai, Z. Kovarik, V. V. Fokin, K. B. Sharpless and P. Taylor, Oxime-assisted acetylcholinesterase catalytic scavengers of organophosphates that resist aging, *J. Biol. Chem.*, 2011, **286**, 29718–29724.
67. Z. Kovarik, Z. Radić, H. A. Berman and P. Taylor, Mutation of acetylcholinesterase to enhance oxime-assisted catalytic turnover of methylphosphonates, *Toxicology*, 2007, **233**, 79–84.
68. O. Mazor, O. Cohen, C. Kronman, L. Raveh, D. Stein, A. Ordentlich and A. Shafferman, Aging-resistant organophosphate bioscavenger based on polyethylene glycol-conjugated F338A human acetylcholinesterase, *Mol. Pharmacol.*, 2008, **74**, 755–763.
69. Z. Radić, T. Dale, Z. Kovarik, S. Berend, E. Garcia, L. Zhang, G. Amitai, C. Green, B. Radić, B. M. Duggan, D. Ajami, J. Rebek and P. Taylor, Catalytic detoxification of nerve agent and pesticide organophosphates by butyrylcholinesterase assisted with non-pyridinium oximes, *Biochem. J.*, 2013, **450**, 231–242.
70. J. Renou, G. Mercey, T. Verdelet, E. Păunescu, E. Gillon, M. Arboléas, M. Loiodice, M. Kliachyna, R. Baati, F. Nachon, L. Jean and P.-Y. Renard, Syntheses and in vitro evaluations of uncharged reactivators for human acetylcholinesterase inhibited by organophosphorus nerve agents, *Chem.-Biol. Interact.*, 2013, **203**, 81–84.
71. R. K. Sit, V. V. Fokin, G. Amitai, K. B. Sharpless, P. Taylor and Z. Radić, Imidazole aldoximes effective in assisting butyrylcholinesterase catalysis of organophosphate detoxification, *J. Med. Chem.*, 2014, **57**, 1378–1389.
72. Y. Ashani, H. Leader, N. Rothschild and C. Dosoretz, Combined effect of organophosphorus hydrolase and oxime on the reactivation rate of diethylphosphoryl-acetylcholinesterase conjugates, *Biochem. Pharmacol.*, 1998, **55**, 159–168.
73. A. Saxena, W. Sun, C. Luo, T. Myers, I. Koplovitz, D. Lenz and B. Doctor, Bioscavenger for protection from toxicity of organosphosphorus compounds, *J. Mol. Neurosci.*, 2006, **30**, 145–147.
74. K. E. LeJeune and A. J. Russell, Biocatalytic nerve agent detoxification in fire fighting foams, *Biotechnol. Bioeng.*, 1999, **62**, 659–665.
75. I. Gill and A. Ballesteros, Degradation of organophosphorous nerve agents by enzyme-polymer nanocomposites: efficient biocatalytic materials for personal protection and large-scale detoxification, *Biotechnol. Bioeng.*, 2000, **70**, 400–410.
76. W. Chen and A. Mulchandani, The use of live biocatalysts for pesticide detoxification, *Trends Biotechnol.*, 1998, **16**, 71–76.
77. L. Merone, L. Mandrich, M. Rossi and G. Manco, A thermostable phosphotriesterase from the archaeon *Sulfolobus solfataricus*: cloning, overexpression and properties, *Extremophiles*, 2005, **9**, 297–305.

78. M. Elias, J. Dupuy, L. Merone, L. Mandrich, E. Porzio, S. Moniot, D. Rochu, C. Lecomte, M. Rossi, P. Masson, G. Manco and E. Chabriere, Structural basis for natural lactonase and promiscuous phosphotriesterase activities, *J. Mol. Biol.*, 2008, **379**, 1017–1028.
79. M. Polhuijs, J. P. Langenberg and H. P. Benschop, New method for retrospective detection of exposure to organophosphorus anticholinesterases: application to alleged sarin victims of japanese terrorists, *Toxicol. Appl. Pharmacol.*, 1997, **146**, 156–161.
80. P. Masson, D. Josse, O. Lockridge, N. Viguié, C. Taupin and C. Buhler, Enzymes hydrolyzing organophosphates as potential catalytic scavengers against organophosphate poisoning, *J. Physiol.*, 1998, **92**, 357–362.
81. P. Masson, F. Nachon, C. A. Broomfield, D. E. Lenz, L. Verdier, L. M. Schopfer and O. Lockridge, A collaborative endeavor to design cholinesterase-based catalytic scavengers against toxic organophosphorus esters, *Chem.-Biol. Interact.*, 2008, **175**, 273–280.
82. R. D. Gupta, M. Goldsmith, Y. Ashani, Y. Simo, G. Mullokandov, H. Bar, M. Ben-David, H. Leader, R. Margalit, I. Silman, J. L. Sussman and D. S. Tawfik, Directed evolution of hydrolases for prevention of G-type nerve agent intoxication, *Nat. Chem. Biol.*, 2011, 7, 120–125.
83. P.-C. Tsai, N. Fox, A. N. Bigley, S. P. Harvey, D. P. Barondeau and F. M. Raushel, Enzymes for the homeland defense: optimizing phosphotriesterase for the hydrolysis of organophosphate nerve agents, *Biochemistry*, 2012, **51**, 6463–6475.
84. C. J. Jackson, C. Scott, A. Carville, K. Mansfield, D. L. Ollis and S. B. Bird, Pharmacokinetics of OpdA, an organophosphorus hydrolase, in the African green monkey, *Biochem. Pharmacol.*, 2010, **80**, 1075–1079.
85. D. G. Ilyushin, I. V. Smirnov, A. A. Belogurov, I. A. Dyachenko, T. I. Zharmukhamedova, T. I. Novozhilova, E. A. Bychikhin, M. V. Serebryakova, O. N. Kharybin, A. N. Murashev, K. A. Anikienko, E. N. Nikolaev, N. A. Ponomarenko, D. D. Genkin, G. M. Blackburn, P. Masson and A. G. Gabibov, Chemical polysialylation of human recombinant butyrylcholinesterase delivers a long-acting bioscavenger for nerve agents in vivo, *Proc. Natl. Acad. Sci. U. S. A.*, 2013, **110**, 1243–1248.
86. M. A. Larson, O. Lockridge and S. H. Hinrichs, Polyproline promotes tetramerization of recombinant human butyrylcholinesterase, *Biochem. J.*, 2014, **462**, 329–335.
87. N. Chilukuri, K. Parikh, W. Sun, R. Naik, P. Tipparaju, B. P. Doctor and A. Saxena, Polyethylene glycosylation prolongs the circulatory stability of recombinant human butyrylcholinesterase, *Chem.-Biol. Interact.*, 2005, **157–158**, 115–121.
88. O. Cohen, C. Kronman, L. Raveh, O. Mazor, A. Ordentlich and A. Shafferman, Comparison of polyethylene glycol-conjugated recombinant human acetylcholinesterase and serum human butyrylcholinesterase as bioscavengers of organophosphate compounds, *Mol. Pharmacol.*, 2006, **70**, 1121–1131.

89. T. Chitlaru, C. Kronman, M. Zeevi, M. Kam, A. Harel, A. Ordentlich, B. Velan and A. Shafferman, Modulation of circulatory residence of recombinant acetylcholinesterase through biochemical or genetic manipulation of sialylation levels, *Biochem. J.*, 1998, **336**, 647–658.
90. J. D. Schneider, S. Marillonnet, A. Castilho, C. Gruber, S. Werner, L. Mach, V. Klimyuk, T. S. Mor and H. Steinkellner, Oligomerization status influences subcellular deposition and glycosylation of recombinant butyrylcholinesterase in Nicotiana benthamiana, *Plant Biotechnol. J.*, 2014, **12**, 832–839.
91. W. Sun, C. Luo, R. S. Naik, B. P. Doctor and A. Saxena, Pharmacokinetics and immunologic consequences of repeated administrations of purified heterologous and homologous butyrylcholinesterase in mice, *Life Sci.*, 2009, **85**, 657–661.
92. B. N. Novikov, J. K. Grimsley, R. J. Kern, J. R. Wild and M. E. Wales, Improved pharmacokinetics and immunogenicity profile of organophosphorus hydrolase by chemical modification with polyethylene glycol, *J. Controlled Release*, 2010, **146**, 318–325.
93. M. Trovaslet-Leroy, L. Musilova, F. Renault, X. Brazzolotto, J. Misik, L. Novotny, M.-T. Froment, E. Gillon, M. Loiodice, L. Verdier, P. Masson, D. Rochu, D. Jun and F. Nachon, Organophosphate hydrolases as catalytic bioscavengers of organophosphorus nerve agents, *Toxicol. Lett.*, 2011, **206**, 14–23.
94. W. Sun, C. Luo, P. Tipparaju, B. P. Doctor and A. Saxena, Effect of polyethylene glycol conjugation on the circulatory stability of plasma-derived human butyrylcholinesterase in mice, *Chem.-Biol. Interact.*, 2013, **203**, 172–176.
95. M. D. Klein and R. Langer, Immobilized enzymes in clinical medicine: an emerging approach to new drug therapies, *Trends Biotechnol.*, 1986, **4**, 179–186.
96. J. Cowan, C. M. Sinton, A. W. Varley, F. H. Wians, R. W. Haley and R. S. Munford, Gene therapy to prevent organophosphate intoxication, *Toxicol. Appl. Pharmacol.*, 2001, **173**, 1–6.
97. A. L. Fu, Y. X. Wang and M. J. Sun, Naked DNA prevents soman intoxication, *Biochem. Biophys. Res. Commun.*, 2005, **328**, 901–905.
98. G. Bradshaw, A. Gutierrez, J. H. Miyake, K. R. Davis, A. C. Li, C. K. Glass, L. K. Curtiss and R. A. Davis, Facilitated replacement of Kupffer cells expressing a paraoxonase-1 transgene is essential for ameliorating atherosclerosis in mice, *Proc. Natl. Acad. Sci. U. S. A.*, 2005, **102**, 11029–11034.
99. M. Miyoshi, Y. Nakano, T. Sakaguchi, H. Ogi, N. Oda, K. Suenari, K. Kiyotani, R. Ozono, T. Oshima, T. Yoshida and K. Chayama, Gene delivery of paraoxonase-1 inhibits neointimal hyperplasia after arterial balloon-injury in rabbits fed a high-fat diet, *Hypertens. Res.*, 2007, **30**, 85–91.
100. P. J. Guns, T. Van Assche, W. Verreth, P. Fransen, B. Mackness, M. Mackness, P. Holvoet and H. Bult, Paraoxonase 1 gene transfer lowers vascular oxidative stress and improves vasomotor function in apolipoprotein E-deficient mice with pre-existing atherosclerosis, *Br. J. Pharmacol.*, 2008, **153**, 508–516.

101. E. G. Duysen, K. Parikh, V. Aleti, V. Manne, O. Lockridge and N. Chilukuri, Adenovirus-mediated human paraoxonase1 gene transfer to provide protection against the toxicity of the organophosphorus pesticide toxicant diazoxon, *Gene Ther.*, 2011, **18**, 250–257.
102. B. Li, E. G. Duysen, L. Y. Poluektova, L. C. Murrin and O. Lockridge, Protection from the toxicity of diisopropylfluorophosphate by adeno-associated virus expressing acetylcholinesterase, *Toxicol. Appl. Pharmacol.*, 2006, **214**, 152–165.
103. N. Chilukuri, E. G. Duysen, K. Parikh, R. diTargiani, B. P. Doctor, O. Lockridge and A. Saxena, Adenovirus-transduced human butyrylcholinesterase in mouse blood functions as a bioscavenger of chemical warfare nerve agents, *Mol. Pharmacol.*, 2009, **76**, 612–617.
104. K. Parikh, E. G. Duysen, B. Snow, N. S. Jensen, V. Manne, O. Lockridge and N. Chilukuri, Gene-delivered butyrylcholinesterase is prophylactic against the toxicity of chemical warfare nerve agents and organophosphorus compounds, *J. Pharmacol. Exp. Ther.*, 2011, **337**, 92–101.
105. Y. Gao, L. Geng, F. Orson, B. Kinsey, T. R. Kosten, X. Shen and S. Brimijoin, Effects of anti-cocaine vaccine and viral gene transfer of cocaine hydrolase in mice on cocaine toxicity including motor strength and liver damage, *Chem.-Biol. Interact.*, 2013, **203**, 208–211.
106. V. Aleti, G. B. Reddy, K. Parikh, P. Arun and N. Chilukuri, Persistent and high-level expression of human liver prolidase in vivo in mice using adenovirus, *Chem.-Biol. Interact.*, 2013, **203**, 191–195.
107. R. C. Gordon, B. P. Doctor, A. Saxena, S. R. Feaster, D. Maxwell, M. Ross, D. Lenz, K. Lejeune and A. Russell, Preparation of enzymatically active sponges or foams for detoxification of hazardous compounds, US Patent No. 6642037 B2, 2003.
108. E. H. Braue, S. T. Hobson, C. Govardhan and N. Khalaf, Active topical skin protectants containing OPAA and CLECS, US Patent No. 6410604 B1, 2002.
109. E. Ghanem and F. M. Raushel, Detoxification of organophosphate nerve agents by bacterial phosphotriesterase, *Toxicol. Appl. Pharmacol.*, 2005, **207**, 459–470.
110. C. Theriot and A. Grunden, Hydrolysis of organophosphorus compounds by microbial enzymes, *Appl. Microbiol. Biotechnol.*, 2011, **89**, 35–43.
111. L. Holm and C. Sander, An evolutionary treasure: unification of a broad set of amidohydrolases related to urease, *Proteins: Struct., Funct., Bioinf.*, 1997, **28**, 72–82.
112. A. N. Bigley and F. M. Raushel, Catalytic mechanisms for phosphotriesterases, *Biochim. Biophys. Acta, Proteins Proteomics*, 2013, **1834**, 443–453.
113. I. Horne, T. D. Sutherland, R. L. Harcourt, R. J. Russell and J. G. Oakeshott, Identification of an OPD (organophosphate degradation) gene in an *Agrobacterium* isolate, *Appl. Environ. Microbiol.*, 2002, **68**, 3371–3376.
114. G. Gotthard, J. Hiblot, D. Gonzalez, M. Elias and E. Chabriere, Structural and enzymatic characterization of the phosphotriesterase OPHC2 from *Pseudomonas pseudoalcaligenes*, *PLoS One*, 2013, **8**, e77995.

115. J. Hiblot, G. Gotthard, E. Chabriere and M. Elias, Structural and Enzymatic characterization of the lactonase *Sis*Lac from Sulfolobus islandicus, *PLoS One*, 2012, **7**, e47028.
116. L. Afriat-Jurnou, C. J. Jackson and D. S. Tawfik, Reconstructing a missing link in the evolution of a recently diverged phosphotriesterase by active-site loop remodeling, *Biochemistry*, 2012, **51**, 6047–6055.
117. X.-J. Luo, X.-D. Kong, J. Zhao, Q. Chen, J. Zhou and J.-H. Xu, Switching a newly discovered lactonase into an efficient and thermostable phosphotriesterase by simple double mutations His250Ile/Ile263Trp, *Biotechnol. Bioeng.*, 2014, **111**, 1920–1930.
118. M. M. Benning, J. M. Kuo, F. M. Raushel and H. M. Holden, Three-dimensional structure of phosphotriesterase: an enzyme capable of detoxifying organophosphate nerve agents, *Biochemistry*, 1994, **33**, 15001–15007.
119. S. D. Aubert, Y. Li and F. M. Raushel, Mechanism for the hydrolysis of organophosphates by the bacterial phosphotriesterase, *Biochemistry*, 2004, **43**, 5707–5715.
120. S.-L. Chen, W.-H. Fang and F. Himo, Theoretical study of the phosphotriesterase reaction mechanism, *J. Phys. Chem. B*, 2007, **111**, 1253–1255.
121. K.-Y. Wong and J. Gao, The reaction mechanism of paraoxon hydrolysis by phosphotriesterase from combined QM/MM simulations, *Biochemistry*, 2007, **46**, 13352–13369.
122. C. J. Jackson, P. D. Carr, H.-K. Kim, J.-W. Liu, P. Herrald, N. Mitić, G. Schenk, C. A. Smith and D. L. Ollis, Anomalous scattering analysis of *Agrobacterium radiobacter* phosphotriesterase: the prominent role of iron in the heterobinuclear active site, *Biochem. J.*, 2006, **397**, 501–508.
123. C. J. Jackson, J.-L. Foo, H.-K. Kim, P. D. Carr, J.-W. Liu, G. Salem and D. L. Ollis, *In crystallo* capture of a michaelis complex and product-binding modes of a bacterial phosphotriesterase, *J. Mol. Biol.*, 2008, **375**, 1189–1196.
124. J. M. Kuo, M. Y. Chae and F. M. Raushel, Perturbations to the active site of phosphotriesterase, *Biochemistry*, 1997, **36**, 1982–1988.
125. D. P. Dumas, H. D. Durst, W. G. Landis, F. M. Raushel and J. R. Wild, Inactivation of organophosphorus nerve agents by the phosphotriesterase from *Pseudomonas diminuta*, *Arch. Biochem. Biophys.*, 1990, **277**, 155–159.
126. F. C. G. Hoskin, J. E. Walker, W.-D. Dettbarn and J. R. Wild, Hydrolysis of tetriso by an enzyme derived from *Pseudomonas diminuta* as a model for the detoxication of *O*-ethyl *S*-(2-diisopropylaminoethyl) methylphosphonothiolate (VX), *Biochem. Pharmacol.*, 1995, **49**, 711–715.
127. V. K. Rastogi, J. J. Defrank, T.-c. Cheng and J. R. Wild, Enzymatic hydrolysis of Russian-VX by organophosphorus hydrolase, *Biochem. Biophys. Res. Commun.*, 1997, **241**, 294–296.
128. C. M. Hill, W.-S. Li, J. B. Thoden, H. M. Holden and F. M. Raushel, Enhanced degradation of chemical warfare agents through molecular engineering of the phosphotriesterase active site, *J. Am. Chem. Soc.*, 2003, **125**, 8990–8991.

129. P.-C. Tsai, A. Bigley, Y. Li, E. Ghanem, C. L. Cadieux, S. A. Kasten, T. E. Reeves, D. M. Cerasoli and F. M. Raushel, Stereoselective hydrolysis of organophosphate nerve agents by the bacterial phosphotriesterase, *Biochemistry*, 2010, **49**, 7978–7987.
130. I. Cherny, P. Greisen, Y. Ashani, S. D. Khare, G. Oberdorfer, H. Leader, D. Baker and D. S. Tawfik, Engineering V-type nerve agents detoxifying enzymes using computationally focused libraries, *ACS Chem. Biol.*, 2013, **8**, 2394–2403.
131. Y.-S. Jeong, J. M. Choi, H.-H. Kyeong, J.-Y. Choi, E.-J. Kim and H.-S. Kim, Rational design of organophosphorus hydrolase with high catalytic efficiency for detoxifying a V-type nerve agent, *Biochem. Biophys. Res. Commun.*, 2014, **449**, 263–267.
132. S. E. Letant, S. R. Kane, B. R. Hart, M. Z. Hadi, T.-C. Cheng, V. K. Rastogi and J. G. Reynolds, Hydrolysis of acetylcholinesterase inhibitors - organophosphorus acid anhydrolase enzyme immobilization on photoluminescent porous silicon platforms, *Chem. Commun.*, 2005, 851–853.
133. C. Karnati, H. Du, H.-F. Ji, X. Xu, Y. Lvov, A. Mulchandani, P. Mulchandani and W. Chen, Organophosphorus hydrolase multilayer modified microcantilevers for organophosphorus detection, *Biosens. Bioelectron.*, 2007, **22**, 2636–2642.
134. F. Worek, T. Seeger, G. Reiter, M. Goldsmith, Y. Ashani, H. Leader, J. L. Sussman, N. Aggarwal, H. Thiermann and D. S. Tawfik, Post-exposure treatment of VX poisoned guinea pigs with the engineered phosphotriesterase mutant C23: a proof-of-concept study, *Toxicol. Lett.*, 2014, **231**, 45–54.
135. D. Jun, K. Kuca, J. Bajgar, M. Hruby, J. Kucka, F. Renault and P. Masson, Phosphotriesterase modified by poly[N-(2-hydroxypropyl)methacrylamide], *Toxicology*, 2007, **233**, 235.
136. I. Petrikovics, D. Papahadjopoulos, K. Hong, T.-C. Cheng, S. I. Baskin, J. Jiang, J. C. Jaszberenyi, B. A. Logue, M. Szilasi, W. D. McGuinn and J. L. Way, Comparing therapeutic and prophylactic protection against the lethal effect of paraoxon, *Toxicol. Sci.*, 2004, **77**, 258–262.
137. R. Parsa and H. Green, Destruction of DFP by organophosphorus acid anhydrase covalently coupled to the cornified layer of human epidermis, *Proc. Int. Symposium on applications of enzymes in chemical and biological defense*, Orlando, FL, 2001, pp. 14–18.
138. C. S. McDaniel, J. McDaniel, M. E. Wales and J. R. Wild, Enzyme-based additives for paints and coatings, *Prog. Org. Coat.*, 2006, **55**, 182–188.
139. X. Wang, N. Wu, J. Guo, X. Chu, J. Tian, B. Yao and Y. Fan, Phytodegradation of organophosphorus compounds by transgenic plants expressing a bacterial organophosphorus hydrolase, *Biochem. Biophys. Res. Commun.*, 2008, **365**, 453–458.
140. E. Efremenko, I. Lyagin, Y. Votchitseva, M. Sirotkina and S. Varfolomeyev, Polyhistidine-containing organophosphorus hydrolase with outstanding properties, *Biocatal. Biotransform.*, 2007, **25**, 103–108.

141. Y. Zhang, J. An, W. Ye, G. Yang, Z.-G. Qian, H.-F. Chen, L. Cui and Y. Feng, Enhancing the promiscuous phosphotriesterase activity of a thermostable lactonase (GkaP) for the efficient degradation of organophosphate pesticides, *Appl. Environ. Microbiol.*, 2012, **78**, 6647–6655.
142. J. Hiblot, G. Gotthard, M. Elias and E. Chabriere, Differential active site loop conformations mediate promiscuous activities in the lactonase *Sso*Pox, *PLoS One*, 2013, **8**, e75272.
143. J. Hiblot, G. Gotthard, C. Champion, E. Chabriere and M. Elias, Crystallization and preliminary X-ray diffraction analysis of the lactonase *Vmo*Lac from *Vulcanisaeta moutnovskia*, *Acta Crystallogr., Sect. F: Struct. Biol. Cryst. Commun.*, 2013, **69**, 1235–1238.
144. E. Porzio, S. Di Gennaro, A. Palma and G. Manco, Mn^{2+} modulates the kinetic properties of an archaeal member of the PLL family, *Chem.-Biol. Interact.*, 2013, **203**, 251–256.
145. J. Bzdrenga, J. Hiblot, G. Gotthard, C. Champion, M. Elias and E. Chabriere, *Sac*Pox from the thermoacidophilic crenarchaeon *Sulfolobus acidocaldarius* is a proficient lactonase, *BMC Res. Notes*, 2014, **7**, 333.
146. C. J. Jackson, K. Weir, A. Herlt, J. Khurana, T. D. Sutherland, I. Horne, C. Easton, R. J. Russell, C. Scott and J. G. Oakeshott, Structure-based rational design of a phosphotriesterase, *Appl. Environ. Microbiol.*, 2009, **75**, 5153–5156.
147. R. Hawwa, S. D. Larsen, K. Ratia and A. D. Mesecar, Structure-based and random mutagenesis approaches increase the organophosphate-degrading activity of a phosphotriesterase homologue from *Deinococcus radiodurans*, *J. Mol. Biol.*, 2009, **393**, 36–57.
148. F. Ely, K. S. Hadler, L. R. Gahan, L. W. Guddat, D. L. Ollis and G. Schenk, The organophosphate-degrading enzyme from *Agrobacterium radiobacter* displays mechanistic flexibility for catalysis, *Biochem. J.*, 2010, **432**, 565–573.
149. L. Merone, L. Mandrich, E. Porzio, M. Rossi, S. Müller, G. Reiter, F. Worek and G. Manco, Improving the promiscuous nerve agent hydrolase activity of a thermostable archaeal lactonase, *Bioresour. Technol.*, 2010, **101**, 9204–9212.
150. T. Naqvi, A. C. Warden, N. French, E. Sugrue, P. D. Carr, C. J. Jackson and C. Scott, A 5000-fold increase in the specificity of a bacterial phosphotriesterase for malathion through combinatorial active site mutagenesis, *PLoS One*, 2014, **9**, e94177.
151. D. Rochu, F. Renault, C. Cléry-Barraud, E. Chabrière and P. Masson, Stability of highly purified human paraoxonase (PON1): association with human phosphate binding protein (HPBP) is essential for preserving its active conformation(s), *Biochim. Biophys. Acta, Proteins Proteomics*, 2007, **1774**, 874–883.
152. R. Morales, A. Berna, P. Carpentier, C. Contreras-Martel, F. Renault, M. Nicodeme, M.-L. Chesne-Seck, F. Bernier, J. Dupuy, C. Schaeffer, H. Diemer, A. Van-Dorsselaer, J. C. Fontecilla-Camps, P. Masson, D. Rochu and E. Chabriere, Serendipitous discovery and X-ray structure of a human phosphate binding apolipoprotein, *Structure*, 2006, **14**, 601–609.

153. H. Diemer, M. Elias, F. Renault, D. Rochu, C. Contreras-Martel, C. Schaeffer, A. Van Dorsselaer and E. Chabriere, Tandem use of X-ray crystallography and mass spectrometry to obtain ab initio the complete and exact amino acids sequence of HPBP, a human 38-kDa apolipoprotein, *Proteins: Struct., Funct., Bioinf.*, 2008, **71**, 1708–1720.
154. A. Berna, K. Scott, E. Chabrière and F. Bernier, The DING family of proteins: ubiquitous in eukaryotes, but where are the genes?, *BioEssays*, 2009, **31**, 570–580.
155. D. Rochu, E. Chabriere, F. Renault, M. Elias, C. Clery-Barraud and P. Masson, Stabilization of the active form(s) of human paraoxonase by human phosphate-binding protein, *Biochem. Soc. Trans.*, 2007, **35**, 1616–1620.
156. O. Khersonsky and D. S. Tawfik, Structure–reactivity studies of serum paraoxonase PON1 suggest that its native activity is lactonase, *Biochemistry*, 2005, **44**, 6371–6382.
157. M. Ben-David, G. Wieczorek, M. Elias, I. Silman, J. L. Sussman and D. S. Tawfik, Catalytic metal ion rearrangements underline promiscuity and evolvability of a metalloenzyme, *J. Mol. Biol.*, 2013, **425**, 1028–1038.
158. A. Smolen, H. W. Eckerson, K. N. Gan, N. Hailat and B. N. La Du, Characteristics of the genetically determined allozymic forms of human serum paraoxonase/arylesterase, *Drug Metab. Dispos.*, 1991, **19**, 107–112.
159. *The paraoxonase: their role in disease development and xenobiotic metabolism*, ed. B. Mackness, M. Mackness, M. Aviram and G. Paragh, Springer, Dordrecht, The Netherlands, 2008, xvi+328 pages.
160. D. Josse, W. Xie, F. Renault, D. Rochu, L. M. Schopfer, P. Masson and O. Lockridge, Identification of residues essential for human paraoxonase (PON1) arylesterase/organophosphatase activities, *Biochemistry*, 1999, **38**, 2816–2825.
161. A. Fokine, R. Morales, C. Contreras-Martel, P. Carpentier, F. Renault, D. Rochu and E. Chabriere, Direct phasing at low resolution of a protein copurified with human paraoxonase (PON1), *Acta Crystallogr., Sect. D: Biol. Crystallogr.*, 2003, **59**, 2083–2087.
162. D. T. Yeung, D. Josse, J. D. Nicholson, A. Khanal, C. W. McAndrew, B. J. Bahnson, D. E. Lenz and D. M. Cerasoli, Structure/function analyses of human serum paraoxonase (HuPON1) mutants designed from a DFPase-like homology model, *Biochim. Biophys. Acta, Proteins Proteomics*, 2004, **1702**, 67–77.
163. M. Harel, A. Aharoni, L. Gaidukov, B. Brumshtein, O. Khersonsky, R. Meged, H. Dvir, R. B. G. Ravelli, A. McCarthy, L. Toker, I. Silman, J. L. Sussman and D. S. Tawfik, Structure and evolution of the serum paraoxonase family of detoxifying and anti-atherosclerotic enzymes, *Nat. Struct. Mol. Biol.*, 2004, **11**, 412–419.
164. V. Katsemi, C. Lücke, J. Koepke, F. Löhr, S. Maurer, G. Fritzsch and H. Rüterjans, Mutational and structural studies of the diisopropylfluorophosphatase from *Loligo vulgaris* shed new light on the catalytic mechanism of the enzyme, *Biochemistry*, 2005, **44**, 9022–9033.

165. M.-M. Blum, F. Löhr, A. Richardt, H. Rüterjans and J. C. H. Chen, Binding of a designed substrate analogue to diisopropyl fluorophosphatase: Implications for the phosphotriesterase mechanism, *J. Am. Chem. Soc.*, 2006, **128**, 12750–12757.
166. T. Wymore, M. J. Field, P. Langan, J. C. Smith and J. M. Parks, Hydrolysis of DFP and the nerve agent (S)-sarin by dfpase proceeds along two different reaction pathways: implications for engineering bioscavengers, *J. Phys. Chem. B*, 2014, **118**, 4479–4489.
167. D. Rochu, E. Chabriere and P. Masson, Human paraoxonase: a promising approach for pre-treatment and therapy of organophosphorus poisoning, *Toxicology*, 2007, **233**, 47–59.
168. F. Worek, T. Seeger, M. Goldsmith, Y. Ashani, H. Leader, J. Sussman, D. Tawfik, H. Thiermann and T. Wille, Efficacy of the rePON1 mutant IIG1 to prevent cyclosarin toxicity in vivo and to detoxify structurally different nerve agents in vitro, *Arch. Toxicol.*, 2014, **88**, 1257–1266.
169. H. G. Davies, R. J. Richter, M. Keifer, C. A. Broomfield, J. Sowalla and C. E. Furlong, The effect of the human serum paraoxonase polymorphism is reversed with diazoxon, soman and sarin, *Nat. Genet.*, 1996, **14**, 334–336.
170. G. Amitai, L. Gaidukov, R. Adani, S. Yishay, G. Yacov, M. Kushnir, S. Teitlboim, M. Lindenbaum, P. Bel, O. Khersonsky, D. S. Tawfik and H. Meshulam, Enhanced stereoselective hydrolysis of toxic organophosphates by directly evolved variants of mammalian serum paraoxonase, *FEBS J.*, 2006, **273**, 1906–1919.
171. Y. Ashani, M. Goldsmith, H. Leader, I. Silman, J. L. Sussman and D. S. Tawfik, *In vitro* detoxification of cyclosarin in human blood pre-incubated *ex vivo* with recombinant serum paraoxonases, *Toxicol. Lett.*, 2011, **206**, 24–28.
172. R. W. James and S. P. Deakin, The importance of high-density lipoproteins for paraoxonase-1 secretion, stability, and activity, *Free Radical Biol. Med.*, 2004, **37**, 1986–1994.
173. L. Gaidukov and D. S. Tawfik, High affinity, stability, and lactonase activity of serum paraoxonase PON1 anchored on HDL with ApoA-I, *Biochemistry*, 2005, **44**, 11843–11854.
174. D. Rochu, E. Chabrière and P. Masson, Paraoxonase-1 and its interactions with HDL: molecular structures of PON-1 and HDL, in *HDL Handbook*, ed. T. Komoda, Academic Press, 2010, pp. 99–132.
175. M. Valiyaveettil, Y. A. Alamneh, B. P. Doctor and M. P. Nambiar, Crossroads in the evaluation of paraoxonase 1 for protection against nerve agent and organophosphate toxicity, *Toxicol. Lett.*, 2012, **210**, 87–94.
176. S. D. Kirby, J. R. Norris, J. Richard Smith, B. J. Bahnson and D. M. Cerasoli, Human paraoxonase double mutants hydrolyze V and G class organophosphorus nerve agents, *Chem.-Biol. Interact.*, 2013, **203**, 181–185.
177. R. D. Gupta, M. Goldsmith, Y. Ashani, Y. Simo, G. Mullokandov, H. Bar, M. Ben-David, H. Leader, R. Margalit, I. Silman, J. L. Sussman and D. S. Tawfik, Directed evolution of hydrolases for prevention of G-type nerve agent intoxication, *Nat. Chem. Biol.*, 2011, **7**, 120–125.

178. M. Goldsmith, Y. Ashani, Y. Simo, M. Ben-David, H. Leader, I. Silman, J. L. Sussman and D. S. Tawfik, Evolved stereoselective hydrolases for broad-spectrum G-type nerve agent detoxification, *Chem. Biol.*, 2012, **19**, 456–466.
179. S. M. Hodgins, S. A. Kasten, J. Harrison, T. C. Otto, Z. P. Oliver, P. Rezk, T. E. Reeves, N. Chilukuri and D. M. Cerasoli, Assessing protection against OP pesticides and nerve agents provided by wild-type HuPON1 purified from Trichoplusia ni larvae or induced *via* adenoviral infection, *Chem.-Biol. Interact.*, 2013, **203**, 177–180.
180. D. G. Mata, P. E. Rezk, P. Sabnekar, D. M. Cerasoli and N. Chilukuri, Investigation of evolved paraoxonase-1 variants for prevention of organophosphorous pesticide compound intoxication, *J. Pharmacol. Exp. Ther.*, 2014, **349**, 549–558.
181. T.-c. Cheng, J. J. DeFrank and V. K. Rastogi, *Alteromonas* prolidase for organophosphorus G-agent decontamination, *Chem.-Biol. Interact.*, 1999, **119–120**, 455–462.
182. C. Theriot, X. Du, S. Tove and A. Grunden, Improving the catalytic activity of hyperthermophilic *Pyrococcus* prolidases for detoxification of organophosphorus nerve agents over a broad range of temperatures, *Appl. Microbiol. Biotechnol.*, 2010, **87**, 1715–1726.
183. C. M. Theriot, R. L. Semcer, S. S. Shah and A. M. Grunden, Improving the catalytic activity of hyperthermophilic *Pyrococcus horikoshii* prolidase for detoxification of organophosphorus nerve agents over a broad range of temperatures, *Archaea*, 2011, **2011**, 565127.
184. R. C. diTargiani, L. Chandrasekaran, T. Belinskaya and A. Saxena, In search of a catalytic bioscavenger for the prophylaxis of nerve agent toxicity, *Chem.-Biol. Interact.*, 2010, **187**, 349–354.
185. M. Costante, L. Biggemann, Y. Alamneh, I. Soojhawon, R. Short, S. Nigam, G. Garcia, B. P. Doctor, M. Valiyaveettil and M. P. Nambiar, Hydrolysis potential of recombinant human skin and kidney prolidase against diisopropylfluorophosphate and sarin by *in vitro* analysis, *Toxicol. In Vitro*, 2012, **26**, 182–188.
186. L. Chandrasekaran, T. Belinskaya and A. Saxena, *In vitro* characterization of organophosphorus compound hydrolysis by native and recombinant human prolidase, *Toxicol. In Vitro*, 2013, **27**, 499–506.
187. P. E. Rezk, P. Zdenka, P. Sabnekar, T. Kajih, D. G. Mata, C. Wrobel, D. M. Cerasoli and N. Chilukuri, An *in vitro* and *in vivo* evaluation of the efficacy of recombinant human liver prolidase as a catalytic bioscavenger of chemical warfare nerve agents, *Drug Chem. Toxicol.*, 2015, **38**, 37–43.
188. Y. Kondo, A. Ishigami, S. Kubo, S. Handa, K. Gomi, K. Hirokawa, N. Kajiyama, T. Chiba, K. Shimokado and N. Maruyama, Senescence marker protein-30 is a unique enzyme that hydrolyzes diisopropyl phosphorofluoridate in the liver, *FEBS Lett.*, 2004, **570**, 57–62.
189. S. Chakraborti and B. J. Bahnson, Crystal structure of human senescence marker protein 30: insights linking structural, enzymatic, and physiological functions, *Biochemistry*, 2010, **49**, 3436–3444.

190. T. Belinskaya, N. Pattabiraman, R. diTargiani, M. Choi and A. Saxena, Differences in amino acid residues in the binding pockets dictate substrate specificities of mouse senescence marker protein-30, human paraoxonase1, and squid diisopropylfluorophosphatase, *Biochim. Biophys. Acta, Proteins Proteomics*, 2012, **1824**, 701–710.
191. K. Karasawa, A. Harada, N. Satoh, K. Inoue and M. Setaka, Plasma platelet activating factor-acetylhydrolase (PAF-AH), *Prog. Lipid Res.*, 2003, **42**, 93–114.
192. G. B. Quistad, K. J. Fisher, S. C. Owen, R. Klintenberg and J. E. Casida, Platelet-activating factor acetylhydrolase: selective inhibition by potent *n*-alkyl methylphosphonofluoridates, *Toxicol. Appl. Pharmacol.*, 2005, **205**, 149–156.
193. G. B. Quistad, C. Barlow, C. J. Winrow, S. E. Sparks and J. E. Casida, Evidence that mouse brain neuropathy target esterase is a lysophospholipase, *Proc. Natl. Acad. Sci. U. S. A.*, 2003, **100**, 7983–7987.
194. T. M. Epstein, U. Samanta, S. D. Kirby, D. M. Cerasoli and B. J. Bahnson, Crystal structures of brain group-VIII phospholipase A2 in nonaged complexes with the organophosphorus nerve agents soman and sarin, *Biochemistry*, 2009, **48**, 3425–3435.
195. J. Järv, Insight into the putative mechanism of esterase acting simultaneously on carboxyl and phosphoryl compounds, in *Enzymes hydrolysing organophosphorus compounds*, ed. E. Reiner, W. N. Aldridge and F. C. G. Hoskin, Ellis Horwood Ltd., Chichester, UK, 1989, pp. 221–225.
196. J. L. Sussman, M. Harel, F. Frolow, C. Oefner, A. Goldman, L. Toker and I. Silman, Atomic structure of acetylcholinesterase from *Torpedo californica*: a prototypic acetylcholine-binding protein, *Science*, 1991, **253**, 872–879.
197. C. B. Millard, O. Lockridge and C. A. Broomfield, Design and expression of organophosphorus acid anhydride hydrolase activity in human butyrylcholinesterase, *Biochemistry*, 1995, **34**, 15925–15933.
198. O. Lockridge, R. M. Blong, P. Masson, M. T. Froment, C. B. Millard and C. A. Broomfield, A single amino acid substitution, Gly117His, confers phosphotriesterase (organophosphorus acid anhydride hydrolase) activity on human butyrylcholinesterase, *Biochemistry*, 1997, **36**, 786–795.
199. P. Masson, F. Nachon and O. Lockridge, Structural approach to the aging of phosphylated cholinesterases, *Chem.-Biol. Interact.*, 2010, **187**, 157–162.
200. C. B. Millard, O. Lockridge and C. A. Broomfield, Organophosphorus acid anhydride hydrolase activity in human butyrylcholinesterase: synergy results in a somanase, *Biochemistry*, 1998, **37**, 237–247.
201. Y. Wang, A. T. Boeck, E. G. Duysen, M. Van Keuren, T. L. Saunders and O. Lockridge, Resistance to organophosphorus agent toxicity in transgenic mice expressing the G117H mutant of human butyrylcholinesterase, *Toxicol. Appl. Pharmacol.*, 2004, **196**, 356–366.
202. L. M. Schopfer, A. T. Boeck, C. A. Broomfield and O. Lockridge, Mutants of human butyrylcholinesterase with organophosphate hydrolase activity; evidence that His117 is a general base catalyst for hydrolysis of echothiophate, *J. Med. Chem. Biol. Radiol. Def.*, 2004, **2**, 1–21.

203. Y. Nicolet, O. Lockridge, P. Masson, J. C. Fontecilla-Camps and F. Nachon, Crystal structure of human butyrylcholinesterase and of its complexes with substrate and products, *J. Biol. Chem.*, 2003, **278**, 41141–41147.
204. T. Poyot, F. Nachon, M. T. Froment, M. Loiodice, S. Wieseler, L. M. Schopfer, O. Lockridge and P. Masson, Mutant of *Bungarus fasciatus* acetylcholinesterase with low affinity and low hydrolase activity toward organophosphorus esters, *Biochim. Biophys. Acta*, 2006, **1764**, 1470–1478.
205. P. Masson, M. T. Froment, E. Gillon, F. Nachon, O. Lockridge and L. M. Schopfer, Hydrolysis of oxo- and thio-esters by human butyrylcholinesterase, *Biochim. Biophys. Acta*, 2007, **1774**, 16–34.
206. F. Nachon, E. Carletti, M. Wandhammer, Y. Nicolet, L. M. Schopfer, P. Masson and O. Lockridge, X-ray crystallographic snapshots of reaction intermediates in the G117H mutant of human butyrylcholinesterase, a nerve agent target engineered into a catalytic bioscavenger, *Biochem. J.*, 2011, **434**, 73–82.
207. M. Amitay and A. Shurki, Hydrolysis of organophosphate compounds by mutant butyrylcholinesterase: a story of two histidines, *Proteins: Struct., Funct., Bioinf.*, 2011, **79**, 352–364.
208. S. V. Lushchekina, P. Masson, F. Nachon, B. L. Grigorenko, A. V. Nemukhin and S. D. Varfolomeev, In Russian: Применение суперкомпьютеров для установления механизмов биохимических реакций (Application of the supercomputers for the enzymology reactions mechanisms identification), *Суперкомпьютерные технологии в науке и образовании (Supercomputer technologies in science, education and industry)*, Moscow State University Publishing, Moscow, 2010, pp. 69–76.
209. Y. Yao, J. Liu and C.-G. Zhan, Why does the G117H mutation considerably improve the activity of human butyrylcholinesterase against sarin? Insights from quantum mechanical/molecular mechanical free energy calculations, *Biochemistry*, 2012, **51**, 8980–8992.
210. P. M. Legler, S. M. Boisvert, J. R. Compton and C. B. Millard, Development of organophosphate hydrolase activity in a bacterial homolog of human cholinesterase, *Front. Chem.*, 2014, **2**, 46.
211. J. Liu and C.-G. Zhan, Reaction pathway and free energy profile for cocaine hydrolase-catalyzed hydrolysis of (−)-cocaine, *J. Chem. Theory Comput.*, 2012, **8**, 1426–1435.
212. M. Zhan, S. Hou, C. G. Zhan and F. Zheng, Kinetic characterization of high-activity mutants of human butyrylcholinesterase for the cocaine metabolite norcocaine, *Biochem. J.*, 2014, **457**, 197–206.
213. M. Dwyer, S. Javor, D. A. Ryan, E. M. Smith, B. Wang, J. Zhang and J. R. Cashman, Novel human butyrylcholinesterase variants: toward organophosphonate detoxication, *Biochemistry*, 2014, **53**, 4476–4487.
214. C. Kronman, B. Velan, D. Marcus, A. Ordentlich, S. Reuveny and A. Shafferman, Involvement of oligomerization, N-glycosylation and sialylation in the clearance of cholinesterases from the circulation, *Biochem. J.*, 1995, **311**(**3**), 959–967.
215. A. Saxena, Y. Ashani, L. Raveh, D. Stevenson, T. Patel and B. P. Doctor, Role of oligosaccharides in the pharmacokinetics of tissue-derived

and genetically engineered cholinesterases, *Mol. Pharmacol.*, 1998, **53**, 112–122.

216. O. Cohen, C. Kronman, A. Lazar, B. Velan and A. Shafferman, Controlled concealment of exposed clearance and immunogenic domains by site-specific polyethylene glycol attachment to acetylcholinesterase hypolysine mutants, *J. Biol. Chem.*, 2007, **282**, 35491–35501.
217. C. Kronman, O. Cohen, L. Raveh, O. Mazor, A. Ordentlich and A. Shafferman, Polyethylene-glycol conjugated recombinant human acetylcholinesterase serves as an efficacious bioscavenger against soman intoxication, *Toxicology*, 2007, **233**, 40–46.
218. C. Kronman, T. Chitlaru, E. Elhanany, B. Velan and A. Shafferman, Hierarchy of Post-translational Modifications Involved in the Circulatory Longevity of Glycoproteins: demonstration of concerted contributions of glycan sialylation and subunit assembly to the pharmacokinetic behavior of bovine acetylcholinesterase, *J. Biol. Chem.*, 2000, **275**, 29488–29502.
219. G. Gregoriadis, A. Fernandes and B. McCormack, Polysialylated proteins. An approach to improving enzyme stability and half-life in the blood circulation, *STP Pharma Sci.*, 1999, **9**, 61–66.
220. R. D. Newcomb, P. M. Campbell, D. L. Ollis, E. Cheah, R. J. Russell and J. G. Oakeshott, A single amino acid substitution converts a carboxylesterase to an organophosphorus hydrolase and confers insecticide resistance on a blowfly, *Proc. Natl. Acad. Sci. U. S. A.*, 1997, **94**, 7464–7468.
221. C. J. Jackson, J.-W. Liu, P. D. Carr, F. Younus, C. Coppin, T. Meirelles, M. Lethier, G. Pandey, D. L. Ollis, R. J. Russell, M. Weik and J. G. Oakeshott, Structure and function of an insect α-carboxylesterase (αEsterase7) associated with insecticide resistance, *Proc. Natl. Acad. Sci. U. S. A.*, 2013, **110**, 10177–10182.
222. A. C. Hemmert, T. C. Otto, R. A. Chica, M. Wierdl, J. S. Edwards, S. L. Lewis, C. C. Edwards, L. Tsurkan, C. L. Cadieux, S. A. Kasten, J. R. Cashman, S. L. Mayo, P. M. Potter, D. M. Cerasoli and M. R. Redinbo, Nerve agent hydrolysis activity designed into a human drug metabolism enzyme, *PLoS One*, 2011, **6**, e17441.
223. K. Fujioka and J. E. Casida, Glutathione S-transferase conjugation of organophosphorus pesticides yields S-phospho-, S-aryl-, and S-alkylglutathione derivatives, *Chem. Res. Toxicol.*, 2007, **20**, 1211–1217.
224. G. Amitai, R. Adani, G. Sod-Moriah, I. Rabinovitz, A. Vincze, H. Leader, B. Chefetz, L. Leibovitz-Persky, D. Friesem and Y. Hadar, Oxidative biodegradation of phosphorothiolates by fungal laccase, *FEBS Lett.*, 1998, **438**, 195–200.
225. M. Trovaslet-Leroy, C. Jolivalt, M.-T. Froment, B. Brasme, B. Lefebvre, D. Daveloose, F. Nachon and P. Masson, Application of laccase-mediator system (LMS) for the degradation of organophosphorus compounds, *Chem.-Biol. Interact.*, 2010, **187**, 393–396.
226. G. Amitai, R. Adani, M. Hershkovitz, P. Bel, I. Rabinovitz and H. Meshulam, Degradation of VX and sulfur mustard by enzymatic haloperoxidation, *J. Appl. Toxicol.*, 2003, **23**, 225–233.

227. A. J. Russell, J. A. Berberich, G. F. Drevon and R. R. Koepsel, Biomaterials for mediation of chemical and biological warfare agents, *Annu. Rev. Biomed. Eng.*, 2003, **5**, 1–27.
228. F. Jovic, L. Louise, C. Mioskowski and P.-Y. Renard, Immunologically driven antibodies chemical engineering: design and synthesis of a hapten aimed at nerve agent hydrolysis, *Tetrahedron Lett.*, 2005, **46**, 6809–6814.
229. I. Smirnov, A. Belogurov Jr, A. Friboulet, P. Masson, A. Gabibov and P.-Y. Renard, Strategies for the selection of catalytic antibodies against organophosphorus nerve agents, *Chem.-Biol. Interact.*, 2013, **203**, 196–201.
230. I. Smirnov, E. Carletti, I. Kurkova, F. Nachon, Y. Nicolet, V. A. Mitkevich, H. Débat, B. Avalle, A. A. Belogurov, N. Kuznetsov, A. Reshetnyak, P. Masson, A. G. Tonevitsky, N. Ponomarenko, A. A. Makarov, A. Friboulet, A. Tramontano and A. Gabibov, Reactibodies generated by kinetic selection couple chemical reactivity with favorable protein dynamics, *Proc. Natl. Acad. Sci. U. S. A.*, 2011, **108**, 15954–15959.
231. I. N. Kurkova, I. V. Smirnov, A. A. Belogurov, Jr., N. A. Ponomarenko and A. G. Gabibov, Creation of catalytic antibodies metabolizing organophosphate compounds, *Biochemistry*, 2012, **77**, 1139–1146.
232. N. Ponomarenko, S. D. Chatziefthimiou, I. Kurkova, Y. Mokrushina, Y. Mokrushina, A. Stepanova, I. Smirnov, M. Avakyan, T. Bobik, A. Mamedov, V. Mitkevich, A. Belogurov, Jr, O. S. Fedorova, M. Dubina, A. Golovin, V. Lamzin, A. Friboulet, A. A. Makarov, M. Wilmanns and A. Gabibov, Role of κ→λ light-chain constant-domain switch in the structure and functionality of A17 reactibody, *Acta Crystallogr., Sect. D: Biol. Crystallogr.*, 2014, **70**, 708–719.
233. R. Ramakrishnan, S. Subramanian, L. Yingjun, R. S. Barhate, L. L. Neeta and S. Ramakrishna, Functionalized polymer nanofibre membranes for protection from chemical warfare stimulants, *Nanotechnology*, 2006, **17**, 2947.
234. M. Zengerle, F. Brandhuber, C. Schneider, F. Worek, G. Reiter and S. Kubik, Highly efficient cyclosarin degradation mediated by a β-cyclodextrin derivative containing an oxime-derived substituent, *Beilstein J. Org. Chem.*, 2011, **7**, 1543–1554.
235. F. Estour, S. Letort, S. Müller, R. K. Kalakuntla, R. Le Provost, T. Wille, G. Reiter, F. Worek, O. Lafont and G. Gouhier, Functionalized cyclodextrins bearing an alpha nucleophile – A promising way to degrade nerve agents, *Chem.-Biol. Interact.*, 2013, **203**, 202–207.
236. R. K. Kalakuntla, T. Wille, R. Le Provost, S. Letort, G. Reiter, S. Müller, H. Thiermann, F. Worek, G. Gouhier, O. Lafont and F. Estour, New modified β-cyclodextrin derivatives as detoxifying agents of chemical warfare agents (I). Synthesis and preliminary screening: evaluation of the detoxification using a half-quantitative enzymatic assay, *Toxicol. Lett.*, 2013, **216**, 200–205.
237. A. Bierwisch, M. Zengerle, H. Thiermann, S. Kubik and F. Worek, Detoxification of alkyl methylphosphonofluoridates by an oxime-substituted β-cyclodextrin – An in vitro structure–activity study, *Toxicol. Lett.*, 2014, **224**, 209–214.

238. S. Müller, F. Estour, R. K. Kalakuntla, R. Le Provost, O. Lafont, F. Worek, H. Thiermann and G. Reiter, New modified β-cyclodextrin derivatives as detoxifying agents of chemical warfare agents (II). In vitro detoxification of cyclosarin (GF): general screening and toxicokinetic aspects of OP scavengers, *Toxicol. Lett.*, 2013, **216**, 206–212.
239. F. Worek, T. Seeger, M. Zengerle, S. Kubik, H. Thiermann and T. Wille, Effectiveness of a substituted β-cyclodextrin to prevent cyclosarin toxicity in vivo, *Toxicol. Lett.*, 2014, **226**, 222–227.
240. A. N. Bigley, C. Xu, T. J. Henderson, S. P. Harvey and F. M. Raushel, Enzymatic neutralization of the chemical warfare agent VX: evolution of phosphotriesterase for phosphorothiolate hydrolysis, *J. Am. Chem. Soc.*, 2013, **135**, 10426–10432.
241. C.-Y. Yang, P. D. Renfrew, A. J. Olsen, M. Zhang, C. Yuvienco, R. Bonneau and J. K. Montclare, Improved stability and half-life of fluorinated phosphotriesterase using Rosetta, *ChemBioChem*, 2014, **15**, 1761–1764.
242. T. C. Otto, J. R. Scott, M. A. Kauffman, S. M. Hodgins, R. C. diTargiani, J. H. Hughes, E. P. Sarricks, G. A. Saturday, T. A. Hamilton and D. M. Cerasoli, Identification and characterization of novel catalytic bioscavengers of organophosphorus nerve agents, *Chem.-Biol. Interact.*, 2013, **203**, 186–190.
243. M. Ferrer, O. Golyshina, A. Beloqui and P. N. Golyshin, Mining enzymes from extreme environments, *Curr. Opin. Microbiol.*, 2007, **10**, 207–214.
244. J. F. Martin and W. W. Troy, Multiscale modeling of nerve agent hydrolysis mechanisms: a tale of two Nobel Prizes, *Phys. Scr.*, 2014, **89**, 108004.
245. S. D. Khare, Y. Kipnis, P. Greisen Jr., R. Takeuchi, Y. Ashani, M. Goldsmith, Y. Song, J. L. Gallaher, I. Silman, H. Leader, J. L. Sussman, B. L. Stoddard, D. S. Tawfik and D. Baker, Computational redesign of a mononuclear zinc metalloenzyme for organophosphate hydrolysis, *Nat. Chem. Biol.*, 2012, **8**, 294–300.
246. V. Murthy, Y. Gao, L. Geng, N. K. LeBrasseur, T. A. White, R. J. Parks and S. Brimijoin, Physiologic and metabolic safety of butyrylcholinesterase gene therapy in mice, *Vaccine*, 2014, **32**, 4155–4162.

CHAPTER 3

Nicotinic Receptors as Targets for Nerve Agent Therapy

JOHN TATTERSALL[a]

[a]Chemical, Biological and Radiological Division, Dstl, Porton Down, Salisbury, SP4 0JQ, UK
*E-mail: jtattersall@dstl.gov.uk

3.1 Introduction

The primary mechanism of the toxic action of organophosphorus (OP) nerve agents and pesticides is inhibition of carboxyl ester hydrolase enzymes, of which acetylcholinesterase (AChE) is the most toxicologically important. AChE (EC 3.1.1.7), also known as true cholinesterase, is a serine protease enzyme that catalyses the hydrolysis of the neurotransmitter acetylcholine (ACh) to choline and acetic acid. AChE is found in the central nervous system (CNS) and peripheral nervous system, neuromuscular junctions (NMJs) and red blood cells (RBCs). Organophosphates inactivate AChE by phosphorylating the serine hydroxyl group located at the active site of the enzyme.

The natural substrate for AChE, ACh, is a neurotransmitter that mediates chemical synaptic transmission at the NMJ, in the peripheral autonomic nervous system and in the CNS. The acute life-threatening toxicity of nerve agents arises from the uncontrolled accumulation of ACh at peripheral and central cholinergic synapses, giving rise to the so-called cholinergic syndrome. This is characterised by peripheral effects [increased secretions, miosis, abdominal cramps, involuntary defecation and urination, changes

Issues in Toxicology No. 27
Chemical Warfare Toxicology, Volume 2: Management of Poisoning
Edited by Franz Worek, John Jenner, and Horst Thiermann

Published by the Royal Society of Chemistry, www.rsc.org

in heart rate, pallor, muscular weakness, fasciculations (localised muscle contraction), muscular paralysis, tachycardia (increased heart rate) and hypertension] and central effects (giddiness, anxiety, headache, impaired memory and alertness, tremor, convulsions, seizures, and respiratory depression).[1,2] Lethality is generally believed to be caused by respiratory paralysis resulting from disruption of the respiratory centres in the brain or from transmission failure at NMJs.[3,4]

The action of ACh is mediated by two main classes of receptors, muscarinic and nicotinic, named after the specific ligands, muscarine and nicotine, that were originally used to distinguish them. The metabotropic muscarinic receptors (mAChRs) are G protein coupled receptors that act through intracellular signal transduction pathways, whereas the ionotropic nicotinic ACh receptors (nAChRs), contain a ligand gated ion channel pore that functions as the transduction mechanism by mediating the flow of ionic currents across the cell membrane. Some authors have attributed the overstimulation of ACh receptors following inhibition of AChE as follows:[5]

1. Muscarinic overstimulation causes bradycardia, bronchorrhea, bronchospasm, diarrhoea, hypotension, lacrimation, miosis, salivation, urination and vomiting;
2. Nicotinic overstimulation in the sympathetic system produces hypertension, mydriasis, sweating and tachycardia;
3. Nicotinic overstimulation in the CNS results in agitation, coma, confusion and respiratory failure;
4. Nicotinic overstimulation at the NMJ causes fasciculations, muscle weakness and paralysis.

The effects of OP anticholinesterases that appear to be most threatening to life are bronchorrhea, bradycardia, hypotension and inhibition of the respiratory centre of the brain.[6,7] These effects are all mediated by muscarinic pathways, hence the requirement for rapid administration of atropine to counter the potentially fatal effects of poisoning. However, paralysis of ventilation through neuromuscular block has also been shown to contribute to respiratory failure caused by OPs, particularly when the muscarinic effects have been mitigated with atropine.[6] The neuromuscular block produced by OP anticholinesterases is mediated *via* nicotinic receptors found on the post-synaptic side of the NMJ.[8–12] Overstimulation and subsequent block of these nicotinic receptors appears to be the most critical nicotinic pathway affected by anticholinesterase agents.[7]

3.2 Current Therapy for Nerve Agent Poisoning

Despite the involvement of nicotinic receptors in many important aspects of nerve agent toxicity, pharmacotherapy focuses only on the muscarinic component, the mainstay of treatment being the competitive mAChR antagonist atropine. The nicotinic effects are treated indirectly, by the use of an oxime to reactivate inhibited AChE; this approach mitigates both nicotinic and muscarinic effects for those nerve agents against which oximes are effective.[13] Oximes are especially useful for treating the nicotinic effects, for which atropine alone is ineffective;[14] however, there is no single, broad spectrum oxime suitable for the antidotal treatment of poisoning with all OP agents. If more than one oxime is available, the choice depends primarily on the identity of the OP compound.[15] For example, pralidoxime is effective against sarin and VX, whilst obidoxime is more effective against tabun.[15] The Hagedorn oximes, such as HI-6 and HLö-7, emerged from the search for reactivators with a greater spectrum of activity, particularly against soman.[15] HI-6 is currently fielded by some nations (*e.g.* Sweden) as a nerve agent antidote and is in development in the UK, Canada, The Netherlands and France. A major consideration in this development is the requirement of a wet–dry autoinjector device, due to the poor stability of HI-6 in aqueous solution. Another bispyridinium oxime, methoxime (MMB-4), is currently in advanced development in the USA.

Despite these efforts, however, the reliance on oxime enzyme reactivators is a fundamental weakness in the search for an improved therapy. The search for the ideal oxime has been hampered by the fact that no single oxime demonstrates adequate reactivating activity against all known nerve agents. Each AChE–OP complex differs chemically and some, after a period of time, undergo ageing (dealkylation of the enzyme–inhibitor complex) and cannot then be reactivated. Whichever oxime is used, it will always be deficient against one or more of the nerve agents, so it is highly unlikely that a generic therapy based on this mechanism will ever be discovered.[16]

3.3 Potential Benefits of Nicotinic Antagonists in Nerve Agent Poisoning

In contrast to the indirect treatment of nicotinic effects by enzyme reactivators, the effectiveness of an appropriate anti-nicotinic drug to treat these effects directly should be independent of the OP nerve agent poison involved, in the same way as that of atropine in antagonising the muscarinic effects. Thus, it would seem appropriate to examine nicotinic antagonists, as well as muscarinic ones, as possible therapeutic agents for anticholinesterase nerve agent toxicity.[13,17] However, nicotinic antagonists are not currently used and they have been largely neglected in published work on nerve agent poisoning.[13,18]

This is probably due, at least in part, to fundamental differences in the structure and function of the two classes of ACh receptors. Muscarinic synapses tend to be involved in regulating rather than instigating neural processes (*e.g.* gastric and glandular secretions, cardiac inhibition and CNS excitation pathways). Although atropine can be very toxic at high concentrations, it offers a sufficient therapeutic index to enable significant benefit in cases of OP poisoning (although it should be noted that atropine is often titrated against signs of poisoning in clinical use, resulting in doses above those that would cause serious adverse effects in unpoisoned individuals). In contrast, many nicotinic antagonists are highly toxic: for example, tubocurarine is the principal component of curare, an arrow poison used in South America. The muscular paralysis produced by tubocurarine induced nicotinic block is extremely potent and very rapid, suggesting that competitive nicotinic antagonists of this type would have a narrow therapeutic index and are unlikely to have utility as a medical therapy for OP poisoning.[17]

Because of the problems associated with nicotinic antagonism, any compound that could have potential as a nerve agent therapy would ideally be required to have minimal physiological effects on unpoisoned NMJs (at therapeutically relevant concentrations), would display antagonism that could not be overcome by high concentrations of ACh in the synapse produced by AChE inhibition and, crucially, would still allow enough current through the ion channel to develop an endplate potential (EPP) capable of triggering an action potential. Competitive nicotinic antagonists do not fulfil these criteria, as their block at low concentrations can be overcome by the build-up of ACh in the synapse caused by AChE inhibition, and they become very toxic at higher concentrations. It has been suggested that large doses of neuromuscular blocking agents could be used in ventilated patients to prevent nAChR mediated damage at the NMJ,[19] but this would not be feasible for immediate first aid or management of mass casualties when ventilation facilities are limited.

Noncompetitive nicotinic antagonists present a more attractive proposition, as their block cannot be overcome by ACh. They could be used to reduce the current flow through the nicotinic channel, thus preventing depolarisation blockade caused by overstimulation of the nicotinic receptors by ACh when AChE is inhibited. Furthermore, antagonism at a level that would have no effect on an unpoisoned NMJ should still antagonise the effect of increasing concentrations of ACh. This is because the proportion blocked should be maintained, irrespective of the concentration of ACh in the synapse, by effectively displaying a use dependent block. This concept is well demonstrated by the effects of MK-801 or memantine at *N*-methyl-D-aspartate (NMDA) receptors, where antagonism is most effective in the face of excessive receptor activation, because statistically more channels are open and available to be blocked.[20,21] The mechanism of inhibition by compounds of this type, whose action is contingent upon prior activation of the receptor by the agonist, is also termed 'uncompetitive' antagonism. In addition to this, as the effects of nicotinic antagonists would occur downstream from the AChE inhibition, they should not suffer from the agent specificity problems that have hampered the development of broad spectrum oximes.

3.4 Nicotinic ACh Receptors

nAChRs are members of the Cys-loop family of neurotransmitter gated ion channels, a family that also includes the γ-aminobutyric acid A (GABA A), strychnine sensitive glycine and 5-hydroxytryptamine 3 (5-HT 3) receptors.[22–26] They are cation selective and share a common basic structure, but their pharmacological and functional properties arise from the wide range of different subunit combinations making up the distinctive subtypes. nAChRs are involved in many physiological functions in the CNS and peripheral nervous system, and are the targets of the widely used drug of abuse nicotine. In humans, nAChRs have been implicated in several neurological and psychiatric disorders, ranging from epilepsy to dementia, and are major targets for pharmaceutical drug discovery. In addition, nAChRs are important targets for neuroactive pesticides in insects and other invertebrates. Historically, nAChRs have been one of the most intensively studied families of neurotransmitter receptors. They were the first neurotransmitter receptors to be biochemically purified and the first to be characterised by molecular cloning and heterologous expression. At present, 17 nicotinic subunits have been cloned, the muscle α1, β1, δ, γ and ε subunits, and the neuronal α2–α10 and β2–β4 subunits.[27,28] With the exception of α8 (avian), all of these are of mammalian origin. Each subunit possesses four transmembrane (TM) domains. The α subunits have two adjacent cysteines essential for ACh binding, but both the α subunit and the non-α subunits contribute to the specificity within each receptor subtype.[29,30] The subunits co-assemble to muscular α1β1γδ and α1β1εδ subtypes and heteromeric and homomeric neuronal nAChRs. The muscle nAChR is described in the next section; neuronal nAChRs are described later in the chapter.

3.5 The Muscle nAChR

The muscle subtype is the best studied nAChR and mediates some of the most important nicotinic effects of OP poisoning, *e.g.* respiratory muscle paralysis. The success of oximes in treating poisoning by reactivatable nerve agents, such as sarin, suggests that peripheral nAChRs, particularly those at the NMJ, play an important role in poisoning. Oximes do not readily cross the blood–brain barrier[31–33] and their effects are therefore confined to the peripheral nervous system.

Muscle nicotinic receptors are cation selective and are found in high concentrations postsynaptically at the motor endplate, where they mediate the transmission of nerve impulses from motor nerves to muscle fibres through the binding of ACh after its release from the nerve terminal into the synaptic cleft. During development, the foetal form of the channel (containing a γ subunit) is replaced by the adult form (containing an ε subunit), which produces a large (290 kDa) glycoprotein consisting of five subunits (α1, ε, α1, β1 and δ) assembled in a ring.[34] The adult muscle α1β1εδ nAChRs preferentially aggregate at the NMJ, are more stable to degradation and have a more rapid response to agonists compared with the α1β1γδ receptor.[30] During immobilisation, denervation or inflammation, however, the γ subunit starts to be re-expressed at the muscle membrane. In animal studies, the neuronal α7 nAChR subtype has also been found in the muscle membrane during development and denervation, suggesting that this receptor subtype might be associated with endplate stabilisation and synaptogenesis.[35–37]

Each of the five subunits has six predicted domains: a large extracellular amino-terminal domain; four membrane spanning segments (M1, M2, M3 and M4); and a long cytoplasmic loop between M3 and M4, giving a total length of about 16 nm.[24] The extracellular domain contains the two ACh binding sites and a long, ~2 nm diameter central or outer vestibule.[38] The ACh binding sites are about 4 nm from the membrane surface on opposite sides of the pore.[39]

Below the outer vestibule, the pore or lumen of the channel narrows through the membrane portion, forming an aqueous path across the membrane. This portion also contains the gate of the channel, which is made by the pore lining M2 segments, and below that is the narrowest part of the open channel, known as the constriction zone.[40] In the closed channel, the M2 helices are not close enough to completely occlude the pore. Instead, they are believed to form a 'hydrophobic girdle', producing an energetic barrier to ionic permeation.[38] Within the intracellular domain there is a smaller inner vestibule that has narrow (0.8–0.9 nm wide) aqueous links to the cell interior. It has been suggested that the vestibule acts as a preselectivity filter for ions, in which the negatively charged groups at the neck and inner walls of the vestibules concentrate the cations they select for, and therefore screen out the anions, or simply guide the cations down the pore by producing an electrostatic field within the vestibule.[41]

The binding of two ACh molecules to the α-subunits causes a dramatic conformational change to the M2 helices that line the pore of the channel in the membrane region. The bends of the helices, instead of pointing towards the axis of the pore, rotate clockwise and away from the constriction zone, opening up the pore.[38] As the pore opens, sodium and calcium ions pass through the channel from the outside to the inside of the cell, and potassium ions move in the opposite direction down their respective electrochemical gradient. The resultant current flow across the membrane is known as the endplate current (EPC) and this produces a rapid depolarisation of the endplate region, which is known as the EPP.[42] The EPP depolarises the endplate region of the muscle fibre over the threshold for induction of a muscle action potential, which then leads to contraction of the muscle fibre.

The nicotinic receptor provides a promiscuous site for antagonists that compete for the natural ligand binding site (competitive antagonists) and those that bind to alternative sites (noncompetitive antagonists). A large range of antagonists interact with the receptor, see reviews by Arias[43] and Sine *et al.*[44] The two natural ligand binding sites present on nicotinic receptors are responsible for many of the pharmacological effects observed in studies of these receptors. One site has a high affinity for the natural ligand (ACh; the site between α and δ subunits) and the other has a low affinity (between α and γ or ε subunits).[45] Agonist binding to these two sites displays positive co-operativity (Hill coefficient of 1.5–3.0), which means that an agonist binding to the first receptor site induces a conformational change in the receptor, increasing the probability of an agonist binding to the second site.[46] Agonists such as ACh trigger the channel to open on binding, while competitive antagonists compete for the same binding site without activating channel opening. Since both α subunits are sequentially identical, the observed high and low affinity for agonists on the receptor results from the interaction of the α subunit with the δ or the ε subunit, respectively (Arias, 2000). The high and low affinity interactions are opposite for competitive antagonists such as D-tubocurarine, which bind with high affinity to the low affinity ACh site and *vice versa*.[47]

The critical portion of the natural ligand binding site is contained in several aromatic residues found in three loop forming binding domains (loops A–C) and in the cysteine pair at residues 192–193.[48] These are found on the α subunit and are known as the principal face. Other residues, such as the negatively charged aspartates and glutamates (loop D), Thr or Tyr (loop E), and Trp (loop F) form four discontinuous loops on non-α subunits that make up the complementary face of the natural ligand binding sites.[49–51] These residues provide the platform for the interaction with ACh and other compounds that bind to the natural ligand binding sites. The ACh molecule comprises a cationic methyl head group, a five atom chain and a tail containing cationic methyl groups. The relative charge and separation of these cationic groups has been shown to be critical in the binding of ACh to the negatively charged residues on the receptor.[52] This concept is also important for the binding of other compounds to the receptor. The poly-bismethonium series of depolarising blockers show increasing potency as the chain length between the charged groups increases up to C10, which declines thereafter.[53] It has been shown that these compounds adopt a rigid conformation, and a molecular length of approximately 20 Å is postulated to provide the best fit to the space available for neuromuscular blocking agents between the receptive sites of the endplate ACh receptor.[54]

The enrichment of aromatic and hydrophobic residues at the ACh binding site was first revealed by mutational analyses and site directed labelling,[55] and later confirmed by the structural determination of the ACh binding protein (AChBP) and the *Torpedo* receptor.[38] (AChBP is a water soluble homologue of the ligand binding domain of nicotinic receptors that is released from molluscan glial cells and modulates ACh mediated synaptic transmission; the crystal structure of AChBP has become an established model for the extracellular domain of pentameric ligand gated ion channels.[56]) Crystal structures of *Lymnaea* AChBP with bound nicotine or carbamylcholine,[57] and more recently of *Aplysia* AChBP with bound lobeline or epibatidine,[58] show that the agonists are fully enveloped by the protein. Stabilisation forces include π-cation, dipole cation, hydrogen bonding and van der Waals interactions. The crystal structure of the extracellular domain of the mouse nicotinic ACh receptor α subunit bound to α-bungarotoxin has also recently been determined at 1.94 Å resolution.[59] A well ordered water molecule and two hydrophilic residues deep in the core of the α-subunit were found. These hydrophilic residues are substituted by large hydrophobic residues (Phe, Leu or Val) in the non-channel homologue AChBPs, suggesting that they have evolved for channel specific functions.[59] Other pharmacologically active compounds that bind to the α subunits include several α-conotoxins, which appear to bind with some overlap to the natural ligand binding site at different locations.[60] Additionally, the α subunits also contain the binding site for certain AChE inhibitors such as physostigmine, which can activate the receptor without interacting with the natural ligand binding sites.[61]

The passage of ions through the channel can be inhibited by noncompetitive antagonists. There are several high affinity luminal binding sites for noncompetitive antagonists found at different rings on the M2 TM domain. Within this domain, the serine ring at the 6 position is the inhibitory locus for chlorpromazine (CPZ),[62] triphenylmethylphosphonium (TPMP+),[63] the local anaesthetic QX-222,[64] phencyclidine (PCP)[65] and trifluoromethyliodophenyldiazirine (TID),[66] which are all noncompetitive antagonists at the nicotinic receptor. TID also binds to the valine ring at the 13 position, which is the postulated site for cembranoids.[67] Additionally, the binding site for the local anaesthetic meproadifen appears to be located at the outer or extracellular ring found at the 20 position,[68] whereas the M2 domain is the locus for endogenous noncompetitive antagonists such as the neuropeptide substance P[69] and the neurotransmitter 5-HT.[70]

Other noncompetitive antagonists bind to non-luminal binding sites around the channel. The quinacrine binding site is a high affinity site located at the lipid–protein interface of the α-M1 domain.[71] Ethidium is believed to interact with the external wall of the vestibule a considerable distance from both the channel lumen and the lipid membrane surface.[72] Additionally, a number of hormones including progesterone, testosterone and glucocorticoids have been postulated to act through interactions with the lipid–protein interface or the extracellular domain of the nicotinic channel.[73–75]

The simplest way to describe the action of luminal antagonists is based on the assumption that these compounds enter the open channel, bind to different rings within the M2 TM domain and inhibit the passage of cations by sterically 'plugging' the receptor pore.[43] The existence of non-luminal antagonist binding sites is not consistent with the open channel blocking mechanism. Instead, the presence of these kinds of sites opens the possibility of the regulation of cation permeation by an allosteric process outside of the pore. In turn, the allosteric mechanism can be viewed as a structural modification of the ion channel by the binding of one antagonist molecule to its specific high affinity binding site.[43]

At high concentrations, ACh itself can inhibit the function of the nicotinic receptor and, thus, auto-inhibit its own function when allowed to build up in the synapse. The low affinity inhibitory binding site for the natural agonist is postulated to be located at or close to the quinacrine locus.[76]

3.6 Blockers of Neuromuscular Transmission

Drugs that block neuromuscular transmission can do so by acting presynaptically to inhibit ACh synthesis or release, by acting postsynaptically to reduce its effects or by enhancing cholinergic transmission unsustainably to disrupt neuromuscular function.[53]

Drugs that act presynaptically can act by inhibiting ACh synthesis (hemicholinium and triethylcholine) or by inhibiting ACh release (botulinum toxin and β-bungarotoxin). Hemicholinium acts as a competitive inhibitor of choline uptake, thereby preventing ACh formation, but is not appreciably taken up itself.[77] Triethylcholine, as well as inhibiting choline uptake, is itself transported and acylated within the terminals, forming acetyltriethylcholine. This is stored in place of ACh and released as a false transmitter, but has no depolarising effect on the postsynaptic membrane.[78] The blocking effect of these drugs develops slowly as the existing stores of ACh become depleted. Vesamicol, which acts by blocking ACh transport into synaptic vesicles, has a similar effect. Quantal ACh release is triggered by the entry of Ca^{2+} into the presynaptic nerve terminal and is therefore blocked by agents that inhibit Ca^{2+} entry, including magnesium ions and some aminoglycoside antibiotics such as streptomycin and neomycin. These drugs occasionally produce muscle paralysis as an unwanted side-effect when used clinically.[79,80] Other blockers of ACh release include the potent neurotoxins botulinum toxin and β-bungarotoxin. These act by disrupting the function of proteins involved in the control of ACh vesicle exocytosis, thereby producing a long lasting block of synaptic function.[81]

The effect of drugs that act presynaptically (either by inhibiting ACh synthesis or release) on neuromuscular function is to reduce the maximum tension that the muscle can develop when it contracts. The amount of ACh released by a nerve impulse normally exceeds by several fold what is needed to elicit an action potential in the muscle fibre; this excess transmitter release is known as the 'safety factor'.[82] As the amount of ACh released per stimulus reduces, the amplitude of the EPP eventually drops below the threshold level required for induction of the muscle action potential. The result of this is that fewer muscle fibres reach the threshold for contraction and so the amplitude of single twitch contractions and the tetanus response reduces. The block produced by hemicholinium is slow in onset, as the preformed stores of ACh have to be exhausted before transmission failure occurs.[83] Botulinum toxin and β-bungarotoxin produce similar effects to hemicholinium on a neuromuscular preparation, but their effects are irreversible.[84]

Drugs that act postsynaptically are more common clinically and generally fall into two categories. Non-depolarising blocking agents (*e.g.* tubocurarine, pancuronium, vecuronium, atracurium, mivacurium and gallamine) act by blocking ACh receptors or the associated ion channel. Depolarising blocking agents (*e.g.* decamethonium and suxamethonium), in contrast, are partial agonists at ACh receptors.

All of the non-depolarising blocking agents used clinically act primarily as competitive receptor antagonists at the nicotinic receptors on the postsynaptic endplate,[53] binding to the natural ligand receptor binding site without activating channel opening. Due to the safety factor, it is necessary to block 70–80% of the receptor sites before transmission actually fails. With sufficient receptor block, the amplitude of the EPP fails to reach the threshold needed to generate an action potential. In any individual muscle fibre, transmission is all or nothing, so graded degrees of blockage represent a varying proportion of muscle fibres failing to respond. In this situation, where the amplitude of the EPP is close to threshold (just above in some muscle fibres, just below in others), small variations in the amount of transmitter released, or in the rate at which it is destroyed, will have a large effect on the proportion of fibres contracting.[82] Other factors that normally have relatively little effect on the efficiency of transmission then become important, such as stimulation frequency, temperature and cholinesterase inhibition.

Some of the non-depolarising blocking agents are also believed to block presynaptic nicotinic receptors, which are involved in a feedback system to regulate the amount of ACh released during repetitive stimulation. Presynaptic ACh receptors have been demonstrated pharmacologically and by molecular biology techniques, but their functions are not well understood when compared with the postsynaptic receptors.[85,86] Presynaptic nAChRs can bind β-bungarotoxin but not α-bungarotoxin, and are inhibited by non-depolarising blocking agents and hexamethonium.[87–89]

There has been much debate about whether this feedback mechanism is positive (ACh release is increased when ACh binds to the presynaptic receptor) or negative (binding of ACh reduces release).[90–95] The historical research was reviewed by Prior *et al.*,[96] who also put forward the hypothesis that tubocurarine enhances ACh release at low frequencies of motor nerve stimulation, whilst depressing release at high frequencies. Therefore, the feedback mechanism would be negative at low stimulation frequencies, but positive at high frequencies. The depression of release at high frequencies is responsible for the typical 'tetanic fade' seen with addition of tubocurarine to a repetitively stimulated diaphragm muscle[97] and the neuronal nAChR subtype on the nerve terminal that mediates this effect has been identified as α3β2.[98] This receptor is inhibited by non-depolarising neuromuscular blocking drugs, but not by suxamethonium at clinically relevant concentrations.[99,100]

Depolarising blocking agents such as suxamethonium and decamethonium act as partial agonists at postjunctional muscle nicotinic receptors, stimulating channel opening and depolarisation of the postsynaptic endplate in a similar way to ACh. Decamethonium is also a potent channel blocker of muscle nicotinic receptors and, therefore, cannot elicit as large an effect as ACh alone.[101] Both compounds are structurally related to ACh but are not rapidly broken down by AChE. This means that that decamethonium and, to a lesser extent, suxamethonium persist at the endplate, where they can continually activate the receptors, causing the channel to remain in an open state and the postsynaptic membrane in a depolarised state. This continual depolarisation leads to inactivation of voltage gated Na^+ channels in the muscle membrane, which are unable to repolarise and produce an action potential when the motor nerve is stimulated and ACh is released across the synaptic cleft.[102] This is known as phase I block. Phase II block is produced by desensitisation of the nicotinic receptors, when these receptors become insensitive to further activation by any agonist.[102] Consequently, the clinical signs of these blocking agents are similar to those seen with anticholinesterase agents at the NMJ: transient twitching of skeletal muscles (fasciculations) is followed by a complete block of neuromuscular function.[97]

3.7 Effects of AChE Inhibitors at the NMJ

Drugs that inhibit AChE at the NMJ initially enhance neuromuscular transmission, before inhibiting it through depolarisation block and desensitisation of the postjunctional nicotinic receptors during repetitive stimulation. The anticholinesterases can be split into three classes: short acting, medium duration and irreversible inhibitors. Edrophonium is a short acting AChE inhibitor: it is readily reversible and its action is very brief.[103] The medium duration inhibitors are the carbamates such as neostigmine, pyridostigmine and physostigmine, which bind to the enzyme in a similar way to ACh, but hydrolysis of these compounds occurs much more slowly. The decarbamoylation of AChE inhibited by these carbamates has a half-life of the order of 30 min.[104,105] The irreversible inhibitors include the OP insecticides and nerve agents.

The effect of anticholinesterases on the phrenic nerve hemidiaphragm preparation is to produce a rapid increase in the amplitude of the single twitch, which can resemble a miniature tetanus. Because the clearance of ACh from the synapse by AChE is reduced, stimulation of the nicotinic receptors by ACh is prolonged, and the amplitude and duration of EPPs are increased.[106] Furthermore, the diffusion of ACh away from receptor sites can lead to antidromic and orthodromic nerve action potentials in some muscle types, which produce repetitive EPPs from a single nerve stimulus.[12] The result of these effects is the recruitment of more muscle fibres, which produces a larger and more sustained contraction.

The block produced by anticholinesterases is initially believed to result from depolarisation block of the muscle membrane. When AChE is inhibited, the duration of the EPPs can extend beyond the duration of the refractory period of the muscle membrane.[107] During a period of repetitive (tetanic) stimulation, the force generated by the muscle is initially very large, but this rapidly fades as the muscle membrane becomes depolarised without a refractory period to allow recovery of voltage gated Na^+ channels. The muscle is unable to respond to new stimuli as it is already in a depolarised state.[108,109]

Then, as desensitisation of the receptor occurs due to the continual presence of ACh, this becomes the dominant method of neuromuscular transmission failure.[107] Continuous stimulation by ACh causes the receptor to become insensitive to ACh binding and the current flow producing the EPP ceases in these receptors.[110,111] More than one desensitisation state exists, dependent on the length of exposure to the agonist,[112] and desensitisation appears to occur much more rapidly in open, activated channels, than in closed or inactivated channels.[113] The potent block during tetanic stimulation and the slight recovery of neuromuscular function during chronic exposure to anticholinesterases can be attributed to different desensitisation states. During a short (*e.g.* 3 s) tetanic stimulation, the desensitisation is rapid and transient and is likely to recover between periods of rapid stimulation separated by several minutes.[113,114] However, a longer lasting desensitisation can occur in receptors chronically exposed to high concentrations of ACh,[112,114] possibly involving other mechanisms, such as receptor phosphorylation[114] and internalisation of the receptors.[115,116]

After a neuromuscular preparation has been exposed to an anticholinesterase for several hours, the ability of the preparation to sustain a tetanic contraction returns slightly. A second dose of an anticholinesterase at this stage has little effect on the response, suggesting that the NMJ has adapted to the conditions created by the inhibited AChE.[117] The mechanism underlying the improved ability of the muscle to sustain tetanic contraction is believed to be chronic desensitisation of the postsynaptic nicotinic receptors, which results in a reduction of the EPP amplitude and duration.[107,117] The muscle membrane is then able to repolarise and undergo a refractory period, restoring contractile function. This will only occur in some fibres, however, so the muscle function as a whole would still be greatly compromised. Meeter[117] suggested that agents that accelerate desensitisation at the NMJ could be useful in the treatment of anticholinesterase poisoning.

The complex nature of the effect of anticholinesterase agents that produces transmission failure at the NMJ makes it particularly intransigent to treatment. Nevertheless, any compound that improves neuromuscular function, however slight, may be of benefit *in vivo* due to the critical outcome expected from block of the NMJ at essential sites.[117,118]

3.8 Anti-Nicotinic Effects of Oximes

During the search for more effective oxime reactivators, it was found that some bispyridinium oximes had other actions in addition to their enzyme reactivating effects.[118] This was shown in studies examining the effects of oximes under conditions when enzyme reactivation did not occur, for example following ageing of the inhibited enzyme, both *in vitro*[119–122] and *in vivo*.[123–125] Furthermore, compounds that lack the oxime reactivating group (*e.g.* SAD-128) were also shown to have efficacy against OP poisoning.[124,126–129] A number of different actions have been postulated to explain the non-reactivating efficacy (the so-called 'direct action') of bispyridinium compounds, including the reversible inhibition of AChE,[130] decreasing the rate of ageing of the OP–AChE complex,[129,131] blockade of muscarinic receptors by both competitive or allosteric means,[132,133] or blocking muscle nicotinic ion channels.[134–141] Of these potential actions, it is the nicotinic antagonist properties of these compounds that are of particular interest for improving the treatment of OP nerve agent poisoning. Decreasing the rate of ageing would carry the same agent specificity problems encountered with the use of oximes, and the other mechanisms are already exploited for treatment.

The therapeutic effects of some oximes against soman poisoning can be demonstrated *in vitro* with the guinea pig phrenic nerve hemidiaphragm preparation.[120–122,138,142] Neuromuscular recovery produced in these experiments is reversed by washing out the oxime and thus appears to be due to a direct pharmacological action. A study by Tattersall[138] showed that a series of structurally related bispyridinium compounds were able to produce varying degrees of recovery in the neuromuscular function of the soman poisoned diaphragm. These compounds produced recovery after ageing (which prevented enzyme reactivation) had occurred. Furthermore, some of these compounds lacked the oxime group that is responsible for reactivating the enzyme. Importantly, the recovery of neuromuscular function in this study correlated with open channel blockade of endplate muscle nicotinic receptors and was achieved at generally lower concentrations than those used in previous studies.

Open channel block, a form of noncompetitive antagonism of the action of ACh at the muscle nAChR, is an attractive concept because the block is use dependent: antagonism becomes greater as activation of the receptor increases. This is the converse of what happens with a competitive antagonist and, at least in principle, appears to be an ideal way of mitigating the effects of OP induced overstimulation of muscle nAChRs.[17] Unlike competitive antagonists, which prevent channel activation, channel blockers are able to modulate rather than eliminate nicotinic receptor function. A competitive antagonist, such as tubocurarine, would counteract the effects of ACh by preventing activation of a proportion of nicotinic receptors, but the antagonism could be overcome by increased concentrations of ACh accumulating at the NMJ and competing with the antagonist. Furthermore, there is a danger that high concentrations of the competitive antagonist would block neuromuscular transmission completely. In contrast to a competitive antagonist, a channel blocker with rapid kinetics would reduce the mean current flowing through a channel without greatly affecting channel activation. Such an action would provide an effective counter to the overstimulation of nicotinic receptors at an endplate subjected to ACh accumulation following inhibition of AChE. Furthermore, because open channel blockade is use dependent, the antagonism would become stronger as more channels were activated. In addition, the rapid cycling of the nicotinic receptor ion channel between blocked and open states could serve as an alternative pathway to protect the receptor from desensitization.[137] A further advantage over competitive antagonists is that high concentrations of such channel blockers would be less likely to block transmission completely.

3.9 Optimisation of the Anti-Nicotinic Properties of Bispyridinium Compounds

Using the bispyridinium structure as a starting point, additional compounds have been synthesised in our laboratory and evaluated for their anti-nicotinic potency and effectiveness in recovering neuromuscular function following soman poisoning. The most studied of these is MB327 (1,1′-(propane-1,3-diyl)bis(4-*tert*-butylpyridinium)diiodide; Scheme 3.1), which was identified as the most effective in a series of *tert*-butyl compounds. It has the same

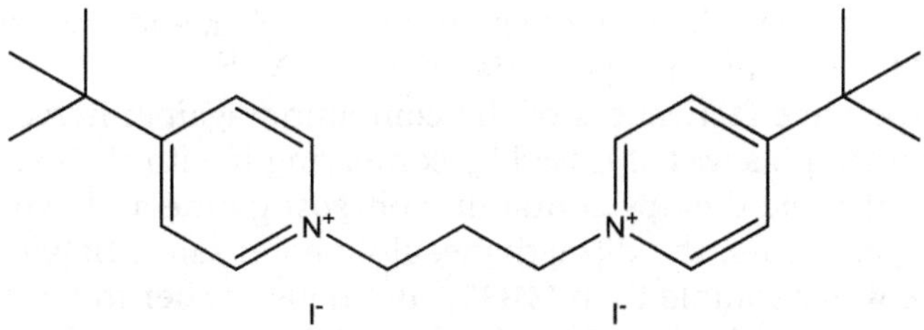

Scheme 3.1 Structure of MB327 (1,1′-(propane-1,3-diyl)bis(4-*tert*-butylpyridinium) diiodide).

tert-butyl groups as SAD-128, but the linker between the two pyridinium moieties has changed from an ether to a hydrocarbon chain, as in TMB-4, which was the most effective compound evaluated by Tattersall.[138]

The ability of MB327 to improve neuromuscular function after soman poisoning was assessed using the guinea pig phrenic nerve hemidiaphragm preparation after ageing of the soman inhibited AChE enzyme had occurred.[143] This ensured that any recovery of the diaphragm function seen was not as a result of reactivation of the AChE enzyme, although none would be expected for a compound lacking the oxime group. During repetitive nerve stimulation at 50 Hz in control conditions, a well maintained, summated muscular contraction was produced. After application of 100 nM soman, typical 'tetanic fade' of the response occurred, resulting in a brief, rapidly decaying contraction as described by Hobbiger.[109] The sequential addition of increasing doses of MB327 (10, 30 and 100 μM) resulted in a concentration dependent recovery of the tetanus shape (but not maximal tension), which was reversed when the MB327 was washed off. The recovery of the response (area under the curve of the response to the tetanic stimulation) was approximately 19% at 30 μM and 30% at 100 μM. At these concentrations, MB327 had no significant effect on unpoisoned diaphragm preparations.

The anti-nicotinic properties of MB327 were evaluated in CN21 cells, derived from the TE671 human rhabdomyosarcoma cell line by stable transfection of the ε subunit to express both the foetal and adult human muscle-type nicotinic receptor.[144] MB327 produced a concentration dependent inhibition of the nicotinic calcium response in these cells, measured using the fluorescent calcium indicator dye Fluo-4.[145] The log half maximal inhibitory concentration (IC_{50}) [M] for this inhibition was −2.86 ± 0.16 (mean ± standard error of the mean) and the Hill slope was −0.89 ± 0.10.

The effect of MB327 on single nicotinic ion channels was assessed in outside-out patches of membrane from CN21 cells, in which channel activity was induced by application of 0.2 μM ACh. Addition of MB327 produced open channel block characterised by a rapid, flickering block of the channels, so that the bursts took the form of a succession of very rapid open and closed events during the burst, instead of the single open events seen in control conditions. The dissociation constant for channel block, K_D, was voltage dependent, characteristic of an open channel blocker, and was estimated as 44.0 ± 2.8 μM at a membrane potential of −100 mV.[145]

The therapeutic effectiveness of the compound against nerve agent poisoning in guinea pigs was assessed by comparing it with the oxime HI-6 as part of a novel triple therapy containing physostigmine and hyoscine.[146,147] For these experiments, the di(methanesulphonate) salt (MB399) was used. This is more water soluble than MB327 and hence easier to formulate, and allowed comparison with an equimolar dose of the same salt of HI-6. Animals were poisoned with 5 × lethal dose, 50% (LD_{50}) of tabun, sarin or soman, and treated 1 min later. When the therapy contained MB399, survival was similar for all three agents.[145,148] In contrast, when MB399 was replaced with HI-6, the survival following tabun poisoning was significantly lower than that following sarin or soman.

HI-6 is a poor reactivator of AChE inhibited by tabun, but effective against sarin and, to a lesser extent, soman. Since the half time of ageing for soman inhibited AChE in the guinea pig is 6–8 min,[143,149] most of the inhibited enzyme would not have aged by the time therapy was given. Had therapy been delayed until ageing had taken place, it is likely that HI-6 would have been less effective. The K_D for MB327 for ion channel blocking was approximately five times smaller than that previously measured for HI-6,[138] indicating that it is a more potent nicotinic antagonist. These results are therefore consistent with the hypothesis that a nicotinic antagonist, by treating the effects of excess ACh, should be effective against all nerve agents, unlike an oxime, which can only reactivate AChE inhibited by certain agents.

MB327 is identical to the compound P62 (diiodide salt) tested by Schoene *et al.*[127] against soman poisoning in mice pretreated with atropine (10 mg kg^{-1}). When given 1 min after a LD_{95} of soman, a dose of 1.76×10^{-5} mol kg^{-1} of P62 reduced the toxic effect to a level of 50% mortality. In the study by Timperley *et al.*,[148] a similar dose of the di(methanesulphonate) salt, MB399 (1.93×10^{-5} mol kg^{-1}), reduced the toxic effect of $5 \times LD_{50}$ of soman to a level of approximately 25% mortality, when administered with physostigmine and hyoscine. A higher dose of MB399 (3.30×10^{-5} mol kg^{-1}) was able to give complete protection against this dose of soman. Schoene *et al.* found that, unlike some of the compounds they tested, P62 had no effect on the inhibition of AChE by soman.[127] This confirms that the protection found for MB399 was not due to interactions with AChE.

These results indicate that substitution of a noncompetitive nicotinic antagonist for the oxime component of therapy is able to protect animals against poisoning by soman, sarin and tabun, and unlike an oxime, is equally effective against all three nerve agents. The effectiveness of the anti-nicotinic against soman, which is difficult to treat because of its rapid ageing and consequent resistance to reactivation by oximes, is particularly significant.

A fundamental question in developing therapies for nerve agent poisoning is whether the effects found in animal studies can be translated to humans; however, since cases of nerve agent poisoning in humans are rare, it is not possible to test this directly. One approach is to study the effects in human tissue, and some studies have been performed using human muscle preparations to test the effects of oximes and related compounds.[120,121,150–152] Disappointingly, these have indicated that the direct effects of HI-6 seen in rodent and marmoset respiratory muscles[138,142,153–156] cannot be verified in human tissue, even if supra-therapeutic HI-6 concentrations are used.[150] For example, Seeger *et al.*[152] found that cumulative HI-6 concentrations up to 1000 μM did not result in an increase of muscle force in soman exposed human intercostal muscles, confirming an earlier study using 600 μM HI-6.[120] This indicates that, although HI-6 has direct effects in animal muscle preparations, it does not act by pharmacological mechanisms other than reactivation of inhibited AChE in human tissue and that these direct effects of HI-6 appear to be without relevance for therapy of humans.

In contrast, the ability of MB327 to restore neuromuscular transmission in rat and guinea pig respiratory muscles has been confirmed in human intercostal muscles at a comparable MB327 concentration.[150] With both rat diaphragm and human intercostal muscle, addition of MB327 following soman poisoning produced a partial recovery of muscle force, which decreased markedly after wash-out of the compound, indicating an effect that was not related to reactivation of soman inhibited AChE. With both species, a concentration dependent recovery of soman impaired neuromuscular transmission by MB327 was demonstrated. The recovery of the muscle force depended on the stimulation frequency and was most pronounced at 25 Hz. With human intercostal muscle preparations, 200 μM MB327 caused a significant recovery of muscle force of 46.5% of control at 25 Hz and of 11.2% of control at 40 Hz. The effect of MB327 (300 μM) was less pronounced in rat diaphragms, reaching 26.3% of control at 25 Hz and 10% of control at 50 Hz. This provides convincing evidence that the therapeutic efficacy of MB327 observed in animals can be extrapolated to humans.

Another crucial aspect for evaluation of the therapeutic application of novel compounds is their potential intrinsic toxicity. Oximes are known to induce a concentration dependent toxic effect, at least partially by reversible inhibition of AChE.[157] MB327 proved to be a weak reversible inhibitor of human AChE, having an IC_{50} of 600 μM[158] and a pronounced therapeutic effect could be achieved with 200 μM MB327 in human muscle preparations.[150] These data indicate that a therapeutic effect can be achieved with MB327 concentrations that do not induce substantial AChE inhibition. Thus, MB327 may be considered as a very promising compound for further development.[150]

3.10 Protection Against Delayed Respiratory Failure

Following organophosphate ingestion and treatment of initial signs of poisoning with atropine, patients may develop muscular paralysis around 1–4 days after the original poisoning. This has been termed the intermediate syndrome (IMS), since it usually follows the acute cholinergic syndrome and occurs earlier than delayed neuropathy.[159,160] IMS is a major cause of morbidity and mortality in patients with acute OP insecticide poisoning. Although the pathophysiology of IMS is not clearly understood, it is generally believed to result from a persistent excess of ACh at the NMJ.[18] Since muscarinic receptors are likely to be blocked with atropine given to patients to control the acute cholinergic syndrome, it seems likely that the neuromuscular dysfunction is due to overstimulation of nicotinic receptors at the NMJ.

Most deaths from respiratory failure have generally been considered to result from one of two distinct clinical syndromes, acute cholinergic respiratory failure or the IMS, but a prospective study of 376 patients with confirmed OP poisoning found that the pattern of failure was variable and overlapped in some cases.[161] There seemed to be two underlying mechanisms (an early acute mixed central and peripheral respiratory failure, and a late peripheral respiratory failure) rather than two distinct clinical syndromes. Delayed failure appeared to be due to respiratory muscle weakness, but its pathophysiology is unclear.

White and Palfreman[19] have proposed the use of large doses of nondepolarising neuromuscular blocking agents in patients requiring ventilation, in order to saturate nicotinic receptor binding sites with the idea of possibly preventing ACh mediated receptor damage at the NMJ. They suggested that this may help shorten the paralysis that occurs during the 'intermediate phase' of recovery from nerve agent poisoning. Small doses of pancuronium have indeed been reported to produce improvements in compound muscle action potentials (CMAP) in patients, albeit when given several days after OP poisoning,[162] supporting the proposition that nAChR antagonists could improve muscle strength after acute OP poisoning.

Recent studies in a minipig model have shown that administration of rocuronium by infusion, sufficient to inhibit NMJ function by about 99%, before administration of dimethoate, reduced neuromuscular damage at 6 h.[163] Rocuronium is a competitive nicotinic antagonist that acts on both pre- and post-synaptic receptors, and may work by protecting these receptors from over-stimulation. This observation has prompted a proof of principle clinical trial (NCT02147054) for therapeutic administration of rocuronium to a small group of OP poisoned patients, who are intubated initially due to reduced consciousness and loss of central respiratory drive. Since neuromuscular blocking agents are not used routinely to aid intubation of such patients, they may safely be given rocuronium to protect the NMJ from overstimulation by ACh. It is hoped that treating a poisoned patient with rocuronium for 2–3 days will prevent the damage that necessitates long term ventilation, reducing the risk of ventilator associated complications.[163]

3.11 Neuronal Nicotinic Receptors

All nAChRs are formed as pentamers of subunits.[164] The neuronal nAChRs include both homomeric and heteromeric receptors, with the α7–9 subunits forming homomeric nAChRs. The heteromeric receptors are formed by a combination of α2–6 and β2–4, most commonly by a single α and a single β subunit, with a stoichiometry of 2α and 3β.[27] By convention, when the precise subunit composition of a nAChR subtype is unknown, this uncertainty is indicated by an asterisk.[22] For example, α4β2* indicates a nAChR that is known to contain α4 and β2 subunits, but may also contain additional subunit types. A summary of subunit combinations identified from studies with native vertebrate AChRs and their distribution in the brain is given by Millar and Gotti.[22]

For α2, α3, α4, β2 and β4 subunits, pairwise combinations of α and β (*e.g.* α3β4, α2β4) are sufficient to form a functional receptor *in vitro*, but more complex isoforms may exist *in vivo*.[165,166] α5 and β3 subunits lack function when expressed alone, or pairwise, but participate in the formation of functional hetero-oligomeric receptors (*e.g.* α4α5β2, α6β2β3) when co-expressed with two other subunits. Incorporation of an accessory subunit can modify the function and pharmacology of heteromeric receptors. For example, incorporation of the α5 subunit with α4β2 nAChRs has been shown to increase Ca^{2+} permeability and confer high affinity sensitivity to the positive allosteric modulator galanthamine.[167] The α6 subunit can form a functional receptor when co-expressed with β4 *in vitro*, but more efficient expression ensues from incorporation of a third partner, such as β3. The α7, α8 and α9 subunits form functional homo-oligomers, but can also combine with a second subunit to constitute a hetero-oligomeric assembly (*e.g.* avian α7α8).[168] For functional expression of the α10 subunit, co-assembly with α9 is necessary. This combination appears to be largely confined to cochlear and vestibular hair cells.[169]

The most abundant nAChR subtypes in the nervous system are homomeric α7 receptors and heteromeric receptors containing only one type of α and one type of β subunit.[23,170,171] The α4β2* receptors account for 90% of the high affinity neuronal nAChRs in the mammalian brain, whereas the α3β4* subtype is predominant in the autonomic ganglia and adrenal medulla, as well as in subsets of neurons in the medial habenula, nucleus interpeduncularis, dorsal medulla, pineal gland and retina; a certain proportion of α3β4* receptors in these tissues also contain accessory subunits.

Besides the widespread α4β2* and more restricted α3β4* subtypes, other native subtypes have been recently identified in specific brain regions. *In situ* hybridisation studies have shown that the α2β2* subtype is highly expressed in many regions of the primate brain,[172,173] whereas its expression in rodents is limited to the retina and interpeduncular nucleus.[174,175]

Although there are many potential combinations of neuronal nAChRs, only a few have been found to be of biological importance. Neuronal nAChRs are widespread in the human body. In the brain, the neuronal α4β2 nAChR is the major nicotinic receptor responsible for addiction to nicotine, whereas α3β4, α3β2 and α7 nAChRs are abundant in autonomic ganglia and in the adrenal medulla. As well as being involved in multiple functions in the CNS, such as behaviour, cognitive function and memory, it is clear that neuronal subtype nAChRs also play an important role in the modulation and regulation of several vital control systems in the peripheral nervous system, such as regulation of breathing, inflammation and in the immune system. Presynaptic nAChRs appear to predominate in the CNS, where they act by regulating the release of other neurotransmitters, either *via* a direct increase of intracellular calcium concentrations or through the depolarisation of the presynaptic bouton (reviewed in ref. 176). Although postsynaptic nAChRs have been detected by physiological methods, they do not seem to play an important role in brain neurotransmission.[171,176,177]

Although some of the neural circuits involved in the acute and chronic effects of nicotine have been identified, much less is known about which native nAChR subtypes are involved in specific physiological functions and pathophysiological conditions.[23] Nicotinic nAChRs are expressed in brainstem and spinal cord regions involved in the control of breathing,[178] where they mediate central cholinergic regulation of respiration and the effects of nicotine on respiratory pattern. Activation of α4* nAChRs in the preBötzinger complex (preBotC), an essential site for normal respiratory rhythm generation in mammals, modulates excitatory glutamatergic neurotransmission and depolarizes preBotC inspiratory neurons, leading to increases in respiratory frequency. nAChRs are also present in motor nuclei innervating respiratory muscles. Activation of post- and/or extra-synaptic α4* nAChRs on hypoglossal (XII) motor neurons depolarises these neurons, potentiating tonic and respiratory related rhythmic activity.[23]

The neuronal nAChR subunits α3–5, α7, β2 and β4 are involved in oxygen signalling from oxygen sensing chemoreceptor type-1 cells in the carotid body.[179] During hypoxia, the neuronal nAChRs form a critical part of the chemoreceptor signal transduction pathway that signals the respiratory circuits of the brain stem, *via* the afferent carotid sinus nerve, to generate a hypoxic ventilatory response.

Recent studies have indicated that many neuronal nAChRs are also expressed in non-neuronal tissue,[27] including skin, leukocytes, kidney, urinary bladder[180–186] and the tegumental cells that line external and internal body surfaces. Bronchial epithelial cells,[187] endothelial cells of blood vessels[188] and skin keratinocytes[189] express neuronal nicotinic receptors composed of α3, α5, β2 and β4 subunits, similar to those expressed in sympathetic ganglia, and neuronal nicotinic receptors composed of α7 subunits.[190] Neuronal nicotinic receptors in tegumental cells are involved in modulating cell shape and motility and therefore in maintaining the integrity of the surfaces lined by those cells. Neuronal nicotinic receptors in non-neuronal tissues may modulate other functions, including cell proliferation and differentiation. The presence of neuronal nicotinic receptors sensitive to nicotine in tissues known to be involved in tobacco toxicity, such as bronchi and blood vessels, raises the possibility that they mediate some of the toxic effects of smoking.[190]

The neuronal α7 nAChR has been localised in macrophages and found to be critical for the cholinergic anti-inflammatory pathway.[191] During inflammation, cytokines activated by pathogens and ischaemia stimulate the afferent vagus nerve to activate a muscarinic (M1) cholinergic brain network *via* the dorsal motor nuclei. Efferent signals from the vagus nerve inhibit cytokine release *via* activation of α7 nAChRs present on macrophages (for a review see ref. 192). An α7 selective partial agonist, GTS-21, has proven to be effective in attenuating the immune response and improving outcomes in animal models of pancreatitis, endotoxaemia, sepsis, acute lung injury and ischaemia reperfusion injury, and has been shown to have a profound anti-inflammatory effect in human leukocytes.[193]

3.12 Drugs Acting at Neuronal Nicotinic Receptors

Recent advances in nAChR biology have identified targets for drug discovery and development for a range of disease indications, including Alzheimer's disease, schizophrenia, pain, depression, smoking cessation and addiction.[194] In parallel, drug discovery efforts over the past 20 years have resulted in the clinical advancement of a number of compounds that exhibit varying ranges of subtype selectivity and target interaction profiles. Although so far only a few nicotinic drugs have been marketed or are in late stage development, progress has been made in the design of novel chemical entities that are being explored for the treatment of various diseases, including addiction, depression, attention deficit hyperactivity disorder, cognitive deficits in schizophrenia and Alzheimer's disease, pain and inflammation.[34] These include agonists, partial agonists, antagonists and allosteric modulators.[195]

Bupropion is one of the few commonly prescribed drugs with significant central anti-nicotinic effects,[196] although it is generally referred to as a dopamine and norepinephrine reuptake inhibitor. Bupropion noncompetitively inhibits several AChRs, including α3β2, α3β4, α4β2, α7 and α1.[197,198] In addition to indications for the management of depression and anxiety, it is also efficacious for smoking cessation.[199] Serious, but rare, side effects include hypertension and seizure.[196,200] Bupropion is contraindicated for patients with serious hypertension, kidney disease, epilepsy or conditions that lower the seizure threshold, such as alcohol withdrawal or eating disorders.

The more recently approved smoking cessation agent varenicline, unlike bupropion, is a partial nicotinic agonist. Varenicline appears to be highly efficacious for smoking cessation, although there are concerns that its use may be associated with an increased risk of behaviour change, agitation, depressed mood and suicidality; however, it is unclear if these effects are secondary to nicotine withdrawal.[201]

Interestingly, the dissociative anaesthetic agent ketamine, which is classified as an NMDA receptor antagonist, also has anti-nicotinic properties at or below the levels used for anaesthesia,[202] and has been investigated as an antidepressant following the observation that a low dose infusion ameliorated mood symptoms in patients being treated for complex regional pain syndrome.[203,204] The role of its anti-nicotinic properties, however, remains unclear.

Mecamylamine hydrochloride (*N*,2,3,3-tetramethyl-bicyclo[2.2.1] heptan-2-amine hydrochloride) was initially developed for its ganglion blocking activity and has been marketed as an antihypertensive agent since the 1950s.[205–207] It is not now widely prescribed, because of its side effects (*e.g.* constipation and gastrointestinal complaints) at antihypertensive doses; however, several other potential therapeutic applications are being investigated, most of them focusing on the drug's ability to cross the blood–brain barrier and selectively antagonise neuronal nAChRs. These include the treatment of a variety of neuropsychiatric conditions, including substance, mood and cognitive disorders, schizophrenia and Tourette's syndrome.[205] Mecamylamine acts as a nonselective antagonist at various nAChRs, both peripherally and centrally, at much lower doses (2.5–10 mg per day) than the effective antihypertensive doses, thus avoiding many of the unwanted side effects associated with the drug's inhibition of parasympathetic activity.[206,207]

Mecamylamine nonselectively and noncompetitively inhibits both peripheral and central nAChRs,[208,209] acting as an open channel blocker.[210] It decreases the duration of the open channel state by interacting with a pore binding site of the open nAChR channel.[206]

3.13 Neuronal Nicotinic Effects in Nerve Agent Poisoning

The central nervous symptoms of nerve agent intoxication have been attributed to an initial effect on muscarinic ACh receptors followed by rapid recruitment of other neurotransmitter systems such as the glutamatergic and the monoaminergic systems (for a review see ref. 211). Activation of nicotinic ACh receptors has not been regarded as a prominent factor in soman intoxication, even though excessive activation of nicotinic receptors by nicotine may precipitate seizures (*e.g.* ref. 212 and 213). Consequently, there have been few studies of the effects of blocking central nAChRs in nerve agent poisoning.

3.13.1 Mecamylamine

Mecamylamine did not have any effect on convulsive activity in rats after soman intoxication[214] and had no effect on soman induced epileptiform discharges in guinea pig hippocampal slices *in vitro*.[215] A lack of effect of mecamylamine has been reported for other models of soman intoxication, including soman induced firing of noradrenergic neurons in the locus coeruleus[216] and soman induced hypothermia.[217]

However, Fleisher *et al.*[218] found that the addition of mecamylamine (1 mg kg^{-1}) to a treatment consisting of atropine (16 mg kg^{-1}) and the AChE reactivator toxogonin (7.5 mg kg^{-1}) improved survival in rats poisoned with sarin, but that mecamylamine was without effect unless toxogonin was included. Subsequently, Heyl *et al.*[219] reported that adding mecamylamine (2 mg kg^{-1}) to a pretreatment consisting of pyridostigmine (0.3 mg kg^{-1}) and atropine (8 mg kg^{-1}) caused a striking improvement in survival in soman intoxicated rabbits.

Doses of mecamylamine used in such studies have varied from as low as 0.8 mg kg^{-1} [220–222] to 20 mg kg^{-1}, which was used by Philippens *et al.*[223] to counteract the effects of the carbamate AChE inhibitor, physostigmine, on the auditory startle reflex in guinea pigs. Dekundy *et al.*[224] found that mecamylamine at 1 mg kg^{-1} diminished seizures induced by the anticholinesterase pesticide methomyl, but not by dichlorvos, and had no effect on lethality of either agent in mice. At a higher dose (10 mg kg^{-1}), mecamylamine decreased the lethality of both anticholinesterases but still had no effect on dichlorvos induced seizures.

Hassel[225] reported that pretreatment with mecamylamine (20 mg kg^{-1}, but not 2 mg kg^{-1}) prolonged survival in mice exposed to soman (1.5 × LD_{50}). Pretreatment with the muscarinic blocker scopolamine (2 or 20 mg kg^{-1}, but not 0.5 mg kg^{-1}) prolonged survival significantly, but the animals displayed immobility, irregular respiration, fasciculations and short episodes of convulsive crawling. These signs of soman poisoning were absent in animals pretreated with scopolamine plus mecamylamine (both drugs 20 mg kg^{-1}), which suggests that they were caused by activation of nicotinic receptors. Administration of mecamylamine (5 mg kg^{-1}) 5 min after soman exposure to scopolamine pretreated animals reduced fasciculations and respiratory irregularities, and prolonged survival compared with scopolamine alone, but a larger dose of mecamylamine (20 mg kg^{-1}), given 10 min after soman exposure, shortened survival. These results suggest that nicotinic activation plays an important role in soman induced signs and lethality, but also that mecamylamine given in large doses after soman exposure may have deleterious effects.

3.13.2 Benthiactzine

Benthiactzine (benzilate thio *S*-2-diethylamino ethyl ester hydrochloride), a drug that blocks both muscarinic and nicotinic ACh receptors, was synthesised by Luo *et al.*[226] as part of a screening programme to identify nicotinic antagonists that might be effective against OP poisoning. Although this compound was found to be much weaker than atropine in binding to mAChRs, it afforded better protection than atropine against VX and sarin poisoning in mice. In SH-EP1 cells stably expressing human nAChRs, benthiactzine inhibited whole cell currents mediated by α4β2 and α4β4 receptors (IC_{50} 4.9 and 7.5 μM, respectively), although it was a less potent antagonist of the α7 mediated response (IC_{50} 92.2 μM). Inhibition of α4β2 and α4β4 receptors, but not of α7 receptors, was voltage and use dependent, suggesting that benthiactzine may block the ion channels of these two receptor subtypes. These results indicate that the anti-nicotinic effects of benthiactzine may provide additional protection against nerve agent poisoning.

3.14 Summary

Although nicotinic receptors are involved in many important aspects of nerve agent toxicity, they have been largely neglected as targets for therapeutic intervention. The principal component of treatment for many years has been the competitive muscarinic antagonist atropine, often supported by an oxime enzyme reactivator and a benzodiazepine anticonvulsant. The lack of interest in specific treatments for the nicotinic effects is at least partly due to the high toxicity of many nicotinic antagonists, but some studies have reported beneficial effects of less toxic anti-nicotinic compounds.

The non-reactivating therapeutic action of certain oximes has been attributed to their anti-nicotinic properties, and we have recently explored this to develop novel noncompetitive nicotinic antagonists that have shown efficacy against nerve agent poisoning in animal studies. Occasional reports have also suggested that the nonselective and noncompetitive nicotinic antagonist mecamylamine may have beneficial effects against OP nerve agent poisoning. A recently synthesised compound, benthiactzine, has been shown to have anti-nicotinic as well as anti-muscarinic activity and to afford better protection than atropine against VX and sarin poisoning.

Historically, nAChRs have been one of the most intensively studied families of neurotransmitter receptors, and recent advances in nAChR biology have identified these receptors as targets for drug development for a range of diseases. Although only a few nicotinic drugs have thus far reached late stage development or marketing, novel chemical entities with nicotinic activity are being explored for the treatment of various diseases, and it is possible that some of these emerging compounds may be found to have beneficial effects in the treatment of poisoning by nerve agents.

References

1. C. H. Gunderson, C. R. Lehmann, F. R. Sidell and B. Jabbari, Nerve Agents – A Review, *Neurology*, 1992, **42**, 946–950.
2. T. C. Marrs, R. L. Maynard and F. R. Sidell, *Organophosphate nerve agents, Chemical Warfare Agents: Toxicology and Treatment*, Wiley, New York, 1996, pp. 83–100.
3. D. L. Rickett, J. F. Glenn and E. T. Beers, Central Respiratory Effects Versus Neuromuscular Actions of Nerve Agents, *Neurotoxicology*, 1986, **7**, 225–236.
4. F. C. T. Chang, R. E. Foster, E. T. Beers, D. L. Rickett and M. G. Filbert, Neurophysiological Concomitants of Soman-Induced Respiratory Depression in Awake, Behaving Guinea-Pigs, *Toxicol. Appl. Pharmacol.*, 1990, **102**, 233–250.
5. T. Leibson and M. Lifshitz, Organophosphate and carbamate poisoning: review of the current literature and summary of clinical and laboratory experience in southern israel, *Isr. Med. Assoc. J.*, 2008, **10**, 767–770.
6. D. Grob, The Manifestations and Treatment of Poisoning Due to Nerve Gas and Other Organic Phosphate Anticholinesterase Compounds, *Arch. Intern. Med.*, 1956, **98**, 221–239.
7. J. H. Wills, in *Pharmacological antagonists of the anticholinesterase agents, Cholinesterases and anticholinesterase agents*, ed. G. B. Koelle, Springer-Verlag, Berlin, 1963, pp. 883–920.
8. J. D. Morrison, The generation of nerve and muscle repetitive activity in the rat phrenic nerve-diaphragm preparation following inhibition of cholinesterase by ecothiopate, *Br. J. Pharmacol.*, 1977, **60**, 45–53.

9. P. F. Heffron and F. Hobbiger, Relationship between inhibition of acetylcholinesterase and response of the rat phrenic nerve-diaphragm preparation to indirect stimulation at higher frequencies, *Br. J. Pharmacol.*, 1979, **66**, 323–329.
10. A. L. Clark, F. Hobbiger and D. A. Terrar, Effects of pancuronium and hexamethonium on paraoxon-induced twitch potentiation and antidromic firing in rat phrenic nerve diaphragm preparations, *Br. J. Pharmacol.*, 1983, **80**, 489–496.
11. A. L. Clark and F. Hobbiger, Twitch potentiation by organophosphate anticholinesterases in rat phrenic nerve diaphragm preparations, *Br. J. Pharmacol.*, 1983, **78**, 239–246.
12. A. L. Clark, F. Hobbiger and D. A. Terrar, Nature of the anticholinesterase-induced repetitive response of rat and mouse striated muscle to single nerve stimuli, *J. Physiol.*, 1984, **349**, 157–166.
13. J. Smythies and B. Golomb, Nerve gas antidotes, *J. R. Soc. Med.*, 2004, **97**, 32.
14. R. S. Wadia, C. Sadagopan, R. B. Amin and H. V. Sardesai, Neurological manifestations of organophosphate insecticide poisoning, *J. Neurol., Neurosurg. Psychiatry*, 1974, **37**, 841–847.
15. J. Kassa, Review of oximes in the antidotal treatment of poisoning by organophosphorus nerve agents, *J. Toxicol., Clin. Toxicol.*, 2002, **40**, 803–816.
16. J. Bajgar, J. Fusek, K. Kuca, L. Bartosova and D. Jun, Treatment of organophosphate intoxication using cholinesterase reactivators: facts and fiction, *Mini-Rev. Med. Chem.*, 2007, **7**, 461–466.
17. R. D. Sheridan, A. P. Smith, S. R. Turner and J. E. H. Tattersall, Nicotinic antagonists in the treatment of nerve agent intoxication, *J. R. Soc. Med.*, 2005, **98**, 114–115.
18. C. Rosenbaum and S. B. Bird, Non-muscarinic therapeutic targets for acute organophosphorus poisoning, *J. Med. Toxicol.*, 2010, **6**, 408–412.
19. S. M. White and T. M. Palfreman, Nicotinic antagonists and nerve gas poisoning, *J. R. Soc. Med.*, 2005, **98**, 336.
20. S. A. Lipton and H. S. Chen, Paradigm shift in NMDA receptor drug development, *Expert Opin. Ther. Targets*, 2005, **9**, 427–429.
21. H. S. Chen, J. W. Pellegrini, S. K. Aggarwal, S. Z. Lei, S. Warach, F. E. Jensen and S. A. Lipton, Open-channel block of N-methyl-D-aspartate (NMDA) responses by memantine: therapeutic advantage against NMDA receptor-mediated neurotoxicity, *J. Neurosci.*, 1992, **12**, 4427–4436.
22. N. S. Millar and C. Gotti, Diversity of vertebrate nicotinic acetylcholine receptors, *Neuropharmacology*, 2009, **56**, 237–246.
23. C. Gotti, F. Clementi, A. Fornari, A. Gaimarri, S. Guiducci, I. Manfredi, M. Moretti, P. Pedrazzi, L. Pucci and M. Zoli, Structural and functional diversity of native brain neuronal nicotinic receptors, *Biochem. Pharmacol.*, 2009, **78**, 703–711.
24. S. M. Sine and A. G. Engel, Recent advances in Cys-loop receptor structure and function, *Nature*, 2006, **440**, 448–455.

25. S. P. H. Alexander, A. Mathie and J. A. Peters, Transmitter-Gated Channels, *Br. J. Pharmacol.*, 2007, **150**, S82–S95.
26. M. O. Ortells and G. G. Lunt, Evolutionary history of the ligand-gated ion-channel superfamily of receptors, *Trends Neurosci.*, 1995, **18**, 121–127.
27. M. J. Fagerlund and L. I. Eriksson, Current concepts in neuromuscular transmission, *Br. J. Anaesth.*, 2009, **103**, 108–114.
28. D. Kalamida, K. Poulas, V. Avramopoulou, E. Fostieri, G. Lagoumintzis, K. Lazaridis, A. Sideri, M. Zouridakis and S. J. Tzartos, Muscle and neuronal nicotinic acetylcholine receptors - Structure, function and pathogenicity, *FEBS J.*, 2007, **274**, 3799–3845.
29. C. W. Luetje and J. Patrick, Both alpha- and beta-subunits contribute to the agonist sensitivity of neuronal nicotinic acetylcholine-receptors, *J. Neurosci.*, 1991, **11**, 837–845.
30. A. C. Missias, G. C. Chu, B. J. Klocke, J. R. Sanes and J. P. Merlie, Maturation of the acetylcholine receptor in skeletal muscle: Regulation of the AChR gamma-to-epsilon switch, *Dev. Biol.*, 1996, **179**, 223–238.
31. T. M. Shih, J. W. Skovira, J. C. O'Donnell and J. H. McDonough, In vivo reactivation by oximes of inhibited blood, brain and peripheral tissue cholinesterase activity following exposure to nerve agents in guinea pigs, *Chem.–Biol. Interact.*, 2010, **1–3**, 207–214.
32. J. W. Skovira, J. C. O'Donnell, I. Koplovitz, R. K. Kan, J. H. McDonough and T. M. Shih, Reactivation of brain acetylcholinesterase by monoisonitrosoacetone increases the therapeutic efficacy against nerve agents in guinea pigs, *Chem.–Biol. Interact.*, 2010, **187**, 318–324.
33. M. J. A. Joosen, M. J. van der Schans, C. G. M. van Dijk, W. C. Kuijpers, H. M. Wortelboer and H. P. M. van Helden, Increasing oxime efficacy by blood-brain barrier modulation, *Toxicol. Lett.*, 2011, **206**, 67–71.
34. R. Hurst, H. Rollema and D. Bertrand, Nicotinic acetylcholine receptors: From basic science to therapeutics, *Pharmacol. Ther.*, 2013, **137**, 22–54.
35. R. A. Corriveau, S. J. Romano, W. G. Conroy, L. Oliva and D. K. Berg, Expression of neuronal acetylcholine-receptor genes in vertebrate skeletal-muscle during development, *J. Neurosci.*, 1995, **15**, 1372–1383.
36. U. Fischer, S. Reinhardt, E. X. Albuquerque and A. Maelicke, Expression of functional alpha 7 nicotinic acetylcholine receptor during mammalian muscle development and denervation, *Eur. J. Neurosci.*, 1999, **11**, 2856–2864.
37. S. J. Romano, P. C. Pugh, J. M. McIntosh and D. K. Berg, Neuronal-type acetylcholine receptors and regulation of alpha 7 gene expression in vertebrate skeletal muscle, *J. Neurobiol.*, 1997, **32**, 69–80.
38. N. Unwin, Refined Structure of the Nicotinic Acetylcholine Receptor at 4 A Resolution, *J. Mol. Biol.*, 2005, **346**, 967–989.
39. J. M. Herz, D. A. Johnson and P. Taylor, Distance between the agonist and noncompetitive inhibitor sites on the nicotinic acetylcholine receptor, *J. Biol. Chem.*, 1989, **264**, 12439–12448.
40. D. Colquhoun, C. Shelley and C. Hatton, Nicotinic acetylcholine receptors, in *Burger's Medicinal Chemistry and Drug Discovery*, ed. D. J. Abraham, John Wiley & Sons, Inc, 6th edn, 2003, pp. 357–405.

41. D. R. Ripoll, C. H. Faerman, P. H. Axelsen, I. Silman and J. L. Sussman, An Electrostatic Mechanism for Substrate Guidance Down the Aromatic Gorge of Acetylcholinesterase, *Proc. Natl. Acad. Sci.*, 1993, **90**, 5128–5132.
42. P. Fatt and B. Katz, An analysis of the end-plate potential recorded with an intra-cellular electrode, *J. Physiol.*, 1951, **115**, 320–370.
43. H. R. Arias, Topology of ligand binding sites on the nicotinic acetylcholine receptor, *Brain Res. Rev.*, 1997, **25**, 133–191.
44. S. M. Sine, H. L. Wang and F. Gao, Toward atomic-scale understanding of ligand recognition in the muscle nicotinic receptor, *Curr. Med. Chem.*, 2004, **11**, 559–567.
45. S. M. Sine, T. Claudio and F. J. Sigworth, Activation of Torpedo Acetylcholine Receptors Expressed in Mouse Fibroblasts - Single Channel Current Kinetics Reveal Distinct Agonist Binding Affinities, *J. Gen. Physiol.*, 1990, **96**, 395–437.
46. S. M. Sine and T. Claudio, Gamma- and delta-subunits regulate the affinity and the cooperativity of ligand binding to the acetylcholine receptor, *J. Biol. Chem.*, 1991, **266**, 19369–19377.
47. S. E. Pedersen and J. B. Cohen, D-Tubocurarine Binding Sites Are Located at Alpha-Gamma and Alpha-Delta Subunit Interfaces of the Nicotinic Acetylcholine Receptor, *Proc. Natl. Acad. Sci. U. S. A.*, 1990, **87**, 2785.
48. J. L. Galzi, F. Revah, A. Bessis and J. P. Changeux, Functional Architecture of the Nicotinic Acetylcholine Receptor - From Electric Organ to Brain, *Annu. Rev. Pharmacol. Toxicol.*, 1991, **31**, 37–72.
49. S. M. Sine, Molecular dissection of subunit interfaces in the acetylcholine receptor: identification of residues that determine curare selectivity, *Proc. Natl. Acad. Sci.*, 1993, **90**, 9436–9440.
50. M. E. O'Leary, G. N. Filatov and M. M. White, Characterization of d-tubocurarine binding site of Torpedo acetylcholine receptor, *Am. J. Physiol.*, 1994, **266**, C648–C653.
51. A. Karlin and M. H. Akabas, Toward a structural basis for the function of nicotinic acetylcholine receptors and their cousins, *Neuron*, 1995, **15**, 1231–1244.
52. F. B. Abramson, R. B. Barlow, M. G. Mustafa and R. P. Stephens, Relationships Between Chemical Structure and Affinity for Acetylcholine Receptors, *Br. J. Pharmacol.*, 1969, **37**, 207–233.
53. W. C. Bowman, Neuromuscular block, *Br. J. Pharmacol.*, 2006, **147**, S277–S286.
54. C. Lee and T. Jones, Molecular conformation-activity relationship of decamethonium congeners, *Br. J. Anaesth.*, 2002, **88**, 692–699.
55. S. M. Sine, The nicotinic receptor ligand binding domain, *J. Neurobiol.*, 2002, **53**, 431–446.
56. A. B. Smit, P. H. N. Celie, I. E. Kasheverov, D. Y. Mordvintsev, P. van Nierop, D. Bertrand, V. Tsetlin and T. K. Sixma, Acetylcholine-binding proteins - Functional and structural hornologs of nicotinic acetylcholine receptors, *J. Mol. Neurosci.*, 2006, **30**, 9–10.

57. P. H. N. Celie, S. E. van Rossum-Fikkert, W. J. van Dijk, K. Brejc, A. B. Smit and T. K. Sixma, Nicotine and carbamylcholine binding to nicotinic acetylcholine receptors as studied in AChBP crystal structures, *Neuron*, 2004, **41**, 907–914.
58. S. B. Hansen, G. Sulzenbacher, T. Huxford, P. Marchot, P. Taylor and Y. Bourne, Structures of Aplysia AChBP complexes with nicotinic agonists and antagonists reveal distinctive binding interfaces and conformations, *EMBO J.*, 2005, **24**, 3635–3646.
59. C. D. Dellisanti, Y. Yao, J. C. Stroud, Z. Z. Wang and L. Chen, Crystal structure of the extracellular domain of nAChR alpha 1 bound to alpha-bungarotoxin at 1.94 A resolution, *Nat. Neurosci.*, 2007, **10**, 953–962.
60. Y. N. Utkin, Y. Kobayashi, F. Hucho and V. I. Tsetlin, Relationship between the binding sites for an alpha-conotoxin and snake venom neurotoxins in the nicotinic acetylcholine receptor from Torpedo californica, *Toxicon*, 1994, **32**, 1153–1157.
61. K. O. Okonjo, J. Kuhlmann and A. Maelicke, A Second Pathway of Activation of the Torpedo acetylcholine Receptor Channel, *Eur. J. Biochem.*, 1991, **200**, 671–677.
62. P. Benoit and J. P. Changeux, Voltage dependencies of the effects of chlorpromazine on the nicotinic receptor channel from mouse muscle cell line So18, *Neurosci. Lett.*, 1993, **160**, 81–84.
63. P. Muhn and F. Hucho, Covalent labeling of the acetylcholine receptor from Torpedo electric tissue with the channel blocker [3H]triphenylmethylphosphonium by ultraviolet irradiation, *Biochemistry*, 1983, **22**, 421–425.
64. E. Neher and J. H. Steinbach, Local anaesthetics transiently block currents through single acetylcholine-receptor channels, *J. Physiol.*, 1978, **277**, 153–176.
65. D. L. Donnelly-Roberts and T. L. Lentz, Binding sites for alpha-bungarotoxin and the noncompetitive inhibitor phencyclidine on a synthetic peptide comprising residues 172-227 of the alpha-subunit of the nicotinic acetylcholine receptor, *Biochemistry*, 1991, **30**, 7484–7491.
66. B. H. White, S. Howard, S. G. Cohen and J. B. Cohen, The hydrophobic photoreagent 3-(trifluoromethyl)-3-m-([125I] iodophenyl) diazirine is a novel noncompetitive antagonist of the nicotinic acetylcholine receptor, *J. Biol. Chem.*, 1991, **266**, 21595–21607.
67. V. A. Eterovic and R. M. Hann, Noncompetitive inhibitors of the acetylcholine receptor help paint a picture of its ion channel, *P. R. Health Sci. J.*, 1995, **14**, 199–209.
68. S. E. Pedersen, S. D. Sharp, W. S. Liu and J. B. Cohen, Structure of the noncompetitive antagonist-binding site of the Torpedo nicotinic acetylcholine receptor. [3H]meproadifen mustard reacts selectively with alpha-subunit Glu-262, *J. Biol. Chem.*, 1992, **267**, 10489–10499.
69. W. B. Stallcup and J. Patrick, Substance P enhances cholinergic receptor desensitization in a clonal nerve cell line, *Proc. Natl. Acad. Sci.*, 1980, **77**, 634–638.
70. J. Garcia-Colunga and R. Miledi, Serotonergic modulation of muscle acetylcholine receptors of different subunit composition, *Proc. Natl. Acad. Sci.*, 1996, **93**, 3990–3994.

71. R. N. Cox, R. R. Kaldany, M. DiPaola and A. Karlin, Time-resolved photolabeling by quinacrine azide of a noncompetitive inhibitor site of the nicotinic acetylcholine receptor in a transient, agonist-induced state, *J. Biol. Chem.*, 1985, **260**, 7186–7193.
72. D. A. Johnson and J. M. Nuss, The histrionicotoxin-sensitive ethidium binding site is located outside of the transmembrane domain of the nicotinic acetylcholine receptor: a fluorescence study, *Biochemistry*, 1994, **33**, 9070–9077.
73. D. Bertrand, S. Valera, S. Bertrand, M. Ballivet and D. Rungger, Steroids inhibit nicotinic acetylcholine receptors, *Neuroreport*, 1991, **2**, 277–280.
74. C. Bouzat and F. J. Barrantes, Modulation of Muscle Nicotinic Acetylcholine Receptors by the Glucocorticoid Hydrocortisone. Possible Allosteric Mechanism of Channel Blockade, *J. Biol. Chem.*, 1996, **271**, 25835–25841.
75. L. Ke and R. J. Lukas, Effects of steroid exposure on ligand binding and functional activities of diverse nicotinic acetylcholine receptor subtypes, *J. Neurochem.*, 1996, **67**, 1100–1112.
76. H. R. Arias and D. A. Johnson, Differential agonist-induced displacement of quinacrine and ethidium from their respective histrionicotoxin-sensitive binding sites on the Torpedo acetylcholine receptor, *Biochemistry*, 1995, **34**, 1589–1595.
77. J. C. Khatter and J. D. Friesen, The effect of hemicholinium-3 on choline and acetylcholine levels in a sympathetic ganglion, *Can. J. Physiol. Pharmacol.*, 1975, **53**, 451–457.
78. G. Buterbauh, P. K. Figge and J. L. Spratt, A comparison of the effects of tetraethylammonium, triethylcholine and hemicholinium on choline uptake by the isolated perfused rabbit heart, *Arch. Int. Pharmacodyn. Ther.*, 1968, **175**, 179–185.
79. J. F. Fiekers, Effects of the aminoglycoside antibiotics, streptomycin and neomycin, on neuromuscular transmission. I. Presynaptic considerations, *J. Pharmacol. Exp. Ther.*, 1983, **225**, 487–495.
80. J. F. Fiekers, Effects of the aminoglycoside antibiotics, streptomycin and neomycin, on neuromuscular transmission. II. Postsynaptic considerations, *J. Pharmacol. Exp. Ther.*, 1983, **225**, 496–502.
81. J. O. Dolly and K. R. Aoki, The structure and mode of action of different botulinum toxins, *Eur. J. Neurol.*, 2006, **13(4)**, 1–9.
82. S. J. Wood and C. R. Slater, Safety factor at the neuromuscular junction, *Prog. Neurobiol.*, 2001, **64**, 393–429.
83. W. C. Bowman and M. J. Rand, Peripheral Autonomic Cholinergic Mechanisms, *Textbook of Pharmacology*, Blackwell Scientific Publications, Oxford, 2nd edn, 1980.
84. C. C. Chang and M. C. Huang, Comparison of the presynaptic actions of botulinum toxin and beta-bungarotoxin on neuromuscular transmission, *Naunyn-Schmiedeberg's Arch. Pharmacol.*, 1974, **282**, 129–142.
85. S. Wonnacott, Presynaptic nicotinic ACh receptors, *Trends Neurosci.*, 1997, **20**, 92–98.

86. W. C. Bowman, Neuromuscular block, *Br. J. Pharmacol.*, 2006, **147**, S277–S286.
87. M. Jonsson, D. Gurley, M. Dabrowski, O. Larsson, E. C. Johnson and L. I. Eriksson, Distinct pharmacologic properties of neuromuscular blocking agents on human neuronal nicotinic acetylcholine receptors, *Anesthesiology*, 2006, **105**, 521–533.
88. J. M. Lindstrom, Nicotinic acetylcholine receptors of muscles and nerves – Comparison of their structures, functional roles, and vulnerability to pathology, in *Myasthenia Gravis and Related Disorders: Biomchemical Basis for Disease of the Neuromuscular Junction*, ed. M. A. Agius, D. P. Richman, R. H. Fairclough and R. A. Maselli, 2003, vol. 998, pp. 41–52.
89. M. J. Fagerlund, M. Dabrowski and L. I. Eriksson, Pharmacological Characteristics of the Inhibition of Nondepolarizing Neuromuscular Blocking Agents at Human Adult Muscle Nicotinic Acetylcholine Receptor, *Anesthesiology*, 2009, **110**, 1244–1252.
90. L. C. Blaber, The prejunctional actions of some non-depolarizing blocking drugs, *Br. J. Pharmacol.*, 1973, **47**, 109–116.
91. W. C. Bowman, Prejunctional and postjunctional cholinoceptors at the neuromuscular junction, *Anesth. Analg.*, 1980, **59**, 935–943.
92. D. F. Wilson, Influence of presynaptic receptors on neuromuscular transmission in the rat, *Am. J. Physiol.*, 1982, **242**, C366.
93. A. Gibb and I. G. Marshall, Nicotinic antagonists produce differing amounts of tetanic fade in the isolated diaphragm of the rat, *Br. J. Pharmacol.*, 1986, **89**, 619–624.
94. C. C. Chang and S. J. Hong, Dissociation of the end-plate potential rundown and the tetanic fade from the postsynaptic inhibition of acetylcholine receptor by alpha-neurotoxins, *Exp. Neurol.*, 1987, **98**, 509–517.
95. W. C. Bowman, I. G. Marshall, A. J. Gibb and A. J. Harborne, Feedback control of neurotransmitter release at the neuromuscular junction, *Trends Pharmacol. Sci.*, 1988, **9**, 16–20.
96. C. Prior, L. Tian, J. Dempster and I. G. Marshall, Prejunctional Actions of Muscle Relaxants: Synaptic Vesicles and Transmitter Mobilization as Sites of Action, *Gen. Pharmacol.*, 1995, **26**, 659–666.
97. W. C. Bowman and M. J. Rand, *Striated Muscle and Neuromuscular Transmission, Textbook of Pharmacology*, Blackwell Scientific Publications, Oxford, 2nd edn, 1980.
98. M. Faria, L. Oliveira, M. A. Timoteo, M. G. Lobo and P. Correia-De-Sa, Blockade of neuronal facilitatory nicotinic receptors containing alpha 3 beta 2 subunits contribute to tetanic fade in the at isolated diaphragm, *Synapse*, 2003, **49**, 77–88.
99. J. A. J. Martyn, M. J. Fagerlund and L. I. Eriksson, Basic principles of neuromuscular transmission, *Anaesthesia*, 2009, **64**, 1–9.
100. M. Jonsson, M. Dabrowski, D. A. Gurley, O. Larsson, E. C. Johnson, B. B. Fredholm and L. I. Eriksson, Activation and inhibition of human muscular and neuronal nicotinic acetylcholine receptors by succinylcholine, *Anesthesiology*, 2006, **104**, 724–733.

101. Y. Liu and J. P. Dilger, Decamethonium is a partial agonist at the nicotinic acetylcholine receptor, *Synapse*, 1993, **13**, 57–62.
102. A. J. Gissen and W. L. Nastuk, Succinylcholine and decamethonium: comparison of depolarization and desensitization, *Anesthesiology*, 1970, **33**, 611–618.
103. D. M. Fisher, Clinical pharmacology of neuromuscular blocking agents, *Am. J. Health-Syst. Pharm.*, 1999, **56**, S4–S9.
104. L. W. Harris, B. G. Talbot, D. R. Anderson, W. J. Lennox and M. D. Green, Oxime-induced decarbamylation and atropine/oxime therapy of guinea pigs intoxicated with pyridostigmine, *Life Sci.*, 1987, **40**, 577–583.
105. S. Eckert, P. Eyer, H. Muckter and F. Worek, Kinetic analysis of the protection afforded by reversible inhibitors against irreversible inhibition of acetylcholinesterase by highly toxic organophosphorus compounds, *Biochem. Pharmacol.*, 2006, **72**, 344–357.
106. H. C. Hartzell, S. W. Kuffler and D. Yoshikami, Post-synaptic potentiation: interaction between quanta of acetylcholine at the skeletal neuromuscular synapse, *J. Physiol. Online*, 1975, **251**, 427–463.
107. R. A. Maselli and C. Leung, Analysis of anticholinesterase-induced neuromuscular transmission failure, *Muscle Nerve*, 1993, **16**, 548–553.
108. L. C. Blaber and W. C. Bowman, Studies on the repetitive discharges evoked in motor nerve and skeletal muscle after injection of anticholinesterase drugs, *Br. J. Pharmacol. Chemother.*, 1963, **20**, 326–344.
109. F. Hobbiger, Pharmacology of anticholinesterase drugs, in *Neuromuscular Junction*, ed. E. Zaimis, Springer-Verlag, Berlin, 1976, pp. 487–581.
110. S. Elenes and A. Auerbach, Desensitization of diliganded mouse muscle nicotinic acetylcholine receptor channels, *J. Physiol.*, 2002, **541**, 367–383.
111. R. Giniatullin, A. Nistri and J. L. Yakel, Desensitization of nicotinic ACh receptors: shaping cholinergic signaling, *Trends Neurosci.*, 2005, **28**, 371–378.
112. R. Reitstetter, R. J. Lukas and R. Gruener, Dependence of Nicotinic Acetylcholine Receptor Recovery from Desensitization on the Duration of Agonist Exposure, *J. Pharmacol. Exp. Ther.*, 1999, **289**, 656–660.
113. A. Auerbach and G. Akk, Desensitization of Mouse Nicotinic Acetylcholine Receptor Channels. A Two-Gate Mechanism, *J. Gen. Physiol.*, 1998, **112**, 181–197.
114. N. D. Boyd, Two distinct kinetic phases of desensitization of acetylcholine receptors of clonal rat PC12 cells, *J. Physiol.*, 1987, **389**, 45–67.
115. A. S. Paul, Agonists cause endocytosis of nicotinic acetylcholine receptors on cultured myotubes, *J. Neurobiol.*, 2001, **49**, 212–223.
116. E. G. Bruneau and M. Akaaboune, The dynamics of recycled acetylcholine receptors at the neuromuscular junction in vivo, *Development*, 2006, **133**, 4485–4493.
117. E. Meeter, Desensitization of the end-plate membrane following cholinesterase inhibition, an adjustment to a new working situation, *Acta Physiol. Pharmacol. Neerl.*, 1969, **15**, 243–258.

118. O. Soukup, D. Jun, G. Tobin and K. Kuca, The summary on non-reactivation cholinergic properties of oxime reactivators: the interaction with muscarinic and nicotinic receptors, *Arch. Toxicol.*, 2013, **87**, 711–719.
119. A. P. Smith and A. W. Muir, Antidotal action of the oxime HS6 at the soman poisoned neuromuscular junction of the rat and guinea pig, *J. Pharm. Pharmacol.*, 1977, **29**, 762–764.
120. A. P. Smith, H. J. van der Wiel and O. L. Wolthuis, Analysis of oxime -induced neuromuscular recovery in guinea pig, rat and man following soman poisoning in vitro, *Eur. J. Pharmacol.*, 1981, **70**, 371–379.
121. O. L. Wolthuis, R. A. P. Van Wersch and H. J. van der Wiel, The efficacy of some bis-pyridinium oximes as antidotes to soman in isolated muscles of several species including man, *Eur. J. Pharmacol.*, 1981, **70**, 355–369.
122. M. C. French, J. R. Wetherell and P. D. T. White, The reversal by oximes and their deoximinomethyl analogues of neuromuscular block produced by soman, *Eur. J. Pharmacol.*, 1983, **91**, 399–409.
123. M. G. Hamilton and P. M. Lundy, HI-6 therapy of soman and tabun poisoning in primates and rodents, *Arch. Toxicol.*, 1989, **63**, 144–149.
124. J. E. S. Stares, Medical protection against chemical-warfare agents, in *Medical Protection Against Chemical-Warfare Agents*, ed. J. E. S. Stares, Almqvist & Wirksell International, Stockholm, 1976, pp. 157–157.
125. H. P. M. van Helden, J. Delange, R. W. Busker and B. P. C. Melchers, Therapy of Organophosphate Poisoning in the Rat by Direct Effects of Oximes Unrelated to Che Reactivation, *Arch. Toxicol.*, 1991, **65**, 586–593.
126. H. Oldiges and K. Schoene, Antidotal effects of pyridinium- and imidazolium salts on soman and paraoxon poisoning in mice. (Pyridinium- und imidazoliumsalze als antidote gegen ber soman- und paraoxonvergiftungen bei mausen), *Arch. Toxicol.*, 1970, **26**, 293–305.
127. K. Schoene, J. Steinhanses and H. Oldiges, Protective activity of pyridinium salts against soman poisoning in vivo and in vitro, *Biochem. Pharmacol.*, 1976, **25**, 1955–1958.
128. R. H. Inns and L. Leadbeater, The efficacy of bispyridinium derivatives in the treatment of organophosphate poisoning in the guinea pig, *J. Pharm. Pharmacol.*, 1983, **35**, 427–433.
129. Z. Grubic and A. Tomazic, Mechanism of action of HI-6 on soman inhibition of acetylcholinesterase in preparations of rat and human skeletal muscle; comparison to SAD-128 and PAM-2, *Arch. Toxicol.*, 1989, **63**, 68–71.
130. L. W. Harris, W. C. Heyl, D. L. Stitcher and C. A. Broomfield, Effects of 1,1'-oxydimethylene bis-(4-tert-butylpyridinium chloride) (SAD-128) and decamethonium on reactivation of soman- and sarin-inhibited cholinesterase by oximes, *Biochem. Pharmacol.*, 1978, **27**, 757–761.
131. K. Schoene, Aging of soman-inhibited acetylcholinesterase: inhibitors and accelerators, *Biochim. Biophys. Acta*, 1978, **525**, 468–471.
132. D. Kuhnen-Clausen, Structure-activity relationship of mono- and bisquaternary pyridines in regard to their parasympathetic effects, *Toxicol. Appl. Pharmacol.*, 1972, **23**, 443–454.

133. Y. Kloog and M. Sokolovsky, Bisquaternary pyridinium oximes as allosteric inhibitors of rat brain muscarinic receptors, *Mol. Pharmacol.*, 1985, **27**, 418–428.
134. J. G. Clement, Toxicology and pharmacology of bispyridinium oximes - insight into the mechanism of action vs. soman poisoning in vivo, *Fundam. Appl. Toxicol.*, 1981, **1**, 193.
135. C.-T. Su, C. P. Tang, C. Ma, Y. S. Shih, C. Y. Liu and M. T. Wu, Quantitative structure-activity relationships and possible mechanisms of action of bispyridinium oximes as antidotes against pinacolyl methylphosphonofluoridate, *Fundam. Appl. Toxicol.*, 1983, **3**, 271–277.
136. C. Caratsch and P. G. Waser, Effects of obidoxime chloride on native and sarin- poisoned frog neuromuscular junctions, *Pflugers Arch.*, 1984, **401**, 84–90.
137. M. Alkondon and E. X. Albuquerque, The nonoxime bispyridinium compound SAD-128 alters the kinetic properties of the nicotinic acetylcholine receptor ion channel - a possible mechanism for antidotal effects, *J. Pharmacol. Exp. Ther.*, 1989, **250**, 842–852.
138. J. E. H. Tattersall, Ion channel blockade by oximes and recovery of diaphragm muscle from soman poisoning in vitro, *Br. J. Pharmacol.*, 1993, **108**, 1006–1015.
139. R. D. Sheridan, D. Beeson and J. E. H. Tattersall, Non-competitive block of the human muscle adult nicotinic acetylcholine receptor (nAChR) ion channel by the bispyridinium compounds, SAD-128, toxogonin and HI-6, *Eur. J. Neurosci. Suppl.*, 2000, **12**, 36.
140. M. Alkondon, K. S. Rao and E. X. Albuquerque, Acetylcholinesterase reactivators modify the functional properties of the nicotinic acetylcholine receptor ion channel, *J. Pharmacol. Exp. Ther.*, 1988, **245**, 543–556.
141. O. Soukup, J. Krusek, M. Kaniakova, U. K. Kumar, M. Oz, D. Jun, J. Fusek, K. Kuca and G. Tobin, Oxime Reactivators and Their in Vivo and in Vitro Effects on Nicotinic Receptors, *Physiol. Res.*, 2011, **60**, 679–686.
142. R. W. Busker, J. J. Zijlstra, H. J. van der Wiel, B. P. C. Melchers and H. P. M. van Helden, Organophosphate poisoning: a method to test therapeutic effects of oximes other than acetylcholinesterase reactivation in the rat, *Toxicology*, 1991, **69**, 331–344.
143. B. G. Talbot, D. R. Anderson, L. W. Harris, L. W. Yarbrough and W. J. Lennox, A comparison of in vivo and in vitro rates of aging of soman-inhibited erythrocyte acetylcholinesterase in different animal species, *Drug Chem. Toxicol.*, 1988, **11**, 289–305.
144. D. Beeson, M. Amar, I. Bermudez, A. Vincent and J. Newsom-Davis, Stable functional expression of the adult subtype of human muscle acetylcholine receptor following transfection of the human rhabdomyosarcoma cell line TE671 with cDNA encoding the epsilon subunit, *Neurosci. Lett.*, 1996, **207**, 57–60.
145. S. R. Turner, J. E. Chad, M. Price, C. M. Timperley, M. Bird, A. C. Green and J. E. H. Tattersall, Protection against nerve agent poisoning by a noncompetitive nicotinic antagonist, *Toxicol. Lett.*, 2011, **206**, 105–111.

146. J. R. Wetherell, M. Price, H. Mumford, S. Armstrong and L. Scott, Development of next generation medical countermeasures to nerve agent poisoning, *Toxicology*, 2007, **233**, 120–127.
147. J. Wetherell, M. Price and H. Mumford, A novel approach for medical countermeasures to nerve agent poisoning in the guinea-pig, *Neurotoxicology*, 2006, **27**, 485–491.
148. C. M. Timperley, M. Bird, A. C. Green, M. Price, J. E. Chad, S. R. Turner and J. E. H. Tattersall, 1,1'-(Propane-1,3-diyl)bis(4-*tert*-butylpyridinium) di(methanesulfonate) protects guinea pigs from soman poisoning when used as part of a combined therapy, *Med. Chem. Commun.*, 2012, **3**, 352–356.
149. L. W. Harris, H. I. Yamamura and J. H. Fleisher, De novo synthesis of acetylcholinesterase in guinea-pig retina after inhibition by pinacolyl methylphosphonofluoridate, *Biochem. Pharmacol.*, 1971, **20**, 2927–2930.
150. T. Seeger, M. Eichhorn, M. Lindner, K. V. Niessen, J. E. H. Tattersall, C. M. Timperley, M. Bird, A. C. Green, H. Thiermann and F. Worek, Restoration of soman-blocked neuromuscular transmission in human and rat muscle by the bispyridinium non-oxime MB327 in vitro, *Toxicology*, 2012, **294**, 80–84.
151. J. E. H. Tattersall, A. P. Smith, K. Waters, R. Mistry and D. Weeden, Therapeutic action of HI-6 against soman poisoning *in vitro*: an interspecies comparison, *Br. J. Pharmacol.*, 1998, **125**, 7P.
152. T. Seeger, K. V. Niessen, P. Langer, J. Gerhardus, F. Worek, H. Friess, R. Bumm, A. L. Mihaljevic and H. Thiermann, Restoration of nerve agent inhibited muscle force production in human intercostal muscle strips with HI 6, *Toxicol. Lett.*, 2011, **206**, 72–76.
153. H. P. M. van Helden, H. J. van der Wiel, J. de Lange, R. W. Busker, B. P. C. Melchers and O. L. Wolthuis, Therapeutic efficacy of HI-6 in soman poisoned marmoset monkeys, *Toxicol. Appl. Pharmacol.*, 1992, **115**, 50–56.
154. B. P. C. Melchers and A. L. van der Laaken, On the mechanism of spontaneous recovery of neuromuscular transmission after acetylcholinesterase inhibition in the rat neuromuscular junction, *Brain Res.*, 1991, **563**, 49–56.
155. H. P. M. van Helden, H. J. van der Wiel, J. de Lange, R. W. Busker, B. P. C. Melchers and O. L. Wolthuis, Therapeutic efficacy of HI-6 in soman poisoned marmoset monkeys, *Toxicol. Appl. Pharmacol.*, 1992, **115**, 50–56.
156. H. P. M. van Helden, R. W. Busker, B. P. C. Melchers and P. L. B. Bruijnzeel, Pharmacological effects of oximes: How relevant are they?, *Arch. Toxicol.*, 1996, **70**, 779–786.
157. T. C. Marrs, Toxicology of oximes used in treatment of organophosphate poisoning, *Adverse Drug React. Toxicol. Rev.*, 1991, **10**, 61–73.
158. K. V. Niessen, J. E. H. Tattersall, C. M. Timperley, M. Bird, A. C. Green, T. Seeger, H. Thiermann and F. Worek, Interaction of bispyridinium compounds with the orthosteric binding site of human α7 and *Torpedo californica* nicotinic acetylcholine receptors (nAChRs), *Toxicol. Lett.*, 2011, **206**, 100–104.

159. P. Jayawardane, A. H. Dawson, V. Weerasinghe, L. Karalliedde, N. A. Buckley and N. Senanayake, The spectrum of intermediate syndrome following acute organophosphate poisoning: A prospective cohort study from Sri Lanka, *PLoS Med.*, 2008, **5**, 1143–1153.
160. N. Senanayake and L. Karalliedde, Neurotoxic effects of organophosphorus insecticides - an intermediate syndrome, *N. Engl. J. Med.*, 1987, **316**, 761–763.
161. M. Eddleston, F. Mohamed, J. O. J. Davies, P. Eyer, F. Worek, M. H. R. Sheriff and N. A. Buckley, Respiratory failure in acute organophosphorus pesticide self-poisoning, *QJM*, 2006, **99**, 513–522.
162. R. Besser, T. Vogt and L. Gutmann, Pancuronium improves the neuromuscular-transmission defect of human organophosphate intoxication, *Neurology*, 1990, **40**, 1275–1277.
163. M. Eddleston, Applied clinical pharmacology and public health in rural Asia—preventing deaths from organophosphorus pesticide and yellow oleander poisoning, *Br. J. Clin. Pharmacol.*, 2013, **75**, 1175–1188.
164. A. Karlin, Emerging structure of the nicotinic acetylcholine receptors, *Nat. Rev. Neurosci.*, 2002, **3**, 102–114.
165. C. Gotti, M. Moretti, A. Gaimarri, A. Zanardi, F. Clementi and M. Zoli, Heterogeneity and complexity of native brain nicotinic receptors, *Biochem. Pharmacol.*, 2007, **74**, 1102–1111.
166. C. Gotti, M. Zoli and F. Clementi, Brain nicotinic acetylcholine receptors: native subtypes and their relevance, *Trends Pharmacol. Sci.*, 2006, **27**, 482–491.
167. A. Kuryatov, J. Onksen and J. Lindstrom, Roles of accessory subunits in alpha 4 beta 2*nicotinic receptors, *Mol. Pharmacol.*, 2008, **74**, 132–143.
168. A. S. Torrao, J. M. Lindstrom and L. R. G. Britto, Distribution of the alpha 2, alpha 3, and alpha 5 nicotinic acetylcholine receptor subunits in the chick brain, *Braz. J. Med. Biol. Res.*, 1997, **30**, 1209–1213.
169. F. Kindt, S. Wiegand, V. Niemeier, J. Kupfer, C. Loser, M. Nilles, H. Kurzen, W. Kummer, U. Gieler and R. V. Haberberger, Reduced expression of nicotinic alpha subunits 3, 7, 9 and 10 in lesional and nonlesional atopic dermatitis skin but enhanced expression of alpha subunits 3 and 5 in mast cells, *Br. J. Dermatol.*, 2008, **159**, 847–857.
170. C. Gotti and F. Clementi, Neuronal nicotinic receptors: from structure to pathology, *Prog. Neurobiol.*, 2004, **74**, 363–396.
171. E. X. Albuquerque, E. F. R. Pereira, M. Alkondon and S. W. Rogers, Mammalian Nicotinic Acetylcholine Receptors: From Structure to Function, *Physiol. Rev.*, 2009, **89**, 73–120.
172. Z. Y. Han, N. Le Novere, M. Zoli, J. A. Hill, N. Champtiaux and J. P. Changeux, Localization of nAChR subunit mRNAs in the brain of Macaca mulatta, *Eur. J. Neurosci.*, 2000, **12**, 3664–3674.
173. Z. Y. Han, M. Zoli, A. Cardona, J. P. Bourgeois, J. P. Changeux and N. Le Novere, Localization of H-3 nicotine, H-3 cytisine, H-3 epibatidine, and I-125 alpha-bungarotoxin binding sites in the brain of Macaca mulatta, *J. Comp. Neurol.*, 2003, **461**, 49–60.

174. M. Moretti, S. Vailati, M. Zoli, G. Lippi, L. Riganti, R. Longhi, A. Viegi, F. Clementi and C. Gotti, Nicotinic acetylcholine receptor subtypes expression during rat retina development and their regulation by visual experience, *Mol. Pharmacol.*, 2004, **66**, 85–96.
175. S. R. Grady, M. Moretti, M. Zoli, M. J. Marks, A. Zanardi, L. Pucci, F. Clementi and C. Gotti, Rodent Habenulo-Interpeduncular Pathway Expresses a Large Variety of Uncommon nAChR Subtypes, But Only the alpha 3 beta 4*and alpha 3 beta 3 beta 4*Subtypes Mediate Acetylcholine Release, *J. Neurosci.*, 2009, **29**, 2272–2282.
176. J. A. Dani and D. Bertrand, Nicotinic acetylcholine receptors and nicotinic cholinergic mechanisms of the central nervous system, *Annu. Rev. Pharmacol. Toxicol.*, 2007, **47**, 699–729.
177. S. Hefft, S. Hulo, D. Bertrand and D. Muller, Synaptic transmission at nicotinic acetylcholine receptors in rat hippocampal organotypic cultures and slices, *J. Physiol.*, 1999, **515**, 769–776.
178. X. M. Shao and J. L. Feldman, Central cholinergic regulation of respiration: nicotinic receptors, *Acta Pharmacol. Sin.*, 2009, **30**, 761–770.
179. M. Shirahata, A. Balbir, T. Otsubo and R. S. Fitzgerald, Role of acetylcholine in neurotransmission of the carotid body, *Respir. Physiol. Neurobiol.*, 2007, **157**, 93–105.
180. L. V. Borovikova, S. Ivanova, M. H. Zhang, H. Yang, G. I. Botchkina, L. R. Watkins, H. C. Wang, N. Abumrad, J. W. Eaton and K. J. Tracey, Vagus nerve stimulation attenuates the systemic inflammatory response to endotoxin, *Nature*, 2000, **405**, 458–462.
181. E. Hagforsen, M. Edvinsson, K. Nordlind and G. Michaelsson, Expression of nicotinic receptors in the skin of patients with palmoplantar pustulosis, *Br. J. Dermatol.*, 2002, **146**, 383–391.
182. H. Kurzen, H. Berger, C. Jager, W. Hartschuh, H. Naher, A. Gratchev, S. Goerdt and M. Deichmann, Phenotypical and molecular profiling of the extraneuronal cholinergic system of the skin, *J. Invest. Dermatol.*, 2004, **123**, 937–949.
183. J. M. Beckel, A. Kanai, S. J. Lee, W. C. de Groat and L. A. Birder, Expression of functional nicotinic acetylcholine receptors in rat urinary bladder epithelial cells, *Am. J. Physiol.: Renal Physiol.*, 2006, **290**, F103–F110.
184. C. R. Gwilt, L. E. Donnelly and D. F. Rogers, The non-neuronal cholinergic system in the airways: An unappreciated regulatory role in pulmonary inflammation?, *Pharmacol. Ther.*, 2007, **115**, 208–222.
185. J. Arredondo, A. I. Chernyavsky, D. L. Jolkovsky, K. E. Pinkerton and S. A. Grando, Receptor-mediated tobacco toxicity: acceleration of sequential expression of alpha 5 and alpha 7 nicotinic receptor subunits in oral keratinocytes exposed to cigarette smoke, *FASEB J.*, 2008, **22**, 1356–1368.
186. A. Wongsriraksa, M. E. Parsons and C. J. Whelan, Characterisation of nicotine receptors on human peripheral blood mononuclear cells (PBMC), *Inflammation Res.*, 2009, **58**, 38–44.

187. D. L. Carlisle, T. M. Hopkins, A. Gaither-Davis, M. J. Silhanek, J. D. Luketich, N. A. Christie and J. M. Siegfried, Nicotine signals through muscle-type and neuronal nicotinic acetylcholine receptors in both human bronchial epithelial cells and airway fibroblasts, *Respir. Res.*, 2004, **5**, 27–28.
188. Y. Wang, E. F. R. Pereira, A. D. J. Maus, N. S. Ostlie, D. Navaneetham, S. Lei, E. X. Albuquerque and B. M. Conti-Fine, Human bronchial epithelial and endothelial cells express alpha 7 nicotinic acetylcholine receptors, *Mol. Pharmacol.*, 2001, **60**, 1201–1209.
189. A. I. Chernyavsky, J. Arredondo, L. M. Marublo and S. A. Grando, Differential regulation of keratinocyte chemokinesis and chemotaxis through distinct nicotinic receptor subtypes, *J. Cell Sci.*, 2004, **117**, 5665–5679.
190. B. M. Conti-Fine, D. Navaneetham, S. Lei and A. D. J. Maus, Neuronal nicotinic receptors in non-neuronal cells: new mediators of tobacco toxicity?, *Eur. J. Pharmacol.*, 2000, **393**, 279–294.
191. J. Viby-Mogensen, Editorial I - Postoperative residual curarization and evidence-based anaesthesia, *Br. J. Anaesth.*, 2000, **84**, 301–303.
192. K. J. Tracey, Physiology and immunology of the cholinergic antiinflammatory pathway, *J. Clin. Invest.*, 2007, **117**, 289–296.
193. M. Kox, J. F. van Velzen, J. C. Pompe, C. W. Hoedemaekers, J. G. van der Hoeven and P. Pickkers, GTS-21 inhibits pro-inflammatory cytokine release independent of the Toll-like receptor stimulated *via* a transcriptional mechanism involving JAK2 activation, *Biochem. Pharmacol.*, 2009, **78**, 863–872.
194. D. Bertrand, M. Gopalakrishnan and D. Donnelly-Roberts, Nicotinic Acetylcholine Receptors as Therapeutic Targets: Emerging Frontiers in Basic Research and Clinical Science-Editorial Perspective, *Biochem. Pharmacol.*, 2009, **78**, 657.
195. D. Guendisch and C. Eibl, Nicotinic acetylcholine receptor ligands, a patent review (2006-2011), *Expert Opin. Ther. Pat.*, 2011, **21**, 1867–1896.
196. J. A. Ascher, J. O. Cole, J. N. Colin, J. P. Feighner, R. M. Ferris, H. C. Fibiger, R. N. Golden, P. Martin, W. Z. Potter, E. Richelson and F. Sulser, Bupropion - a review of its mechanism of antidepressant activity, *J. Clin. Psychiatry*, 1995, **56**, 395–401.
197. J. E. Slemmer, B. R. Martin and M. I. Damaj, Bupropion is a nicotinic antagonist, *J. Pharmacol. Exp. Ther.*, 2000, **295**, 321–327.
198. H. R. Arias, Is the inhibition of nicotinic acetylcholine receptors by bupropion involved in its clinical actions?, *Int. J. Biochem. Cell Biol.*, 2009, **41**, 2098–2108.
199. A. I. Herman and M. Sofuoglu, Comparison of Available Treatments for Tobacco Addiction, *Curr. Psychiatry Rep.*, 2010, **12**, 433–440.
200. J. V. Fleet, P. J. Manberg, L. L. Miller, N. Hartotruax, T. Sato, R. J. Fleck, W. C. Stern and A. E. Cato, Overview of clinically significant adverse reactions to bupropion, *J. Clin. Psychiatry*, 1983, **44**, 191–196.

201. K. Cahill, L. Stead and T. Lancaster, A Preliminary Benefit-Risk Assessment of Varenicline in Smoking Cessation, *Drug Saf.*, 2009, **32**, 119–135.
202. J. O. Udesky, N. Z. Spence, R. Achiel, C. Lee and P. Flood, The role of nicotinic inhibition in ketamine-induced behavior, *Anesth. Analg.*, 2005, **101**, 407–411.
203. G. E. Correll and G. E. Futter, Two case studies of patients with major depressive disorder given low-dose (subanesthetic) ketamine infusions, *Pain Med.*, 2006, **7**, 92–95.
204. C. A. Zarate, J. B. Singh, P. J. Carlson, N. E. Brutsche, R. Ameli, D. A. Luckenbaugh, D. S. Charney and H. K. Manji, A randomized trial of an N-methyl-D-aspartate antagonist in treatment-resistant major depression, *Arch. Gen. Psychiatry*, 2006, **63**, 856–864.
205. P. Gerretsen and B. G. Pollock, Drugs with anticholinergic properties: a current perspective on use and safety, *Expert Opin. Drug Saf.*, 2011, **10**, 751–765.
206. J. M. Young, R. D. Shytle, P. R. Sanberg and T. P. George, Mecamylamine: New therapeutic uses and toxicity/risk profile, *Clin. Ther.*, 2001, **23**, 532–565.
207. I. Bacher, B. Wu, D. R. Shytle and T. P. George, Mecamylamine - a nicotinic acetylcholine receptor antagonist with potential for the treatment of neuropsychiatric disorders, *Expert Opin. Pharmacother.*, 2009, **10**, 2709–2721.
208. R. A. Giniatullin, E. M. Sokolova, S. Di Angelantonio, A. Skorinkin, M. V. Talantova, V. Talantova and A. Nistri, Rapid relief of block by mecamylamine of neuronal nicotinic acetylcholine receptors of rat chromaffin cells in vitro: An electrophysiological and modeling study, *Mol. Pharmacol.*, 2000, **58**, 778–787.
209. R. L. Papke, P. R. Sanberg and R. D. Shytle, Analysis of mecamylamine stereoisomers on human nicotinic receptor subtypes, *J. Pharmacol. Exp. Ther.*, 2001, **297**, 646–656.
210. W. A. Varanda, Y. Aracava, S. M. Sherby, W. G. Vanmeter, M. E. Eldefrawi and E. X. Albuquerque, The acetylcholine-receptor of the neuromuscular-junction recognizes mecamylamine as a noncompetitive antagonist, *Mol. Pharmacol.*, 1985, **28**, 128–137.
211. J. H. McDonough and T.-M. Shih, Neuropharmacological mechanisms of nerve agent induced seizures and neuropathology, *Neurosci. Biobehav. Rev.*, 1997, **21**, 559–579.
212. M. I. Damaj, W. Glassco, M. Dukat and B. R. Martin, Pharmacological characterization of nicotine-induced seizures in mice, *J. Pharmacol. Exp. Ther.*, 1999, **291**, 1284–1291.
213. S. Roshan-Milani, L. Ferrigan, M. J. Khoshnood, C. H. Davies and S. R. Cobb, Regulation of epileptiform activity in hippocampus by nicotinic acetylcholine receptor activation, *Epilepsy Res.*, 2003, **56**, 51–65.
214. T. Shih, J. H. McDonough, Jr. and I. Koplovitz, Anticonvulsants for soman-induced seizure activity, *J. Biomed. Sci.*, 1999, **6**, 86–96.

215. P. K. Harrison, R. D. Sheridan, A. C. Green, I. R. Scott and J. E. H. Tattersall, A guinea pig hippocampal slice model of organophosphate-induced seizure activity, *J. Pharmacol. Exp. Ther.*, 2004, **310**, 678–686.
216. M. Ennis and M. T. Shipley, Tonic activation of locus-ceruleus neurons by systemic or intracoerulear microinjection of an irreversible acetylcholinesterase inhibitor - increased discharge rate and induction of c-fos, *Exp. Neurol.*, 1992, **118**, 164–177.
217. J. G. Clement, Pharmacological nature of soman-induced hypothermia in mice, *Pharmacol. Biochem. Behav.*, 1993, **44**, 689–702.
218. J. H. Fleisher, L. W. Harris, G. R. Miller, N. C. Thomas and W. J. Cliff, Antagonism of sarin poisoning in rats and guinea-pigs by atropine oximes and mecamylamine, *Toxicol. Appl. Pharmacol.*, 1970, **16**, 40–47.
219. W. C. Heyl, L. W. Harris and D. L. Stitcher, Effects of carbamates on whole-blood cholinesterase activity - chemical protection against soman, *Drug Chem. Toxicol.*, 1980, **3**, 319–332.
220. L. Harris and D. Stitcher, Protection against diisopropylfluorophosphate intoxication by pyridostigmine and physostigmine in combination with atropine and mecamylamine, *Naunyn-Schmiedeberg's Arch. Pharmacol.*, 1984, **327**, 64–69.
221. W. J. Lennox, L. W. Harris, B. G. Talbot and D. R. Anderson, Relationship between reversible acetylcholinesterase inhibition and efficacy against soman lethality, *Life Sci.*, 1985, **37**, 793–798.
222. T. M. Shih, J. H. McDonough and I. Koplovitz, Anticonvulsants for soman-induced seizure activity, *J. Biomed. Sci.*, 1999, **6**, 86–96.
223. I. Philippens, B. Olivier and B. P. C. Melchers, Effects of physostigmine on the startle in guinea pigs: Two mechanisms involved, *Pharmacol., Biochem. Behav.*, 1997, **58**, 909–913.
224. A. Dekundy, R. M. Kaminski and W. A. Turski, Dizocilpine improves beneficial effects of cholinergic antagonists in anticholinesterase-treated mice, *Toxicol. Sci.*, 2003, **72**, 289–295.
225. B. Hassel, Nicotinic mechanisms contribute to soman-induced symptoms and lethality, *Neurotoxicology*, 2006, **27**, 501–507.
226. W. Luo, X. Ge, W. Cui and H. Wang, Targeting Cholinesterase Inhibitor Poisoning with a Novel Blocker Against Both Nicotinic and Muscarinic Receptors, *Neurotoxic. Res.*, 2010, **18**, 173–186.

CHAPTER 4

Mustard: Pathophysiology and Therapeutic Approaches

DIRK STEINRITZ*[a], FRANK BALSZUWEIT[a], HORST THIERMANN[a], AND KAI KEHE[a]

[a]Bundeswehr Institute of Pharmacology and Toxicology, Neuherbergstraße 11, 80937 Munich, Germany
*E-mail: dirksteinritz@bundeswehr.org

4.1 Introduction

Sulfur mustard (SM) or mustard gas [bis(2-chloroethyl)sulphide; CASRN: 505-60-2] was first synthesized by Despretz in 1822, and was rediscovered later by Guthrie and Niemann.[1,2] The latter researchers noted the typical vesicant properties of SM and there is some evidence that Niemann suffered from pulmonary late effects resulting in an early death.

Meyer synthesized SM of higher purity, which was an important step towards the production of large quantities of this compound.[3] SM toxicity and its easy synthesis were the main reasons why the German chemists Lommel and Steinkopf made the decision to use this substance as a chemical warfare agent. Although SM was first used in the last year of World War I (WWI), it achieved the title "king of chemical warfare agents". The mortality of SM is comparatively low, but the burden to the medical system is high. Many victims need long lasting medical care after exposure. After the Iraq–Iran war (1980–1988), nearly 30 000 Iranian victims still suffer from late effects.

Issues in Toxicology No. 27
Chemical Warfare Toxicology, Volume 2: Management of Poisoning
Edited by Franz Worek, John Jenner, and Horst Thiermann

Published by the Royal Society of Chemistry, www.rsc.org

There is no other chemical substance that is so closely related to chemical warfare as SM. Nearly 100 years of ongoing research into medical countermeasures against SM have not resulted in an effective antidote against this poison. Beside this, SM and related compounds were tested as treatments against various diseases (psoriasis, skin cancer and for tattoo removal). In the 1940s, Goodman and colleagues successfully used nitrogen mustards as effective treatments against several forms of leukemia. The disclosure of this research at the end of WWII was recognized as the first pharmacological treatment of cancer and a significant milestone in pharmacology.[4]

Nowadays, most nations have signed the Chemical Weapons Convention (CWC). The task of the intergovernmental Organization for Prohibition of Chemical Weapons (OPCW) is to verify the adherence of nations to the CWC. The OPCW was awarded the 2013 Nobel Peace Prize for its "extensive work to eliminate chemical weapons".

As a consequence of the CWC, the member states agreed to destroy their stockpiles of chemical weapons. Syria was the most recent accessory state to sign the CWC, and a great number of chemical weapons is currently being destroyed offshore in a safe procedure, completely preventing the release of residual SM into the environment. Unfortunately, in previous decades, the destruction of chemical weapons was less sophisticated. Several sea areas are contaminated with dumped chemical ammunition from WWII. In recent years, fishermen have occasionally been exposed to SM from broken shells in their fishing nets and military duty personnel have been exposed while demilitarizing old chemical warfare munitions.[5,6]

4.2 Chemistry

At room temperature, SM is an oily, lipophilic liquid with no specific odor. However, technical impurities result in a marked mustard or garlic like smell, after which this agent was named: mustard gas. SM has a higher specific weight than water. Therefore, sea dumped SM remains on the sea bed. SM hydrolyzes by a S_N1 mechanism in two steps (Figure 4.1). Estimated rate constants for the two steps are $(2.93 \pm 0.15) \times 10^{-3}$ and $(3.87 \pm 0.14) \times 10^{-3}\ s^{-1}$ in water at 25 °C.[7] The resulting products are thiodiglycol and hydrochloric acid. Thus, chloride ion concentration and pH determine the speed of hydrolysis. As mentioned before, SM is an oily liquid. Therefore, the reaction of SM in water will only take place at the surface of the SM drop. Therefore, SM released from old ammunition on the sea bed will remain active for decades.

4.3 Toxicokinetics

SM can enter the body *via* the skin, lungs, eyes or after ingestion. It has been assumed that the effect of SM on organs follows Haber's law ($c \times t$ = constant), where c is concentration and t time. A recent reevaluation of existing human data based on the ten Berge model ($c^n \times t$ = constant) calculated n values of

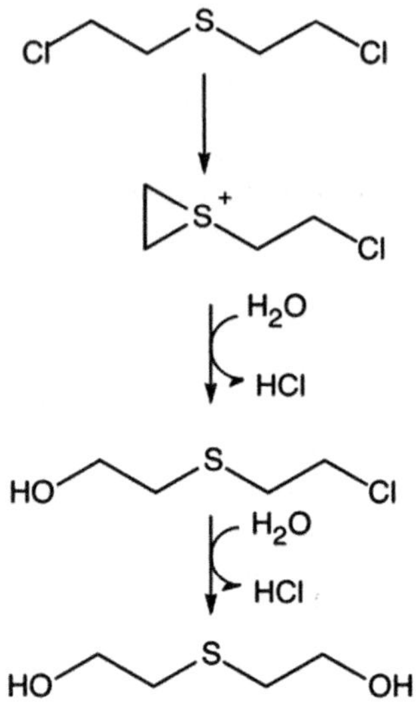

Figure 4.1 Primary hydrolysis pathway of SM in an aqueous environment.

0.96 and 1.11.[8] The penetration rate of liquid SM through human skin *in vivo* has been estimated as 60–240 μg cm^{-2} h^{-1}.[9] Skin absorption rates are influenced by anatomical localization (skin thickness), hair density and moistness of the skin. Under non-occlusive conditions, 80% of topically applied SM evaporates and only 20% is absorbed. Between 10 and 20% of this fraction is fixed to macromolecules and 80% reaches blood circulation.[9,10] A depot of active (unhydrolyzed) SM has been identified within the lipid rich *stratum corneum*.[10]

The distribution of SM can be described by a two compartment model with two half times (initial α and terminal β). Half times of SM were calculated as $t_{1/2}\alpha = 5.56$ min and $t_{1/2}\beta = 3.59$ h, with a distribution volume in the *steady state* of 74.4 l kg^{-1}.[11] The high distribution volume can be explained by distribution within lipid rich tissues (fat and brain). This experimental finding correlates with clinical observations. High amounts of unhydrolyzed SM have been detected in the fat tissue of a victim.[12] The increase in SM hemoglobin adducts over several days is probably due to SM redistribution from deep depots (Figure 4.2).[13]

SM metabolites were found to be eliminated through the renal route; 98% of the radioactivity from ^{14}C-labeled SM was found in the urine, whereas only 3% was in the intestine in rats. The total clearance was 21 l kg^{-1} h^{-1}.[11] Glutathione (GSH) conjugates of SM and the sulfone as well as thiodiglycol were detected in the urine. Thiodiglycol and thiodiglycol sulfoxide are also detectable in the urine in trace amounts under normal conditions. Thus, their specificity is limited. However, large amounts are detectable after exposure.[14,15] More reliable metabolites derive from the β-lyase pathway, which shows no background.[16]

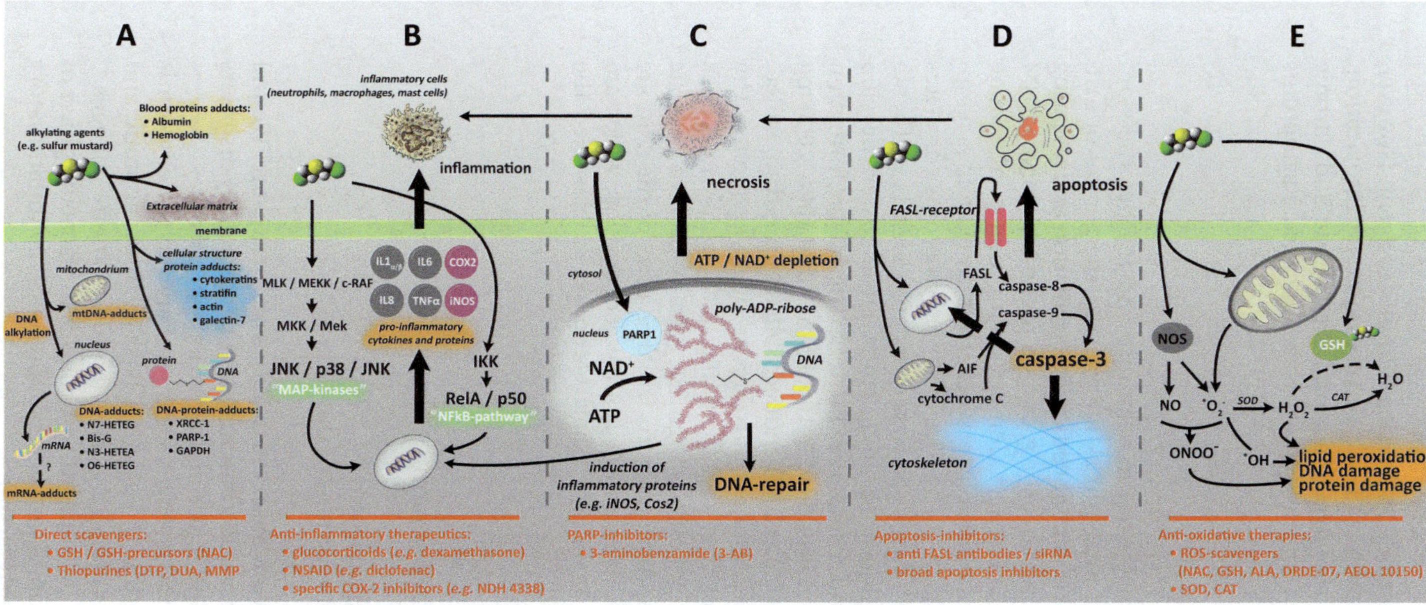

Figure 4.2 Schematic overview of the pathophysiology of SM and therapeutic approaches (red text). (A) SM adduct formation with intra- and extra-cellular components and proteins. SM is able to react with blood proteins (albumin and hemoglobin), resulting in fingerprint adducts. In addition, the extracellular matrix components and intracellular proteins can be covalently modified. The DNA/RNA alkylating properties of SM are well established. SM is a bi-functional agent that is able to crosslink proteins to proteins and also proteins to DNA. (B) Inflammatory response due to SM exposure. Exposure to SM activates MAP kinases and NF-κB pathways resulting in the induction of pro-inflammatory cytokines and proteins leading to an inflammatory response. (C) SM induced PARP activation and its role in necrosis. PARP-1 is activated after SM exposure. As a result, PAR is linked to the alkylation sites of the DNA. This modification is considered to play a crucial role in DNA repair, but also contribute to ATP/NAD^+ depletion resulting in necrosis. In addition, PARylation of DNA induces pro-inflammatory cytokines. (D) SM induced apoptosis. After SM exposure, both intrinsic and extrinsic apoptosis are initiated. A common endpoint is the activation of caspase-3. Apoptosis in general is not accompanied by severe inflammation. However, apoptosis is an active process that can switch to rather uncontrolled necrosis. (E) Formation of ROS/RNS due to SM exposure. SM exposure results in the formation of highly reactive oxygen and nitrogen species. In addition, covalent binding of SM to GSH diminishes the GSH pool, thus enhancing ROS/RNS. Lipid peroxidation, DNA and protein damage will occur.

4.4 Clinical Picture

In a military context, SM is classified as a vesicant or blister agent. However, SM enters the body through various routes and causes systemic intoxication. The main affected organs are the skin, lungs and eyes. Acute and chronic symptoms have been described. In the following sections, acute symptoms are the main focus.

4.4.1 Skin

SM vapor diffuses rapidly through normal clothing and reaches the skin. SM penetrates especially moist and thin skin areas, *e.g.* the genital or axillae region.[17,18] Physical stress with enhanced blood circulation and sweating as well as local mechanical shear stress (*e.g.* from a backpack) enhance SM penetration through the skin. SM penetration does not produce immediate cutaneous symptoms. Erythema and blisters occur typically after a symptom free period of several hours (3–24 h). The onset of symptoms correlates inversely with the resorbed SM dose. The first cutaneous sign is erythema (vapor: 100–300 mg min m^{-3}, liquid: 10–20 μg cm^{-2}). Little blisters develop later, which commonly fuse and form larger blisters. The blister formation threshold dose for SM vapor and liquid is 20–100 μg cm^{-2} and 1000–2000 mg min m^{-3}, respectively.[19,20] The typical SM induced blisters are thin walled, contain a clear, yellowish liquid, and are surrounded by an erythema. The Nikolsky I and II signs are: positive, slight rubbing of the skin can induce blisters that can be moved.[21] Nikolsky's sign is typically present in toxic epidermal necrolysis and pemphigus vulgaris. If large areas of the skin are contaminated with high doses, deep and necrotic ulcers develop, which are characterized by slow wound healing.[17,22] Balali-Mood *et al.* classified the cutaneous skin lesions:

1. Erythematous form
2. Pigmentary exfoliation
3. Superficial vesicular to bullous form
4. Bullous necrotization
5. Deep necrotizing non-bullous form
6. Allergic and toxic contact reactions of the skin.

The most clinical symptoms are observed 3–4 days after exposure. Wound healing is delayed and secondary infections may occur. Pigmentary disorders are typical late effects. Hypo- and hyper-pigmentation can occur.[23]

Microscopy of affected lesions reveals a clear cut between the epidermis and dermis. Keratinocytes within the stratum basale show apoptotic and necrotic cell death. Cell nuclei present karyolytic and pyknotic changes.[24] Dermal capillaries are dilated, including thrombosis.[25] In the acute phase of SM injury, a massive infiltration of leukocytes represents the inflammatory response in the histopathological picture.[21]

4.4.2 Lungs

The respiratory tract is more susceptible than the skin. Ten fold smaller concentrations of SM vapor (12–70 mg min m^{-3}) induce the first symptoms,[26] which are observed after a symptomless period of several hours. The onset of symptoms correlates inversely with the inhaled SM dose. The earlier the symptoms are observed, the more severe the lungs are damaged. One has to keep in mind that not only the SM concentration in the air is relevant, but also respiration rate and tidal volume determine the amount of inhaled SM dose.

Respiratory symptoms start with a sore throat, hoarseness, coughing and sneezing. Several hours later, tracheitis, bronchitis, bronchial necrosis and pneumonia develop. Epithelial sheets from the trachea and bronchial tract (pseudomembranes) can detach from the wall and lead to severe obstruction of deeper airways.[17,22] Even the collapse of a lung has been described.[27] SM induced pulmonary lesions are the main reasons for lethal outcomes and the most severe late effects.[28] In a study of 62 patients who died after SM inhalation, 62% showed initial signs of fibrinous bronchopneumonia, 66% develop lung abscesses and 5% lung gangrene within 2 weeks after SM inhalation. With respect to these clinical observations, Koch and Aschoff classified the SM induced injuries of the respiratory tract:[27]

1. Catarrhal phase
2. Pseudomembranous laryngotracheitis
3. Pseudomembranous bronchitis and bronchopneumonia
4. Lung abscesses and gangrene

Severe SM inhalatory trauma affects deep lung structures and can cause alveolar edema.[25]

Only limited data are available concerning the histopathological changes after SM inhalation. Published observations from WWI and Iraq–Iran war victims clearly revealed that SM affects primarily the upper respiratory tract and only in severe intoxications the alveolae.[27,29,30] Pseudomembranes were often found one day after exposure. These membranes consist of fibrin, necrotic epithelia, cellular debris and infiltrated neutrophils. Extensive necrotic changes of respiratory epithelia from the uvula down to the bronchi are observable 3–6 days after SM exposure, resulting in a thick pseudomembranous membrane covering the upper respiratory tract.[31]

4.4.3 Eyes

Due to their thin epithelial layer, eyes are very susceptible towards SM vapor. Thus, eye symptoms are most likely to be observed first. In cases of exposure to high SM concentrations, symptoms have been described after only 30 min.[32] The possibility of irritating technical impurities has to be taken into account. Mild symptoms (*e.g.* mild ocular irritation) are observed at low SM concentrations of 12–70 mg min m^{-3}. Conjunctivitis (irritation) was described at SM concentrations of 50–100 mg min m^{-3}. Corneal edema, photophobia and blepharospasmus are frequently observed at SM concentrations above 200 mg min m^{-3}.[24,33] Victims suffer from severe blepharospasm, perceived as blindness. Although permanent loss of vision is rare, recovery takes 4–5 weeks.[17,23,33]

4.5 Therapeutic Interventions for SM Injury in Correlation with the Molecular Pathology

Considering the pathology of SM injury, which is highly complex on the molecular level and even more complex when considering cell to cell interactions, it is hardly surprising that no causative antidote against SM poisoning exists. Therapeutic efforts after SM exposure are aimed at:

1. Limitation of symptoms, in particular, pain and inflammation
2. Life-saving interventions in the case of critical complications, in particular pseudomembrane formation and secondary infections
3. Rapid elimination of residual agent, both externally and internally
4. Debridement of cells and tissues that have been irreversibly damaged, wherever possible
5. Skin grafting surgery to replace destroyed or debrided skin

Many of these interventions have no pharmacological mechanism of action, but instead a surgical or other physical mechanism. This initial overview will outline the non-pharmacological interventions against SM injury. Afterwards, current and potential future pharmacological therapies will be described. The outlook will be focused on the future use of stem cells and tissue engineering to restore the functionality of tissues that have been damaged by SM.

The first and foremost rule for medical personnel and all first responders in the case of a suspected or confirmed SM exposure is to implement adequate means of self-protection. This is of particular importance as SM—unlike acid and alkaline burns—does not cause immediate pain that might warn the exposed person, but causes severe injury after a latency period of several hours (in some cases, more than 24 h). When signs and symptoms of SM injury do appear, they preclude the exposed person from performing any duties that involve manual interaction, *i.e.* in a worst case scenario, the medical personnel are no longer able to care for their patients, instead, they become casualties and patients themselves. The ultimate consequence might be the absence or limitation of care for patients suffering from SM exposures and/or other illnesses and injuries. This is a critical risk, especially during deployed military operations, but also in the case of a civilian mass casualty scenario when the number of patients might overwhelm the capabilities of the medical system.

A key component of adequate self-protection is casualty decontamination. Removal of contaminated clothing is a simple intervention that is able to eliminate more than 90% of any particular agent, including SM. When the location of SM (or any other chemical warfare agent) contamination is known, spot decontamination can be performed, using the CE-certified skin decontaminant, reactive skin decontamination lotion (RSDL), if available. While RSDL does not chemically react to inactivate SM—it does chemically inactivate a variety of nerve agents—it is able to physically dissolve and remove SM. RSDL has been proven to be safe for use on human skin and even though it is not meant to be purposefully applied to wounds, it is known to be tolerated in them.

When RSDL is not available or large areas of skin are suspected of contamination, water is to be used for decontamination. This is also true in the case of suspected contaminations of the eyes; RSDL and other reactive solutions must not be applied to the eyes under any circumstances. A low concentration of chloride ions rapidly accelerates the hydrolysis and inactivation of SM. The most rapid hydrolysis occurs in distilled water and, if available, its use on the skin can be considered. However, rapid decontamination takes priority and immediate use of tap water in excess is preferred over any delay in the search for "better" means of decontamination.

Oxidizing solutions, including hypochlorite solutions, are highly efficient to decontaminate materials but should not be used for casualty decontamination as severe side effects to the human skin can occur. Under no circumstances should they be applied to wounds or eyes.

Even when all of the SM has been removed from or inactivated on the surface, there is a considerable risk that free SM may form depots in lipophilic tissues of the organism. An initial depot may form in the stratum corneum, the layer of cornified keratinocytes that constitutes the skin's primary mechanical and chemical barrier. The extent and relevance of a cutaneous SM depot has been described recently[34] and it has been concluded that the amount of SM deposited per cm^2 of skin was at least 20 fold that of an acute toxic dose. Autopsy and forensic analysis from a deceased patient demonstrated that SM depots were not limited to the skin, but formed in a number of organs, including the liver and brain.[35,36] These depots can cause a threat to surgeons or pathologists.

The SM depot in the stratum corneum can be removed by surgical wound debridement, using either mechanical means or laser. Graham *et al.* (2009) demonstrated that early laser debridement significantly reduced scar formation and other long term adverse effects of SM exposure.[37] The effects of laser debridement may partially be attributed to the removal of SM depots in the skin. Another mechanism might be the elimination of cells that had been irreversibly damaged by SM. If those cells were permitted to survive, they might actually amplify the damage to neighboring tissues by producing pro-apoptotic and pro-inflammatory cytokines. It has also been shown that the beneficial effects of laser debridement were even more pronounced when this procedure was followed by topical application of an aqueous solution of nutrients, including monosaccharides, nucleotides and amino acids.[37]

To date, the beneficial mechanism of that solution has not been studied or understood in detail, but it might be plausible to assume that those nutrients facilitate the repair process in cells that received reversible SM damage and help to overcome a potential cellular energy crisis.

Topical formulations have an important role in the treatment of skin after SM injury. Along with active pharmacological compounds, the entire composition of those topical formulations has a pronounced effect. Lipophilic ointments have to be avoided in the first few days after SM exposure. As mentioned before, SM may form a depot in the lipophilic strata of the skin. Covering skin with a lipophilic ointment or cream will block transpiration, creating an environment known as an "occlusion". Without transpiration, water will be deposited in the stratum corneum, making it more permeable. Studies by Chilcott *et al.* (2000) have shown that the systemic resorption of SM from its depot may be amplified significantly under occluded conditions.[9]

In contrast, hydrophilic formulations, including gels, lotions and—after an initial period—hydrophilic creams do not block transpiration. Water from those formulations can evaporate, creating a cooling effect that reduces pain and discomfort and may even slow down the course of detrimental secondary effects in damaged tissues.

4.5.1 Search for Novel Therapies, the Animal Efficacy Rule, Regulatory Requirements and Their Effect on Research Strategies

The following sections will present an overview of pharmacological treatment strategies currently being discussed or investigated for use after SM injury. Most of these studies rely almost exclusively on animal and *in vitro* data. Fortunately, cases of human exposure to SM have been rare since the end of the Iran–Iraq war in the 1980s. In some cases, experience gained from the long-term treatment of Iranian veterans, suffering from chronic illness years and decades after exposure, helped to initiate research programs to understand the protective mechanisms of apparently beneficial treatments, *e.g.* macrolide antibiotics.

For obvious ethical reasons, a purposeful exposure of humans to SM or in fact to any noxious agent cannot be considered and, thus, with the above-mentioned exception of clinical experience from the treatment of chronic SM induced injuries, the efficacy of antidotes has to be demonstrated in animal studies. Regulatory agencies have thus developed the so-called animal efficacy rule: when efficacy studies in humans cannot be done, animal studies can be accepted as evidence for efficacy to allow regulatory approval of a new antidote. However, inter-species differences do exist. A strategy to address this issue is to demonstrate efficacy both in animal models and in cell culture studies, using primary cells and/or cell lines of human origin. Cell culture studies are also useful to rapidly acquire research data on the efficacy of potential antidotes, reduce the number of animal studies and focus the necessary animal experiments on the most promising candidate compounds.

Prior to regulatory approval, the safety and pharmacokinetic profile of any new drug, including antidotes, have to be investigated in clinical studies, *i.e.* in humans. This effort can mostly be avoided for drugs that are already approved for different indications. Not surprisingly, a lot of the research efforts to improve therapy for SM injuries have been focused on approved drugs and, in some cases, compounds isolated from plants (*e.g.* curcumin) that are inherently assumed to be safe.

4.5.2 Alkylation

Although SM has been known for almost 200 years (first synthesized by Depretz in 1822), knowledge about the molecular pathology—especially in low dose exposure scenarios—is limited. The alkylating properties of mustard agents (sulfur and nitrogen mustards) are well known: after internal cycling and formation of a sulfonium ion intermediate, one of the chlorine atoms functions as a leaving group, thus forming a highly reactive carbenium ion.[38] Due to its high reactivity, this carbenium ion is capable of reacting with a variety of cellular components. Probably best investigated are the alkylation reactions with nucleic acids that occur both *in vitro* and *in vivo*.[39–44] This pioneering work is based on the experiments conducted by Lawley and Brookes, who demonstrated that SM binds covalently to highly electronegative sites in DNA bases.[44] It was shown *in vitro* that alkylation of guanine bases at *N*7 is the most frequent adduct resulting in the formation of *N*7-[2-[(2-hydroxyethyl)thio]ethyl]guanine (*N*7-HETEG), followed by the inter- and intra-strand di-adduct between two guanine bases resulting in bis[2-(guanine-7-yl)ethyl]sulfide (Bis-G), and *N*3-[2-[(2-hydroxyethyl)thio]ethyl]adenine (*N*3-HETEA) was shown to be another major adduct.[41] The frequency of these major adducts may vary to some extent, but in general the *N*7-guanine mono-adduct represents about 60% of all observed adducts, followed by the *N*3-adenine mono-adduct making up about 15% and the formation of *N*7-guanine di-adduct observed in 10%.[40,41] A less abundant but biologically highly relevant adduct is the alkylation product of guanine at the *O*6 residue resulting in the formation of *O*6-[2-[(2-hydroxyethyl)thio]ethyl]guanine (*O*6-HETEG). This adduct was found to account for only approximately 0.1% of all adducts, but apparently this lesion cannot be repaired *via* DNA alkyltransferases and thus has to be considered as mutagenic.[40] Recent studies based on ultrahigh performance liquid chromatography and tandem mass spectrometry revealed a much higher rate of bifunctional adducts after SM exposure both *in vitro* and *in vivo*. It was shown *in vivo* that *N*7-HETEG was formed in 64–81%, Bis-G in 18–42%, *N*3-HETEA in 1.3–4.6% and *O*6-HETEG in 0.04–0.62%.[45] Interestingly, the ratio between the adduct species *in vitro* was dependent on the exposure concentration: with increasing concentrations of SM an increased formation of the main adduct *N*7-HETEG was observed, while bifunctional adducts were less abundant; whereas *N*3-HETEA and *O*6-HETEG adduct formation was only slightly dependent on the SM concentration.[45] However, this effect was not evident *in vivo*. Here, a linear relationship between the exposure dosage and the amount of DNA adduct formation was observable. Beside nuclear alkylation of nuclear DNA, SM may affect several other cellular targets and can form conjugates with a variety of proteins. Although it is well established that SM affects mitochondrial function, there is only one report about alkylation of mitochondrial DNA (mtDNA).[46] Remarkably, mtDNA lesions induced by SM were much fewer compared with nuclear lesions, and showed different kinetics. Guanine and adenine nucleotides are also common in RNA species, including mRNA, tRNA and rRNA. Thus, alkylation of RNA by SM is conceivable and has been discussed,[47] but has not been explored so far. Moreover, the biological relevance of RNA alkylation is controversial, as DNA alkylation was found to have more pronounced effects on protein synthesis (due to impaired transcription) *in vitro* in relation to RNA alkylation and impaired translation.[48,49] On the other hand, RNA repair mechanisms do not exist, thus RNA alkylation might have a substantial impact.

SM is well known to form adducts with a number of blood proteins as well as cellular proteins. Proteomic experiments conducted with radioactive C^{14}-labeled SM in human keratinocytes revealed direct alkylation of several cytokeratins, stratifin, actin and galectin-7,[50] although the direct covalent modification sites were not investigated. It is conceivable that due to covalent protein modifications, the biological function of affected proteins is impaired, which may influence cell signaling. In addition to a loss of protein function due to covalent modification, proteins may be fixed intracellularly by bifunctional alkylating agents, which will result in a functional loss of the protein even though the protein function itself might be unaffected. An excellent example is given by the cross-linking and immobilization of DNA repair enzymes to DNA in the presence of nitrogen mustards.[51] Of special interest is the covalent binding and immobilization of XRCC-1, poly(ADP-ribose) polymerase (PARP)-1 and GAPDH to *N*7-guanine moieties in DNA by nitrogen mustards[52] as these enzymes are considered to play a pivotal role in SM pathophysiology.[53,54] Cells—especially basal keratinocytes—are in close contact with the extracellular matrix (ECM) at the epidermal–dermal junction. Disturbance of this junction after exposure to SM is thought to rely on ECM modifications caused by alkylation. Again, it was shown that SM is able to directly alkylate the ECM, which might destabilize the epidermal–dermal junction and contribute to vesication.[55] Alkylation of ECM components might also affect cell migration as processing of the ECM is key during cell migration.

Interactions of SM with macromolecules, especially with plasma proteins such as hemoglobin and albumin, have been described[13,56,57] and are used as biomarkers to indicate systemic uptake of SM. Multiple alkylated species have been observed in hemoglobin after SM exposure using matrix-assisted laser desorption/ionization–time of flight/mass spectrometry.[57] Regarding albumin, alkylated cysteine and valine residues have been reported, and can even be detected days after the exposure.[13]

4.5.3 Direct SM Scavengers

Due to the high reactivity of the positively charged carbenium ion intermediate, there have been attempts to use negatively charged compounds to directly scavenge SM, thus preventing cell damage.

Gross *et al.* used the GSH precursor L-oxothiazolidine 4-carboxylate to counteract SM toxicity and demonstrated that pre-treatment of human peripheral blood lymphocytes with that compound led to some protection after SM exposure.[58] However, the effect was moderate to weak and post-treatment was ineffective.

Thiopurines have been shown to react with a wide range of electrophilic toxicants. Liu *et al.* reported direct scavenging properties of thiopurines against different half-mustards.[59] *The investigated compounds*, 2,6-dithiopurine (DTP), 2,6-dithiouric acid (DUA) and 9-methyl-6-mercaptopurine (MMP), were superior to *N*-acetylcysteine (NAC) and GSH in the authors' experiments. Powell *et al.* demonstrated that DTP blocked the toxicity and mutagenesis of SM in human skin cells.[60] Remarkably, Boulware *et al.* reported that post-treatment with DTP, beginning 1 h after 2-chloroethyl ethyl sulfide (CEES) exposure, was able to abolish the CEES induced increase in mutation frequency in mice.[61] These findings suggest the possibility that DTP, previously shown to be non-toxic in mice, may be useful as a therapeutic agent in accidental or malicious human exposures to SM.[61]

4.5.4 Inflammation

Acute SM injury is almost inevitably accompanied by a strong inflammation that contributes to pain and discomfort, and may even aggravate secondary damage. It is important to note that SM exposure will results in both pro-inflammatory but also anti-inflammatory cellular responses. A plethora of *in vitro* and *in vivo* studies revealed a rise in inflammatory cytokines in response to SM exposure. IL-1(α/β), IL-6, IL-8 and TNF-α are considered key cytokines in the pro-inflammatory response[38,62–66] and are released shortly after SM exposure. Dermal exposure of mice to nitrogen mustard resulted in the recruitment of inflammatory cells (neutrophils, macrophages and mast cells), confirming the results so far.[67] The release of inflammatory cytokines is regulated by MAP kinases and the NF-κB pathway. NF-κB is the hypernym for the NF-κB/Rel family, which consists of five proteins [NF-κB1 (p50), NF-κB2 (p52), RelA (p65), RelB and c-Rel]. Most commonly, a heterodimer between p50 and p65 is formed and this is a major mediator of inflammatory processes.[68] Once activated by receptor activated catalytic kinases (IKK), resulting in the degradation of IkBα, released NF-κB translocates into the nucleus and acts as a transcription factor for the abovementioned cytokines IL-6, IL-8 and TNF-α. Rebholz *et al.* demonstrated that SM exposure induced canonical NF-κB pathways in keratinocytes.[69] Recently, it was also shown that SM activates RelA in neutrophils with the subsequent release of IL-6, IL-8 and TNF-α.[70] In line with this finding were the results from Yazdani *et al.* who showed that NF-κB pathways are upregulated in SM exposed patients.[71] Beside NF-κB induced release of inflammatory cytokines, the induction of COX-2, in particular, and other inflammatory proteins has been described.[72–76] MAP kinases (p38, JNK and ERK1/2) are also directly involved in the regulation of cytokine production. It has been reported that SM activates all three MAP kinases together with the upstream kinases. A direct link between MAP kinase activation and cytokine regulation after SM exposure has been described.[69,70,77]

4.5.5 Anti-Inflammatory Therapy

Anti-inflammatory therapy should be a key component of any treatment of SM injury. In general, both glucocorticoids and non-steroidal anti-inflammatory "drugs" (NSAIDs) may be considered for the treatment of SM injury. Glucocorticoids modify gene expression and thus have the opportunity to influence (*i.e.* reduce) inflammation at a very early stage. Within the group of glucocorticoids, there are some highly potent compounds, *e.g.* dexamethasone, that exert an anti-inflammatory effect at concentrations in the low micromolar range or even lower.

NSAIDs do not have the immunosuppressive effects of glucocorticoids, reducing the risk of—potentially serious—secondary infections in the affected skin areas. They may thus have an advantage over glucocorticoids or at least contribute to the anti-inflammatory effect—allowing a dose reduction and safer use of glucocorticoids.

However, relatively few studies have been conducted to investigate the effects of anti-inflammatory drugs in general. Panahi *et al.* (2011) tested betamethasone, along with doxepin, for the topical treatment of chronic SM skin injuries in Iranian veterans several years after SM exposure.[78] Both compounds successfully reduced pruritus, burning sensation, skin dryness and skin scaling, and the Dermatology Life Quality Index improved.

Young *et al.* (2012) tested a number of pro-drugs of NSAIDs in a mouse ear vesicant model. They found a reduction of CEES induced inflammation and edema after treatment with the pro-drugs diclofenac, indomethacin and naproxen, while notably, ibuprofen amplified the inflammation.[79]

Similar findings had already been reported by Amitai *et al.* (2006), who found that a diclofenac pro-drug reduced mouse ear edema after SM exposure, whereas ibuprofen did not.[80]

Recently, Chang *et al.* (2014) reported highly protective effects of a novel COX-2 specific compound and its pro-drug, NDH 4338, in mice after exposure to SM. This might indicate that partial or full COX-2 specific inhibitors might be more effective and/or safer after SM exposure.[81]

Summarizing the current state of knowledge, comparatively little is known about the efficacy and safety of anti-inflammatory drugs after SM exposure—despite the fact that these compounds are likely to be used whenever medical personnel are confronted with SM injury and the inevitable inflammation. Glucocorticoids appear to provide a benefit, possibly at the cost of unwanted immunosuppression. Regarding NSAIDs, differences between the compounds in this group exist and current data suggest diclofenac may be among the more beneficial compounds. Some findings suggest ibuprofen should be used with caution. The most recent findings on novel COX-2 selective drugs may not immediately improve therapeutic options, considering the time and effort required to obtain regulatory approval. They might, however, help us to understand why some NSAIDs may be more beneficial than others. COX-2 selective inhibitors that are already approved for clinical use may be of interest for future research efforts. In general, the efficacy and safety of anti-inflammatory compounds after SM exposure need to be investigated with a broadened scope and in further detail.

4.5.6 Repair of SM Induced DNA Lesions with a Focus on PARP

Alkylation of DNA nucleotides represents a severe cellular state that is a crossroads with regard to cell fate. Already in 1948 it was assumed that DNA was a major target in SM toxicity.[82] Decades later, it was recognized that DNA lesions can be repaired and that recovery in bacteria suffering from SM lesions is associated with resistance to the cytotoxic effects of mustards, but the underlying mechanisms were still unclear at that time.[83] Early *in vitro* experiments with primary rat keratinocytes revealed that within 1 h of a low dose (0.1 μM) SM exposure, DNA structure was compromised.[84] However, even after exposure with 5 μM of SM, a complete restoration of the gross DNA structural integrity was observed. Nevertheless, this repair process was inefficient as thymidine incorporation into the DNA was compromised.[84] Although this first study did not elucidate the possible underlying mechanisms, it clearly demonstrates that DNA alkylation is not a one-way road. Nowadays, it is a well established concept that after alkylation, activation of repair pathways can be observed.

A milestone with regard to DNA repair mechanisms associated with DNA damaging agents was the work by Berger *et al.* in 1979: for the first time it was shown that DNA damage in response to UV light and DNA strand breaks induced the formation of PAR. Later on, Berger formulated his well-known "suicide hypothesis", which correlates cell death to the depletion of cofactors (*i.e.* NAD) during PARylation of DNA strand breaks.[85] Depletion of NAD and the consequential decrease of energy equivalents (*i.e.* ATP) was attributed to rapid cell death (necrosis) before DNA repair takes place. According to the proposed mechanism, PARP inhibitors were used to counteract cofactor depletion and—in theory—allow DNA repair.

The physiological role of poly-PARylation (including in DNA repair) is complex and not fully understood even today. Poly(ADP-ribosyl)ation is a post-translational protein modification induced by various stimuli.[54] PARylation is mediated by PARPs, of which two family members (PARP-1 and PARP-2) are activated by DNA strand breaks.[54] Beside DNA PARylation, a number of proteins (including p53, NF-κB, histones and DNA topoisomerases) undergo PARylation,[54,86] which is thought to have a regulatory function in this context.

PARPs might orchestrate the delicate balance between survival and death signaling.[86] Probably the most accepted role of PARylation with regard to DNA damage is as a sensor and marker of DNA lesions and inducer of DNA repair.[54,86] Beyond its role in DNA repair, PARP-1 is involved in the upregulation of inflammatory cytokines (*e.g.* TNF-α) and proteins (*e.g.* iNOS) *via* NF-κB pathways.[87]

The role of PARylation in SM injury is well established.[38,53,54,88–92] The first link between PARP-1 and SM toxicity was reported by Papirmeister *et al.* in 1985: based on Berger's suicide hypothesis,[85] Papirmeister and colleagues demonstrated the occurrence of DNA strand breaks as repair intermediates after SM exposure, which led to excessive PARP-1 activation and subsequent loss of NAD and ATP.[20] But unfortunately, although PARP inhibitors showed pronounced effects in preserving NAD levels after SM exposure,[93] the overall toxicity remained unaffected. It was found that due to PARP inhibition a shift from necrosis to apoptosis occurred.[53,94,95] Furthermore, due to blockage of base excision repair mechanisms, cells are unable to repair DNA lesion at all (even at low concentrations of the DNA damaging agent), which will then accumulate to a critical level. Thus, PARP inhibition might even aggravate cytotoxicity in this scenario. Moreover, mutagenic lesions might persist due to PARP blocking and DNA repair inhibition, which may account for the observed tumorgenesis.

Thus, in our view, PARP inhibitors should be considered with caution and should not be considered as a first line therapy for SM injury.

4.5.7 PARP Inhibitors

PARP is a family of enzymes that have an essential role in the cellular response to genomic stress, *i.e.* noxae that might damage DNA integrity. PARP forms macromolecules of PAR in the vicinity of damaged DNA, which in turn attract repair enzymes that often reverse DNA damage. Unfortunately, excessive PARP activation after SM exposure has often been associated with necrotic cell death, *e.g.* by Meier and Millard (1998),[96] Hinshaw *et al.* (1999)[88] and Bhat *et al.* (2000).[89] The monomeric molecule from which PAR is formed is $NADH^+$ and thus PARP over-activation may deplete the affected cell of $NADH^+$, resulting in a severe energy crisis, leading to necrotic cell death. As necrosis, the uncontrolled form of cell death, is associated with a pro-inflammatory response, it is usually considered the least desirable pathway of cell death. A shift from necrotic to apoptotic cell death is considered beneficial.

PARP inhibitors in theory may have the potential to prevent $NADH^+$ depletion and necrotic cell death, and were thus considered for the treatment of SM injuries. However, Bhat *et al.* (2006)[97] cautioned that PARP was essential for SM induced DNA damage repair. PARP inhibition might thus also prevent DNA repair in cells affected by moderate, *i.e.* reversible, DNA damage. Even though apoptosis might be the predominant pathway of cell death, the overall damage to cells and tissues might actually increase. Another risk from

PARP inhibition and impaired DNA repair might be the survival of cells with damaged DNA, some of which might ultimately result in tumor formation.

Kehe *et al.* (2007)[53] have shown that the PARP inhibitor 3-aminobenzamide (3-AB) did not affect overall cell viability after SM exposure, although 3-AB could induce a shift from necrotic to apoptotic cell death. $NADH^+$ depletion, the primary mechanism of PARP mediated necrosis after SM exposure, was only observed after exposure to 1000 μM SM and above. However, at the cellular level, 1000 μM SM constitutes a near-catastrophic exposure and cells affected by this concentration would inevitably die, with little chance for pharmacological intervention. In neighboring tissues that are suffering from moderate SM exposure and potentially reversible DNA damage, PARP inhibition and impaired DNA repair might ultimately do more harm than good.

The potential use of PARP inhibitors as a therapeutic strategy after SM exposure is still under discussion and research efforts are underway to clarify the issue. Considering the abovementioned findings, it may not be the most promising approach and caution is definitely advised.

4.5.8 SM and Cell Death

After exposure to SM both necrotic and apoptotic cell death can be observed.[38,91,95,98–100] Necrosis is considered to be a less controlled mode of cell death that is linked to severe cellular dysfunction, which prevents a controlled mode of cell death, namely apoptosis. It is plausible that a high dose exposure to SM predominantly results in necrosis (*via* PARP activation, NAD and subsequent energy depletion). *In vitro* experiments revealed that necrosis was not evident in endothelial cells after lower dose exposure scenarios (concentrations below 250 μM), whereas concentrations above 500 μM strongly increased necrosis.[101] Remarkably, even at high concentrations of SM, apoptosis was still evident. This finding was proven in animal experiments that revealed both apoptosis and necrosis occurring side by side after SM exposure.[102,103] This effect is most likely to be class specific, as nitrogen mustard (*i.e.* HN2) revealed comparable effects.[104] In general, necrosis has to be considered as a "worst-case scenario" with regard to cell death: while apoptosis can be influenced to a certain degree [but can also proceed to (apo) necrosis], necrosis is considered as the irreversible and uncontrolled loss of cell membrane integrity and subsequent uncontrolled release of cell content causing an inflammatory response. Thus, necrosis will always be involved in a SM exposure and has to be considered as an uncontrollable and thus unwanted process.

Apoptosis, however, is a controlled mode of cell death in which acute cellular injury or a cellular response to stress trigger well orchestrated multiform signaling cascades that result in cell suicide.[105] While necrosis was considered as the predominant mode of action in toxicology in the past, apoptosis as a "programmed cell death" is nowadays regarded as a key process in toxicology.[106] In short, activation of effector caspases (cysteine dependent aspartate directed proteases), in particular caspase-3, -6 and -7, leads to cleavage of numerous proteins located in the cytoskeleton, cytoplasm and nucleus,[105,106] resulting in the formation of apoptotic bodies (cell blebs with intact membrane) containing the cellular remnants. These blebs will be taken up by neighboring cells through phagocytosis. Phagocytosis of apoptotic cell remnants is specifically termed efferocytosis. In contrast to necrosis, the inflammatory response is low as there is only marginal release of cytoplasmic contents into the extracellular space. An increase of intracellular calcium, generation of ROS, mitochondrial dysfunction and activation of death receptors on the cell surface are important inducers of apoptosis. With regard to SM toxicity, apoptosis has been investigated in detail. Death receptor mediated apoptosis (also called "extrinsic apoptosis") is initiated by binding of specific ligands to their designated receptors. Alkylating agents were shown to activate extrinsic apoptotic pathways.[90,107] SM increased levels of both Fas receptor and Fas ligand in human epidermal keratinocytes, which resulted in cleavage of pro-caspase-8 and later pro-caspase-9. Caspase-9 activation, in particular, is associated with mitochondrial stress reactions and mitochondrial mediated apoptosis (*e.g.* a decrease in Bcl-2, and release of AIF and cytochrome C).[108] Finally, executive caspases (*i.e.* caspase-3) are activated and induce protein fragmentation (*e.g.* cleavage of PARP) as well as DNA condensation and fragmentation. Finally, non-vital cells are recognized by macrophages and are cleared by efferocytosis.[106] Keratinocytes that lack the Fas associated death domain were shown to be less sensitive to SM exposures: *in vitro* the processing and thereby activation of pro-caspase-3, -7 and -8 was evident in normal human keratinocytes whereas in knockdown cells DNA cleavage and caspase-6 mediated nuclear lamin cleavage was diminished.[107] *In vivo* experiments revealed that after exposure to SM in rats a distinct increase in Fas ligand levels was observed in the bronchoalveolar lavage fluid,[109] giving further evidence that extrinsic apoptotic pathways are involved in the molecular pathology of SM poisoning. Blocking of Fas ligand associated pathways was beneficial in a number of studies; however, complete protection against SM induced cell damage was not achieved by inhibition of Fas pathways.

In contrast to extrinsic apoptosis, which relies on an extracellular signal to induce apoptosis, intrinsic apoptosis is triggered by intracellular events and is closely related to mitochondria. Release of pro-apoptotic proteins from the intermembrane proteins into the cytosol activates the caspase machinery. This process is well orchestrated and under the control of proteins from the Bcl-2 family. Another possible mechanism of apoptotic cell death initiated by mitochondria is the release and translocation of AIF into the cytoplasm and nucleus, resulting in DNA fragmentation.[106] Both apoptotic pathways are described after SM exposure and have been targeted by therapeutic measures. However, although caspase inhibitors showed some beneficial effects, up to now, no reliable therapeutic measures targeting apoptosis are available. Inhibition of apoptotic pathways resulted in a shift from apoptosis to necrosis without affecting overall cell vitality.[53]

4.5.9 Limitation of Extrinsic Apoptosis

Apoptosis is a key mechanism of SM induced cytotoxicity and, in particular, extrinsic apoptosis has a very important role. As extrinsic apoptosis may also affect cells that have not (or have only reversibly) been affected by SM, limitation of extrinsic apoptosis may be one of the most promising therapeutic strategies against SM injury. This would be an effective way to avoid excessive apoptosis and subsequent tissue damage, while intrinsic apoptosis could still eliminate cells that had been irreversibly damaged.

A number of studies have identified the Fas ligand as a key mediator of extrinsic apoptosis after SM exposure. Initial evidence for the role of the Fas ligand was presented, by Rosenthal *et al.* (2003).[107] Antibodies against Fas ligand reduced SM toxicity in human keratinocytes. When cells expressed a domain-negative Fas associated death domain (FADD-DN), a pronounced reduction of apoptosis was observed. Results were confirmed in mice that had received human keratinocyte grafts expressing FADD-DN.

The clinical relevance of the Fas ligand was first shown by Ghazanfari *et al.* (2009),[110] who found elevated Fas ligand levels in the serum of patients with chronic pulmonary illness after SM exposure. A study by Pirzad *et al.* (2010)[111] confirmed these findings, demonstrating elevated Fas ligand levels in bronchoalveolar lavage fluid. Both studies show that the relevance of Fas ligand mediated extrinsic apoptosis extends far beyond the acute injury into the stage of chronic illness.

A potential therapeutic strategy against excessive extrinsic apoptosis, mediated through Fas ligand was presented by Keyser *et al.* (2013),[109] who used small interfering RNA (siRNA) to block the expression of the Fas receptor. A significant reduction of necrosis and apoptosis was observed in normal human bronchial/tracheal epithelial (NHBE) cells, even when siRNA was used as a post-exposure intervention.

Other pathways of extrinsic apoptosis do exist and, possibly, a therapeutic strategy should not be limited to target a single mediator. Inhibition of caspase-8 may potentially counteract extrinsic apoptosis, induced by a variety of mediators. However, caution needs to be exercised because apoptosis, including extrinsic apoptosis, is a continuous process within the human body and necessary to maintain homeostasis and clinical health. Systemic suppression of extrinsic apoptosis may have serious adverse effects, including the survival of malignant and dysfunctional cells, and consequences including, but not limited to, cancer development. In contrast, topical application of compounds that antagonize extrinsic apoptosis at the affected areas of skin or respiratory system may be a highly promising approach.

4.5.10 Reactive Species Formation After SM Exposure

Superoxide (O^{*}_{2-}) and hydroxyl radicals (OH*) are the two major reactive intermediates derived from oxygen that are known as ROS. ROS are formed under physiological conditions and play an important role in cell signaling.

However, increased levels of ROS of various origins can result in significant cell damage.

There is strong agreement that SM induces cellular stress, including the formation of reactive species. The first direct evidence that radicals are involved in SM toxicity was provided by Anderson *et al.*, who showed with electron paramagnetic resonance that free radical and lipid peroxidation occurred *in vivo* just 1 h after pulmonary exposure to SM vapor. Later on, it was found by Brimfield *et al.* that SM leads to the formation of carbon based radicals, which in turn results in the formation of superoxide, peroxyl and hydroxyl radicals.[112] Superoxide dismutase (SOD) or catalase (CAT) were both able to eliminate ROS formation. Conjugation of SM with GSH can cause the loss of a significant number of anti-oxidative compounds, thus resulting in an oxidative stress response.[113] Furthermore, SM was shown to inhibit activities of several antioxidant enzymes *in vivo*,[114] thus aggravating ROS induced cell damage. Peroxynitrite, the reactive product between O^{*}_{2-} and NO, interacts with lipids, DNA and proteins, thereby causing massive cell damage.[115] There are numerous reports that show the involvement of NO/NO synthases (NOS) in SM toxicity.[116–121] Increased expression of NOS [*i.e.* inducible NOS (iNOS)] and activation of endothelial NOS have been demonstrated after SM exposure.[120] However, although protein expression or activation was evident after SM exposure, a reliable increase in NO formation was not evident. Catalytic decoupling of NOS (thereby producing ROS instead of NO) that could be counteracted with BH_4 has been discussed.[120]

Recent work has demonstrated that mitochondrial dysfunction and mitochondrial derived ROS stress are important events in SM pathophysiology.[121–125]

4.5.11 Anti-Oxidative Interventions

Oxidative stress is known to be a key factor in SM toxicity. In particular, due to altered gene expression and dysfunctional enzymes, cells are slowly, but increasingly overburdened by ROS and RNS. A number of therapeutic interventions have been attempted to reverse these effects.

Therapeutic approaches using SOD to counteract SM induced toxicity revealed that SOD can provide significant protective effects *in vivo* when administered prophylactically.[47] However, in the study conducted by Eldad *et al.* no protection was evident when SOD was administered after SM exposure.

NAC and GSH, a physiological anti-oxidative tri-peptide, have often been discussed as a means of intervention after SM injury. There was, however, often an assumption that their beneficial effect originated largely or even exclusively from a chemical scavenging reaction with free SM, often leading to the conclusion that they were useful as pre-treatments only.

Ghanei *et al.* (2004) successfully used a combination of NAC and clarithromycin in patients with chronic lung injury after SM exposure.[126] In this case, there was some uncertainty as to whether the clinical improvement could be attributed to NAC, clarithromycin or the combination thereof.

However, recently, Jugg *et al.* (2013) demonstrated that nebulized NAC was highly effective to reduce pulmonary symptoms after SM vapor exposure in large swine.[127] They showed that survival improved, along with oxygen saturation and membrane integrity.

Mukhopadhyay *et al.* (2009) used liposomes to transport NAC, along with vitamin E and related compounds (tocopherol α, γ and δ), to the CEES exposed lungs of guinea pigs.[128] While the activation of MAP kinase family enzymes was not changed by therapeutic intervention, the CEES induced activation of AP-1 transcription factors and the corresponding increase in the protein levels of Fos, ATF and Jun family members was counteracted by this anti-oxidative therapy. CEES induced inflammation and infiltration of neutrophils, eosinophils and erythrocytes into the alveolar space were also reduced. A subsequent study by Mukhopadhyay *et al.* (2010) also confirmed a decrease in CEES induced activation of pro-inflammatory cytokines IL-1β and IL-6.[129]

Tewari-Singh *et al.* (2011) investigated GSH pre-treatment in HaCaT cells, mouse epidermal cells and living mice. GSH reversed the CEES induced decrease in cell viability and DNA synthesis.[130] A dose of 300 mg kg^{-1} body weight, administered orally prior to topical exposure to CEES reduced the CEES induced increase of skin bifold and epidermal thickness, apoptotic cell death, and myeloperoxidase activity.

Steinritz *et al.* (2010) tested the antioxidants NAC and α-linolenic acid for their ability to restore wound healing in a mouse embryoid body model and found temporary, but not permanent, protective effects.[131] However, α-linolenic acid, in particular, was found to improve migration of early endothelial cells by protecting mitochondrial function.[122]

As an alternative anti-oxidant, Anand *et al.* (2011) suggested the use of *S*-2(2-aminoethylamino) ethyl phenyl sulfide, termed DRDE-07, and initially found a reduction of liver toxicity in mice that had been percutaneously exposed to 1 LD_{50} of SM.[132] However, unlike NAC or GSH, DRDE-07 has no well established safety record and the application of 20% of the LD_{50} of the antidote prior to a potential exposure certainly has no relevance in future clinical applications. An alternative application of DRDE-07 with some potential relevance was presented by Lomash *et al.* (2012), who used topical formulations of that compound, following dermal exposure of mice to SM and reported accelerated wound healing.[133]

A particularly novel approach to reduce oxidative stress after SM injury is the use of catalytic antioxidants. These compounds facilitate the reaction and inactivation of ROS and RNS in a redox reaction. Subsequently, the catalytic antioxidant is restored to its original state. For this reason, much smaller quantities of the active compound are able to significantly reduce oxidative stress, potentially allowing anti-oxidative interventions in a faster and safer way. Currently, the manganoporphyrin AEOL 10150 is among the most studied catalytic antioxidants, including as a potential therapeutic for SM injury.

An initial study in rats by O'Neill *et al.* (2010) investigated the protective effects of AEOL 10150 after CEES inhalation and found that a number of pathological parameters that increase after CEES inhalation (lactate dehydrogenase activity, protein, IgM, red blood cells and neutrophils in bronchoalveolar lavage fluid, lung myeloperoxidase activity, as well as lung oxidative stress markers 8-OHdG and 4-HNE) were decreased by AEOL 10150 treatment.[125] A subsequent study by O'Neill *et al.* (2011) confirmed that reduction of ROS and RNS was the actual mechanism behind the protective effects.[121]

Tewari-Singh *et al.* (2014) tested AEOL 10150 in mice epidermal cells, human HaCaT cells and living mice, and established a combination of a subcutaneous injection (5 mg kg^{-1} body weight) and a topical formulation of AEOL 10150 that is capable of reducing CEES induced symptoms by more than 50%, as assessed by epidermal thickness, myeloperoxidase activity and DNA oxidation.[123]

Pohanka *et al.* (2011) used melatonin in SM exposed rats to activate the endogenous anti-oxidative system. Melatonin treatment successfully enhanced the production of low molecular weight antioxidants, reduced lipid peroxidation and SM induced protein carbonylation.[134]

An anti-oxidative strategy beyond the classic pharmacological interventions was suggested by Ishida *et al.* (2012), who demonstrated accelerated healing of scratch wounds in cultures of human keratinocytes following gene transfer of iNOS to overcome SM induced inhibition of that enzyme.[135] This most interesting paper, introducing gene therapy strategies into medical chemical defense research, certainly highlights the important role of iNOS; clinical application, however, may be difficult. Gene transfer deeply and irreversibly interferes with the target cells and, as such, is associated with inherent risks. While pharmacological interventions, *i.e.* drugs, can be discontinued if patients may not tolerate them, gene transfer is permanent. Application of gene transfer will require years of research, in particular, into safety issues, and may constitute a last resort option if and when oxidative stress cannot be controlled by pharmacological means.

In summary, anti-oxidative therapy continues to be an important perspective in the therapy of SM injuries. The physiological anti-oxidant GSH and its well-known precursor NAC with their excellent safety records remain compounds of interest, in particular with increasing evidence of their efficacy in post-exposure therapy and innovative means to topically deliver high concentrations of anti-oxidants to the affected areas. Catalytic antioxidants may significantly contribute to therapeutic success and accelerate the elimination of excessive concentrations of ROS and RNS. Strategies of gene therapy are important to further understand the mechanisms of oxidative stress in SM exposed cells, but their clinical application may be limited and will require additional research.

4.5.12 Other Therapeutic Approaches

4.5.12.1 Macrolide Antibiotics

Initial observations on the protective effects of macrolide antibiotics in patients after SM injuries were first described by Ghanei *et al.* (2004), who had noticed a benefit in patients suffering from chronic pulmonary diseases several years after SM exposure.[126] These patients, who had not shown improvement after glucocorticoid and immunosuppressive therapy, responded well to a combined therapy of NAC and clarithromycin. Doses of clarithromycin were below those used for antibiotic treatment and the mechanism of action was obviously independent from any antibiotic effect. The protective mechanisms of clarithromycin and related compounds have been studied since then.

Gao *et al.* (2007) investigated the effects of roxithromycin in a human respiratory epithelial cell line and observed significant reductions of necrosis and inflammation.[136] In particular, reduced expression of IL-1β, IL-6, IL-8 and TNF-α was shown. Over-expression of iNOS was also reversed by roxithromycin treatment. A subsequent study by Gao *et al.* (2008) focused on the reversal of iNOS over-expression and excessive nitric oxide production.[137] Along with roxithromycin, azithromycin, clarithromycin and erythromycin were also tested and found to be effective.

A novel protective mechanism of macrolide antibiotics was identified by Gao *et al.* (2009): the phagocytotic and chemotactic activity of THP-1 cells, an immunocompetent monocytic cell line, was successfully restored by a 10 μM treatment with any of the following macrolide antibiotics: azithromycin, clarithromycin, erythromycin and roxithromycin.[138]

In line with previous findings, production of pro-inflammatory cytokines and over-production of iNOS were also reduced.

In vivo data on the efficacy of macrolide antibiotics, in particular, roxithromycin, were presented by Gao *et al.* (2011). Rats were exposed to a respiratory SM challenge. Either 10, 20 or 40 mg kg^{-1} roxithromycin was administered prior to exposure and again afterwards in 24 h intervals.[139] Tissue damage was significantly reduced by 20 and 40 mg kg^{-1} roxithromycin, with the 40 mg kg^{-1} dose exhibiting the most pronounced effect.

In summary, the efficacy of macrolide antibiotics in the case of SM injury is supported by clinical, animal and *in vitro* data. Their protective effect in patients with chronic respiratory illness from SM exposure might be of particular interest and could be attributed to the restoration of chemotaxis and phagocytosis of immune cells. Zarin *et al.* (2010) identified functional phagocytotic removal of apoptotic bodies as a key mechanism to mitigate chronic illness after SM exposure.[140]

Macrolide antibiotics are approved drugs and known to be safe. In order to apply for regulatory approval for their use for treatment of acute or chronic SM injuries, more *in vivo* data, using different species, might be necessary. *In vitro* studies with more complex cell culture models of human cell lines might also facilitate the extrapolation of animal data to a clinical situation in humans. Even though protective effects were found with a variety of macrolide compounds, the most in-depth investigation, including dose–effect relationships in animal studies, has focused on roxithromycin, possibly identifying this as the most promising compound.

A potential risk of prolonged therapy using macrolide antibiotics at sub-antibiotic doses may be the development of resistant bacteria strains. Nevertheless, pronounced clinical improvement may outweigh this risk. Therapeutic guidelines, however, should select alternative antibiotics to be used in the case of bacterial infection and nursing procedures should be adjusted to avoid or minimize the spread of resistant bacteria strains.

4.5.12.2 Silibinin

Silibinin is the lead compound isolated from the seeds of milk thistle, *Silybum marianum*. It has been known for many years and is approved for clinical use, both as a specific antidote against green death cap (*Amanita phalloides*) poisoning and for liver protection against unspecific noxae, including nutritive stress, alcohol and infections. While its efficacy as an antidote against *Amanita phalloides* is exerted through a highly specific receptor interaction, protection against the abovementioned variety of noxae is considered the result of pleiotropic effects, a synergism of multiple mechanisms that help to protect and sustain at a cellular level. Silibinin stabilizes bio-membranes, enhancing protein synthesis and reducing oxidative stress.

These multiple protective effects should also be beneficial against SM toxicity. Stabilization of bio-membranes might reduce uncontrolled disintegration of damaged cells (*i.e.* necrosis). Reduction of oxidative stress might be a key to ensure the mid to long term survival of cells that have received moderate yet reversible damage from SM. Enhanced *de novo* synthesis of proteins should help to replace alkylated, dysfunctional enzyme and membrane proteins with the intact, fully functional structures and, thus, facilitate cell survival.

The protective effects of silibinin against alkylating substances, *i.e.* analogs of SM, were first shown in two studies by Tewari-Singh *et al.*, in rabbit corneal cultures, mice skin cells and mice skin (*in vivo*).[72,74] In both studies, similar substances were used, *i.e.* nitrogen mustard in the rabbit cornea culture studies and CEES (hemi-mustard) in the mice cells and living mice.

The efficacy of silibinin against SM itself was demonstrated by Balszuweit *et al.* (2013), using immortalized human keratinocytes (HaCaT cells).[141] This study also demonstrated for the first time that the water soluble pro-drug of silibinin, silibinin bis-succinate, was metabolized by HaCaT cells into free silibinin, and application of the pro-drug in 50–100 μM concentrations, known to be safe and effective in the case of *Amanita phalloides* poisoning, exerted significant protective effects. At the same time, in severely poisoned cells, apoptosis was slightly amplified, which may be a useful mechanism to eliminate cells with irreversible damage to their DNA, thus reducing the risk of cancer formation from SM injuries.

Due to its ability to counteract several aspects of SM toxicity and to significantly reduce cell necrosis—along with its favorable regulatory status as an approved drug—silibinin or, more specifically, silibinin bis-succinate probably constitutes one of the most promising approaches to improve therapy for SM injury in the near future. Subsequent research efforts should test the compound in more complex cell culture models and in animals. Animal studies could also clarify the issue as to whether or not direct topical delivery of silibinin bis-succinate to injured skin areas might be more beneficial than systemic administration. When these issues have been successfully addressed, regulatory approval for the use of silibinin bis-succinate against SM injury may be sought.

4.5.12.3 Phytopharmaceuticals

While most of the previously discussed compounds and therapeutic strategies have been subjected to systematic investigation over several years and often by multiple working groups, independent of each other, there are also a number of compounds that have been investigated in a single study. Many of these compounds are phytopharmaceuticals, plant derived compounds with moderate pharmacological activity used as food or traditional herbal medicines.

Often, these compounds are considered inherently safe. There is, however, some need to exercise caution. SM poisoning is an extreme situation, already at the molecular and cellular level, triggering a number of cytotoxic and highly complex processes. The risk that an otherwise safe and beneficial compound might actually accelerate, for example, inflammation or apoptosis in SM exposed cells and tissues cannot be ruled out *a priori*. This is not meant to discourage research into phytopharmaceuticals—to the contrary, comprehensive data on their efficacy and safety will be needed before considering their clinical use.

Tekiner *et al.* (2009) demonstrated that proanthocyanidin, administered orally at a dose of 100 mg kg^{-1} per day after a respiratory exposure to nitrogen mustard reduced neuro-degeneration in the rat brain.[142] A subsequent study by Tekiner *et al.* (2011) revealed strengthened anti-oxidative defenses as a potential mechanism of this protective effect.[143]

Pohanka *et al.* (2011) attempted to use 10 or 20 mg of epigallocatechin gallate to improve anti-oxidative defenses prior to a 20 or 80 mg SM exposure in rats. Even though a slight anti-apoptotic effect of epigallocatechin gallate was observed, most of the results were rather inconclusive, and the authors summarized that there were difficulties in antioxidant therapy as prophylaxis for the oxidative stress related toxins.[144]

Boskabady *et al.* (2011) investigated extracts from *Nigella sativa* in comparison to and in combination with dexamethasone in SM exposed guinea pigs for their effects on the course of lung injury.[145] *Nigella sativa* extracts decreased tracheal responsiveness to methacholine and the number of invading neutrophils, partly reversing the effects of SM exposure. However, *Nigella sativa* extracts alone had no effect on monocytes and eosinophils, found in bronchoalveolar lavage solutions. IL-4, an anti-inflammatory cytokine was elevated, both by dexamethasone and *Nigella sativa*.

Boskabady *et al.* (2012) demonstrated that vitamin E reduced tissue damage in the liver and kidney of guinea pigs after respiratory SM exposure.[146]

Panahi *et al.* (2012) presented a clinical, double blinded trial demonstrating the reduction of pruritus by curcumin treatment.[147] A dose of 1 g curcumin per day, used as a nutritional supplement, reduced pruritus, improved quality of life and also had a significant effect on several parameters of oxidative stress, including substance P, SOD, GSH peroxidase and catalase. In a separate paper, Panahi *et al.* (2012) also demonstrated the anti-inflammatory effects of curcumin supplementation: serum levels of IL-8 and C-reactive protein decreased; however, IL-6 remained largely unchanged.[148]

Sahebkar (2012) discussed baicalin, a bioactive flavonoid from the roots of *Scutellaria* spp., as a potentially promising drug for the management of SM induced cutaneous complications.[149] This assessment, however, was made on the theoretical evaluation of molecular mechanisms. There are currently no related experimental or clinical data for baicalin in the literature.

In summary, research into phytopharmaceuticals for the treatment of acute or chronic SM injuries has revealed some interesting results, but certainly no "miracle compound" capable of dramatically reversing SM induced pathology. Currently, the most successful strategies in this regard have been curcumin (supported by clinical data) and possibly proanthocyanidin, which exhibited some neuro-protective effects. Subsequent research may potentially reveal a more pronounced benefit from high dose therapy and further details of the mechanisms of action. Phytopharmaceuticals may not necessarily be the key pillars of future therapy of SM injury, but may have a useful, supportive role, in particular in the long term treatment of chronic injury.

4.5.12.4 Cell Therapies

As SM injuries often result in permanently damaged and/or dysfunctional tissues, a solely pharmacological therapy is unable to reverse those effects. Cell therapies, use of stem cells or even tissue engineering have often been discussed as a novel therapeutic strategy, potentially capable of fully restoring health after SM injury. Regrettably, however, most of these approaches are in their early experimental stages. This section will provide an overview of cell therapies and grafting techniques that have either been used successfully in patients or shown very promising results in animal models.

Graham *et al.* (2009) tested an autologous cell harvesting device in a domestic swine model, used in combination with laser debridement, vacuum closure and application of an oxygenized nutrient solution.[37] The authors found that harvest and transfer of autologous cells contributed significantly to wound healing, in some cases without visible scarring.

A deficit or dysfunction of limbal corneal stem cells is one of the reasons for the chronic pathological processes after SM exposure to the eye. The late effects of SM injury may become evident years to decades after the exposure and have proved very difficult to treat. An increasingly eroding cornea, along with uncontrolled neovascularization may often result in blindness. Kadar *et al.* (2014) tested bevacizumab in a rabbit eye model and were able to symptomatically reduce corneal neovascularization, whereas no effect on stem cell deficits was observed.[150]

Javadi *et al.* (2011) surveyed the success and failure of several limbal stem cell transplantation techniques in survivors of SM attacks and found that keratolimbal allograft (KLAL) and lamellar keratoplasty (LK) were by far superior methods, resulting in rejection-free graft survival rates of 80% in the KLAL group and 90% in the LK group 40 and 28 months after surgery, respectively.[151] Living related conjunctival limbal allograft (lrCAL) and penetrating keratoplasty (PK) were less successful, with approximately 39% rejection free survival at the time of observation.

Recently, Dachir *et al.* (2014) demonstrated that intra-dermal injections of activated human macrophages in SM exposed guinea pigs decreased the wound area, improved barrier function and accelerated wound healing.[152]

Research into mesenchymal stem cells and their potential use in the long term therapy of SM injury is in progress. Schmidt *et al.* (2013) have shown that mesenchymal stem cell cells were able to survive surprisingly high concentrations of SM and retain their ability to differentiate. Migratory ability, however, was impaired by very low SM concentrations.[153]

In summary, some cell transplantation techniques have already demonstrated their ability to restore, to a significant degree, the health of patients suffering from the long term effects of SM exposure, or to prevent severe late effects, such as blindness. More research effort is needed, in particular in the field of stem cell therapy. In the long term, however, cell therapies may have the potential to allow restoration of health. The probable role of pharmacological interventions will be to minimize the damage in the acute stage of SM induced injury and to slow down any destructive or detrimental processes in the chronic stage.

4.6 Summary and Outlook

Almost a century of medical experience with the consequences of SM exposure and the advancement in life sciences in the past three decades have not revealed a causative therapy against SM injuries. The situation, however, is far from being hopeless. Supportive therapy, by general means of intervention (wound debridement, cooling *etc.*), prevention or therapy of infections, and anti-inflammatory therapy can help to ensure survival and restore, to a significant degree, quality of life in patients after light to moderate exposures. Cell transplantation techniques have been successfully used to avoid blindness.

Significant advances in the understanding of SM induced pathology have the potential to improve therapeutic options in the near to medium term future. Key pillars of a successful therapy will be to control or antagonize the excessive inflammation and extrinsic apoptosis, to alleviate the oxidative stress and turn the reaction towards SM injury of the systemic immune system from an aggravating to a mitigating response. Improved phagocytosis, *e.g.* by macrolide antibiotics and reduction of the systemic poison load may be an important factor to achieve that aim. Silibinin, due to its pleiotropic activity that helps to control many aspects of molecular SM toxicity, may have another important role to improve therapy for SM injuries.

Improving and accelerating wound healing after SM exposure remains a challenge and it is currently difficult to predict whether pharmacological interventions or (possibly autologous) cell transplants will ultimately be the key.

In summary, however, there is hope and realistic prospects to offer effective and significantly improved therapy to the potential victims of this hideous chemical weapon.

References

1. F. Guthrie, Ueber einige Derivate der Kohlenwasserstoffe C nHn, *Ann. Chem. Pharm.*, 1860, 266.
2. A. Niemann, Ueber die Einwirkung des braunen Chlorschwefels auf Elaylgas, *Ann. Chem. Pharm.*, 1860, **113**, 288.
3. V. Meyer, Ueber Thiodiglykolverbindungen, *Ber. Dtsch. Chem. Ges.*, 1886, **19**, 3259.
4. L. S. Goodman, M. M. Wintrobe, W. Dameshek, M. J. Goodman, A. Gilman and M. T. McLennan, Landmark article Sept. 21, 1946: nitrogen mustard therapy. Use of methyl-bis(beta-chloroethyl)amine hydrochloride and tris(beta-chloroethyl)amine hydrochloride for Hodgkin's disease, lymphosarcoma, leukemia and certain allied and miscellaneous disorders. By Louis S. Goodman, Maxwell M. Wintrobe, William Dameshek, Morton J. Goodman, Alfred Gilman and Margaret T. McLennan, *JAMA, J. Am. Med. Assoc.*, 1984, **251**, 2255.
5. H. Q. Le and S. J. Knudsen, Exposure to a First World War blistering agent, *Emerg. Med. J.*, 2006, **23**, 296.
6. J. Newmark, J. M. Langer, B. Capacio, J. Barr and R. G. McIntosh, Liquid SM exposure, *Mil. Med.*, 2007, **172**, 196.
7. R. I. Tilley, The hydrolysis of bis(2-chlorethyl) sulfide (sulfur mustard) in aqueos mixtures of ethanol, acetone and dimethyl sulfoxide, *Aust. J. Chem.*, 1993, **46**, 293.
8. A. Watson, D. Opresko, R. Young and V. Hauschild, Development and Application of Acute Exposure Guideline Levels (AEGLs) for Chemical Warfare Nerve and Sulfur Mustard Agents, *J. Toxicol. Environ. Health, Part B*, 2006, **9**, 173.
9. R. P. Chilcott, J. Jenner, W. Carrick, S. A. Hotchkiss and P. Rice, Human skin absorption of Bis-2-(chloroethyl)sulphide (sulphur mustard) in vitro, *J. Appl. Toxicol.*, 2000, **20**, 349.
10. H. Cullumbine, Medical Aspects of mustard gas poisoning, *Nat. Publishing Group*, 1947, **159**, 151.
11. A. Maisonneuve, I. Callebat, L. Debordes and L. Coppet, Biological fate of sulphur mustard in rat: toxicokinetics and disposition, *Xenobiotica*, 1993, **23**, 771.
12. W. Eisenmenger, G. Drasch, C. M. von, E. Kretschmer and G. Roider, Clinical and morphological findings on mustard gas [bis(2-chloroethyl) sulfide] poisoning, *J. Forensic Sci.*, 1991, **36**, 1688.
13. D. Noort, A. Fidder, C. E. Degenhardt-Langelaan and A. G. Hulst, Retrospective detection of sulfur mustard exposure by mass spectrometric analysis of adducts to albumin and hemoglobin: an in vivo study, *J. Anal. Toxicol.*, 2008, **32**, 25.

14. R. M. Black and R. W. Read, Biological fate of sulphur mustard, 1,1'-thiobis(2-chloroethane): identification of beta-lyase metabolites and hydrolysis products in human urine, *Xenobiotica*, 1995, **25**, 167.
15. R. M. Black, An overview of biological markers of exposure to chemical warfare agents, *J. Anal. Toxicol.*, 2008, **32**, 2.
16. C. L. Young, D. Ash and W. J. Driskell, *et al.*, A rapid, sensitive method for the quantitation of specific metabolites of sulfur mustard in human urine using isotope-dilution gas chromatography-tandem mass spectrometry, *J. Anal. Toxicol.*, 2004, **28**, 339.
17. M. Balali-Mood and M. Hefazi, Comparison of early and late toxic effects of sulfur mustard in Iranian veterans, *Basic Clin. Pharmacol. Toxicol.*, 2006, **99**, 273.
18. K. J. Smith, C. G. Hurst, R. B. Moeller, H. G. Skelton and F. R. Sidell, Sulfur mustard: its continuing threat as a chemical warfare agent, the cutaneous lesions induced, progress in understanding its mechanism of action, its long-term health effects, and new developments for protection and therapy, *J. Am. Acad. Dermatol.*, 1995, **32**, 765.
19. S. M. Nagy, C. Golumbic, W. H. Stein, J. S. Fruton and M. Bergmann, The penetration of vesicant vapours into human skin, *J. Gen. Physiol.*, 1946, **29**, 441.
20. B. Papirmeister, C. L. Gross, H. L. Meier, J. P. Petrali and J. B. Johnson, Molecular basis for mustard-induced vesication, *Fundam. Appl. Toxicol.*, 1985, **5**, S134.
21. Z. S. Naraghi, P. Mansouri and M. Mortazavi, A clinicopathological study on acute cutaneous lesions induced by sulfur mustard gas (yperite), *Eur. J. Dermatol.*, 2005, **15**, 140.
22. M. Balali-Mood and M. Hefazi, The pharmacology, toxicology, and medical treatment of sulphur mustard poisoning, *Fundam. Clin. Pharmacol.*, 2005, **19**, 297.
23. M. Balali-Mood, M. Hefazi and M. Mahmoudi, *et al.*, Long-term complications of sulphur mustard poisoning in severely intoxicated Iranian veterans, *Fundam. Clin. Pharmacol.*, 2005, **19**, 713.
24. J. L. Willems, Clinical management of mustard gas casualties, *Ann. Med. Militaris*, 1989, **3**, 1.
25. F. Flury and H. Wieland, Über Kampfgasvergiftungen. VII. Die pharmakologische Wirkung des Dichloräthylsulfids, *Z. Gesamte. Exp. Med.*, 1921, **13**, 367.
26. B. Papirmeister, *Medical defense against mustard gas*, 1991, 1. Introduction, p. 1.
27. W. Koch, L. Aschoff and O. von Schjerning, D. Direkte Kriegserkrankung durch Einwirkung chemischer Mittel, *Pathol. Anat.*, 1921, 526.
28. M. Ghanei, M. Mokhtari, M. M. Mohammad and J. Aslani, Bronchiolitis obliterans following exposure to sulfur mustard: chest high resolution computed tomography, *Eur. J. Radiol.*, 2004, **52**, 164.
29. C. Guignabert, L. Taysse and J. H. Calvet, *et al.*, Effect of doxycycline on sulfur mustard-induced respiratory lesions in guinea pigs, *Am. J. Physiol.: Lung Cell. Mol. Physiol.*, 2005, **289**, L67.

30. M. Hochmeister and W. Vycudilik, Morpho-toxicologic findings following war gas effect (S-Lost), *Beitr. Gerichtl. Med.*, 1989, **47**, 533.
31. O. Heitzmann, öber Kampfgasvergiftungen. VIII. Die pathologisch-anatomischen VerÑnderungen nach Vergiftung mit DichlordiÑthylsulfid unter BerÅcksichtigung der Tierversuche, *Z. Gesamte. Exp. Med.*, 1921, **13**, 484.
32. Y. Solberg, M. Alcalay and M. Belkin, Ocular injury by mustard gas, *Surv. Ophthalmol.*, 1997, **41**, 461.
33. W. J. Geeraets, S. Abedi and R. V. Blanke, Acute corneal injury by mustard gas, *South Med. J.*, 1977, **70**, 348.
34. I. J. Hattersley, J. Jenner, C. Dalton, R. P. Chilcott and J. S. Graham, The skin reservoir of sulphur mustard, *Toxicol. In Vitro*, 2008, **22**, 1539.
35. G. Drasch, G. Kretschmer, L. Kauert and L. Von Meyer, Concentration of mustard gas [bis(2-chloroethyl)sulfide] in the tissues of a victim of a vesicant exposure, *J. Forensic Sci.*, 1987, **32**, 1788.
36. K. Kehe, H. Thiermann, F. Balszuweit, F. Eyer, D. Steinritz and T. Zilker, Acute effects of sulfur mustard injury-Munich experiences, *Toxicology*, 2009, **263**, 3.
37. J. S. Graham, R. S. Stevenson and L. W. Mitcheltree, *et al.*, Medical management of cutaneous sulfur mustard injuries, *Toxicology*, 2009, **263**, 47.
38. K. Kehe, F. Balszuweit, D. Steinritz and H. Thiermann, Molecular toxicology of sulfur mustard-induced cutaneous inflammation and blistering, *Toxicology*, 2009, **263**, 12.
39. D. B. Ludlum, W. P. Tong, J. R. Mehta, M. Kirk and B. Papirmeister, Formation of O6-ethylthioethyldeoxyguanosine from the reaction of chloroethyl ethyl sulfide with deoxyguanosine, *Cancer Res.*, 1984, **44**, 5698.
40. D. B. Ludlum, S. Kent and J. R. Mehta, Formation of O6-ethylthioethylguanine in DNA by reaction with the sulfur mustard, chloroethyl sulfide, and its apparent lack of repair by O6-alkylguanine-DNA alkyltransferase, *Carcinogenesis*, 1986, **7**, 1203.
41. A. Fidder, G. W. Moes and A. G. Scheffer, *et al.*, Synthesis, characterization, and quantitation of the major adducts formed between sulfur mustard and DNA of calf thymus and human blood, *Chem. Res. Toxicol.*, 1994, **7**, 199.
42. P. Brookes and P. D. Lawley, The reaction of mustard gas with nucleic acids in vitro and in vivo, *Biochem. J.*, 1960, **77**, 478.
43. P. Brookes and P. D. Lawley, The reaction of mono- and di-functional alkylating agents with nucleic acids, *Biochem. J.*, 1961, **80**, 496.
44. P. D. Lawley and P. Brookes, Interstrand cross-linking of DNA by difunctional alkylating agents, *J. Mol. Biol.*, 1967, **25**, 143.
45. L. Yue, Y. Wei and J. Chen, *et al.*, Abundance of four sulfur mustard-DNA adducts ex vivo and in vivo revealed by simultaneous quantification in stable isotope dilution-ultrahigh performance liquid chromatography-tandem mass spectrometry, *Chem. Res. Toxicol.*, 2014, **27**, 490.

46. S. Shahin, C. Cullinane and P. J. Gray, Mitochondrial and nuclear DNA damage induced by sulphur mustard in keratinocytes, *Chem.-Biol. Interact.*, 2001, **138**, 231.
47. K. A. Kreuter, S. B. Mahon and D. S. Mukai, *et al.*, Detection and monitoring of early airway injury effects of half-mustard (2-chloroethylethylsulfide) exposure using high-resolution optical coherence tomography, *J. Biomed. Opt.*, 2009, **14**, 044037.
48. A. Masta, P. J. Gray and D. R. Phillips, Nitrogen mustard inhibits transcription and translation in a cell free system, *Nucleic Acids Res.*, 1995, **23**, 3508.
49. A. Masta, P. J. Gray and D. R. Phillips, Molecular basis of nitrogen mustard effects on transcription processes: role of depurination, *Nucleic Acids Res.*, 1994, **22**, 3880.
50. M. A. E. Mol, R. M. van den Berg and H. P. Benschop, Proteomic assessment of sulfur mustard-induced protein adducts and other protein modifications in human epidermal keratinocytes, *Toxicol. Appl. Pharmacol.*, 2008, **230**, 97.
51. R. Loeber, E. Michaelson, Q. Fang, C. Campbell, A. E. Pegg and N. Tretyakova, Cross-linking of the DNA repair protein Omicron6-alkylguanine DNA alkyltransferase to DNA in the presence of antitumor nitrogen mustards, *Chem. Res. Toxicol.*, 2008, **21**, 787.
52. E. D. Michaelson-Richie, X. Ming and S. G. Codreanu, *et al.*, Mechlorethamine-induced DNA-protein cross-linking in human fibrosarcoma (HT1080) cells, *J. Proteome Res.*, 2011, **10**, 2785.
53. K. Kehe, K. Raithel, H. Kreppel, M. Jochum, F. Worek and H. Thiermann, Inhibition of poly(ADP-ribose) polymerase (PARP) influences the mode of sulfur mustard (SM)-induced cell death in HaCaT cells, *Arch. Toxicol.*, 2007, 1.
54. M. Debiak, K. Kehe and A. Bürkle, Role of poly(ADP-ribose) polymerase in sulfur mustard toxicity, *Toxicology*, 2009, **263**, 20.
55. Z. Zhang, B. P. Peters and N. A. Monteiro-Riviere, Assessment of sulfur mustard interaction with basement membrane components, *Cell Biol. Toxicol.*, 1995, **11**, 89.
56. D. Noort, E. R. Verheij, A. G. Hulst, L. P. de Jong and H. P. Benschop, Characterization of sulfur mustard induced structural modifications in human hemoglobin by liquid chromatography–tandem mass spectrometry, *Chem. Res. Toxicol.*, 1996, **9**, 781.
57. E. O. Price, J. R. Smith, C. R. Clark, J. J. Schlager and M. L. Shih, MALDI-ToF/MS as a diagnostic tool for the confirmation of sulfur mustard exposure, *J. Appl. Toxicol.*, 2000, **20**(**suppl. 1**), S193.
58. C. L. Gross, K. C. Giles and W. J. Smith, L-oxothiazolidine 4-carboxylate pretreatment of isolated human peripheral blood lymphocytes reduces sulfur mustard cytotoxicity, *Cell Biol. Toxicol.*, 1997, **13**, 167.
59. J. Liu, K. L. Powell, H. D. Thames and M. C. MacLeod, Detoxication of sulfur half-mustards by nucleophilic scavengers: robust activity of thiopurines, *Chem. Res. Toxicol.*, 2010, **23**, 488.

60. K. L. Powell, S. Boulware, H. Thames, K. M. Vasquez and M. C. MacLeod, 2,6-Dithiopurine blocks toxicity and mutagenesis in human skin cells exposed to sulfur mustard analogues, 2-chloroethyl ethyl sulfide and 2-chloroethyl methyl sulfide, *Chem. Res. Toxicol.*, 2010, **23**, 497.
61. S. Boulware, T. Fields and E. McIvor, *et al.*, 2,6-Dithiopurine, a nucleophilic scavenger, protects against mutagenesis in mouse skin treated in vivo with 2-(chloroethyl) ethyl sulfide, a mustard gas analog, *Toxicol. Appl. Pharmacol.*, 2012, **263**, 203.
62. C. M. Arroyo, R. J. Schafer, E. M. Kurt, C. A. Broomfield and A. J. Carmichael, Response of normal human keratinocytes to sulfur mustard: cytokine release, *J. Appl. Toxicol.*, 2000, **20**(**suppl. 1**), S63.
63. C. L. K. Sabourin, J. V. Rogers and Y. W. Choi, *et al.*, Time- and dose-dependent analysis of gene expression using microarrays in sulfur mustard-exposed mice, *J. Biochem. Mol. Toxicol.*, 2004, **18**, 300.
64. J. V. Rogers, Y. W. Choi and R. C. Kiser, *et al.*, Microarray analysis of gene expression in murine skin exposed to sulfur mustard, *J. Biochem. Mol. Toxicol.*, 2004, **18**, 289.
65. C. L. Sabourin, J. P. Petrali and R. P. Casillas, Alterations in inflammatory cytokine gene expression in sulfur mustard-exposed mouse skin, *J. Biochem. Mol. Toxicol.*, 2000, **14**, 291.
66. P. W. Wentz, J. Savory and R. E. Cross, Improved method for measurement of inorganic phosphate in serum with a centrifugal analyzer, *Clin. Chem.*, 1976, **22**, 257.
67. A. K. Jain, N. Tewari-Singh, S. Inturi, D. J. Orlicky, C. W. White and R. Agarwal, Histopathological and immunohistochemical evaluation of nitrogen mustard-induced cutaneous effects in SKH-1 hairless and C57BL/6 mice, *Exp. Toxicol. Pathol.*, 2014, **66**, 129.
68. A. Mantovani, Molecular pathways linking inflammation and cancer, *Curr. Mol. Med.*, 2010, **10**, 369.
69. B. Rebholz, K. Kehe, T. Ruzicka and R. A. Rupec, Role of NF-kappaB/RelA and MAPK pathways in keratinocytes in response to sulfur mustard, *J. Invest. Dermatol.*, 2008, **128**, 1626.
70. H.-Y. Ham, C.-W. Hong, S.-N. Lee, M.-S. Kwon, Y.-J. Kim and D.-K. Song, Sulfur mustard primes human neutrophils for increased degranulation and stimulates cytokine release *via* TRPM2/p38 MAPK signaling, *Toxicol. Appl. Pharmacol.*, 2012, **258**, 82.
71. S. Yazdani, M. H. Karimfar and A. A. Imani Fooladi, *et al.*, Nuclear factor κB1/RelA mediates the inflammation and/or survival of human airway exposed to sulfur mustard, *J. Recept. Signal Transduction Res.*, 2011, **31**, 367.
72. N. Tewari-Singh, A. K. Jain, S. Inturi, C. Agarwal, C. W. White and R. Agarwal, Silibinin attenuates sulfur mustard analog-induced skin injury by targeting multiple pathways connecting oxidative stress and inflammation, *PLoS One*, 2012, **7**, e46149.
73. A. K. Jain, N. Tewari-Singh, S. Inturi, D. J. Orlicky, C. W. White and R. Agarwal, Myeloperoxidase deficiency attenuates nitrogen mustard-induced skin injuries, *Toxicology*, 2014, **320**, 25.

74. N. Tewari-Singh, A. K. Jain and S. Inturi, *et al.*, Silibinin, dexamethasone, and doxycycline as potential therapeutic agents for treating vesicant-inflicted ocular injuries, *Toxicol. Appl. Pharmacol.*, 2012, **264**, 23.
75. A. T. Black, P. J. Hayden and R. P. Casillas, *et al.*, Expression of proliferative and inflammatory markers in a full-thickness human skin equivalent following exposure to the model sulfur mustard vesicant, 2-chloroethyl ethyl sulfide, *Toxicol. Appl. Pharmacol.*, 2010, **249**, 178.
76. U. Wormser, R. Langenbach, S. Peddada, A. Sintov, B. Brodsky and A. Nyska, Reduced sulfur mustard-induced skin toxicity in cyclooxygenase-2 knockout and celecoxib-treated mice, *Toxicol. Appl. Pharmacol.*, 2004, **200**, 40.
77. E. C. K. Yego and J. F. Dillman, Cytokine regulation by MAPK activated kinase 2 in keratinocytes exposed to sulfur mustard, *Toxicol. In Vitro*, 2013, **27**, 2067.
78. Y. Panahi, S. M. Davoudi, F. Beiraghdar and M. Amiri, Doxepin cream vs. betamethasone cream for treatment of chronic skin lesions due to sulfur mustard, *Skinmed*, 2011, **9**, 152.
79. S. C. Young, K. M. Fabio and M.-T. Huang, *et al.*, Investigation of anticholinergic and non-steroidal anti-inflammatory prodrugs which reduce chemically induced skin inflammation, *J. Appl. Toxicol.*, 2012, **32**, 135.
80. G. Amitai, R. Adani, E. Fishbein, H. Meshulam, I. Laish and S. Dachir, Bifunctional compounds eliciting anti-inflammatory and anti-cholinesterase activity as potential treatment of nerve and blister chemical agents poisoning, *J. Appl. Toxicol.*, 2006, **26**, 81.
81. Y.-C. Chang, J. D. Wang and R. A. Hahn, *et al.*, Therapeutic potential of a non-steroidal bifunctional anti-inflammatory and anti-cholinergic agent against skin injury induced by sulfur mustard, *Toxicol. Appl. Pharmacol.*, 2014, **280**, 236.
82. R. M. Herriott and W. H. Price, The formation of bacterial viruses in bacteria rendered nonviable by mustard gas, *J. Gen. Physiol.*, 1948, **32**, 63.
83. M. Fox and D. Scott, The genetic toxicology of nitrogen and sulphur mustard, *Mutat. Res.*, 1980, **75**, 131.
84. P. L. Ribeiro, R. S. Mitra and I. A. Bernstein, Assessment of the role of DNA damage and repair in the survival of primary cultures of rat cutaneous keratinocytes exposed to bis(2-chloroethyl)sulfide, *Toxicol. Appl. Pharmacol.*, 1991, **111**, 342.
85. N. A. Berger, Poly(ADP-ribose) in the cellular response to DNA damage, *Radiat. Res.*, 1985, **101**, 4.
86. A. Chiarugi, Poly(ADP-ribose) polymerase: killer or conspirator? The "suicide hypothesis" revisited, *Trends Pharmacol. Sci.*, 2002, **23**, 122.
87. F. J. Oliver, J. Ménissier-de Murcia and C. Nacci, *et al.*, Resistance to endotoxic shock as a consequence of defective NF-kappaB activation in poly (ADP-ribose) polymerase-1 deficient mice, *EMBO J.*, 1999, **18**, 4446.
88. D. B. Hinshaw, I. J. Lodhi, L. L. Hurley, K. B. Atkins and M. I. Dabrowska, Activation of poly [ADP-Ribose] polymerase in endothelial cells and keratinocytes: role in an in vitro model of sulfur mustard-mediated vesication, *Toxicol. Appl. Pharmacol.*, 1999, **156**, 17.

89. K. R. Bhat, B. J. Benton, D. S. Rosenthal, M. E. Smulson and R. Ray, Role of poly(ADP-ribose) polymerase (PARP) in DNA repair in sulfur mustard-exposed normal human epidermal keratinocytes (NHEK), *J. Appl. Toxicol.*, 2000, **20**(**suppl. 1**), S13.
90. D. S. Rosenthal, C. M. Simbulan-Rosenthal, S. Iyer, W. J. Smith, R. Ray and M. E. Smulson, Calmodulin, poly(ADP-ribose)polymerase and p53 are targets for modulating the effects of sulfur mustard, *J. Appl. Toxicol.*, 2000, **20**(**suppl. 1**), S43.
91. D. S. Rosenthal, C. M. Simbulan-Rosenthal and W. F. Liu, *et al.*, PARP determines the mode of cell death in skin fibroblasts, but not keratinocytes, exposed to sulfur mustard, *J. Invest. Dermatol.*, 2001, **117**, 1566.
92. K. R. Bhat, B. J. Benton and R. Ray, Poly (ADP-ribose) polymerase (PARP) is essential for sulfur mustard-induced DNA damage repair, but has no role in DNA ligase activation, *J. Appl. Toxicol.*, 2006, **26**, 452.
93. H. L. Meier, C. L. Gross and B. Papirmeister, 2,2'-Dichlorodiethyl sulfide (sulfur mustard) decreases NAD+ levels in human leukocytes, *Toxicol. Lett.*, 1987, **39**, 109.
94. H. L. Meier, C. B. Millard and J. Moser, Poly(ADP-ribose) polymerase inhibitors regulate the mechanism of sulfur mustard-initiated cell death in human lymphocytes, *J. Appl. Toxicol.*, 2000, **20**(**suppl. 1**), S93.
95. D. Steinritz, J. Emmler and M. Hintz, *et al.*, Apoptosis in sulfur mustard treated A549 cell cultures, *Life Sci.*, 2007, **80**, 2199.
96. H. L. Meier and C. B. Millard, Alterations in human lymphocyte DNA caused by sulfur mustard can be mitigated by selective inhibitors of poly(ADP-ribose) polymerase, *Biochim. Biophys. Acta*, 1998, **1404**, 367.
97. K. R. Bhat, B. J. Benton and R. Ray, DNA ligase I is an in vivo substrate of DNA-dependent protein kinase and is activated by phosphorylation in response to DNA double-strand breaks, *Biochemistry*, 2006, **45**, 6522.
98. R. Ray, C. M. Simbulan-Rosenthal and B. M. Keyser, *et al.*, Sulfur mustard induces apoptosis in lung epithelial cells *via* a caspase amplification loop, *Toxicology*, 2010, **271**, 94.
99. R. Ray, B. Keyser, B. Benton, A. Daher, C. M. Simbulan-Rosenthal and D. S. Rosenthal, Sulfur mustard induces apoptosis in cultured normal human airway epithelial cells: evidence of a dominant caspase-8-mediated pathway and differential cellular responses, *Drug Chem. Toxicol.*, 2008, **31**, 137.
100. D. S. Rosenthal, C. M. Simbulan-Rosenthal and S. Iyer, *et al.*, Sulfur mustard induces markers of terminal differentiation and apoptosis in keratinocytes *via* a Ca2+-calmodulin and caspase-dependent pathway, *J. Invest. Dermatol.*, 1998, **111**, 64.
101. M. I. Dabrowska, L. L. Becks, J. L. J. Lelli, M. G. Levee and D. B. Hinshaw, Sulfur mustard induces apoptosis and necrosis in endothelial cells, *Toxicol. Appl. Pharmacol.*, 1996, **141**, 568.
102. K. J. Smith, J. S. Graham, R. B. Moeller, C. V. Okerberg, H. Skelton and C. G. Hurst, Histopathologic features seen in sulfur mustard induced cutaneous lesions in hairless guinea pigs, *J. Cutaneous Pathol.*, 1995, **22**, 260.

103. K. J. Smith, H. G. Skelton, D. W. Hobson, F. M. Reid, J. A. Blank and C. G. Hurst, Cutaneous histopathologic features in weanling pigs after exposure to three different doses of liquid sulfur mustard, *Am. J. Dermatopathol.*, 1996, **18**, 515.
104. J. H. Calvet, M. Feuermann, B. Llorente, F. Loison, A. Harf and F. Marano, Comparative toxicity of sulfur mustard and nitrogen mustard on tracheal epithelial cells in primary culture, *Toxicol. In Vitro*, 1999, **13**, 859.
105. D. R. Green, *Means to an End*, 2011.
106. S. Orrenius, P. Nicotera and B. Zhivotovsky, Cell death mechanisms and their implications in toxicology, *Toxicol. Sci.*, 2011, **119**, 3.
107. D. S. Rosenthal, A. Velena and F.-P. Chou, *et al.*, Expression of dominant-negative Fas-associated death domain blocks human keratinocyte apoptosis and vesication induced by sulfur mustard, *J. Biol. Chem.*, 2003, **278**, 8531.
108. M. Sourdeval, C. Lemaire and A. Deniaud, *et al.*, Inhibition of caspase-dependent mitochondrial permeability transition protects airway epithelial cells against mustard-induced apoptosis, *Apoptosis*, 2006, **11**, 1545.
109. B. M. Keyser, D. K. Andres and E. Nealley, *et al.*, Postexposure application of Fas receptor small-interfering RNA to suppress sulfur mustard-induced apoptosis in human airway epithelial cells: implication for a therapeutic approach, *J. Pharmacol. Exp. Ther.*, 2013, **344**, 308.
110. T. Ghazanfari, Z. Sharifnia and R. Yaraee, *et al.*, Serum soluble Fas ligand and nitric oxide in long-term pulmonary complications induced by sulfur mustard: Sardasht-Iran Cohort Study, *Int. Immunopharmacol.*, 2009, **9**, 1489.
111. G. Pirzad, M. Jafari and S. Tavana, *et al.*, The Role of Fas-FasL Signaling Pathway in Induction of Apoptosis in Patients with Sulfur Mustard-Induced Chronic Bronchiolitis, *J. Toxicol.*, 2010, **2010**, 373612.
112. A. A. Brimfield, S. D. Soni, K. A. Trimmer, M. A. Zottola, R. E. Sweeney and J. S. Graham, Metabolic activation of sulfur mustard leads to oxygen free radical formation, *Free Radicals Biol. Med.*, 2012, **52**, 811.
113. V. Paromov, Z. Suntres, M. Smith and W. L. Stone, Sulfur mustard toxicity following dermal exposure: role of oxidative stress, and antioxidant therapy, *J. Burns Wounds*, 2007, **7**, e7.
114. K. Husain, S. N. Dube, K. Sugendran, R. Singh, S. Das Gupta and S. M. Somani, Effect of topically applied sulphur mustard on antioxidant enzymes in blood cells and body tissues of rats, *J. Appl. Toxicol.*, 1996, **16**, 245.
115. P. Pacher, J. S. Beckman and L. Liaudet, Nitric oxide and peroxynitrite in health and disease, *Physiol. Rev.*, 2007, **87**, 315.
116. T. W. Sawyer and D. Risk, Effects of selected arginine analogues on sulphur mustard toxicity in human and hairless guinea pig skin keratinocytes, *Toxicol. Appl. Pharmacol.*, 2000, **163**, 75.
117. T. W. Sawyer, Characterization of the protective effects of L-nitroarginine methyl ester (L-NAME) against the toxicity of sulphur mustard in vitro, *Toxicology*, 1998, **131**, 21.

118. T. W. Sawyer, Modulation of sulfur mustard toxicity by arginine analogues and related nitric oxide synthase inhibitors in vitro, *Toxicol. Sci.*, 1998, **46**, 112.
119. T. W. Sawyer, P. M. Lundy and M. T. Weiss, Protective effect of an inhibitor of nitric oxide synthase on sulphur mustard toxicity in vitro, *Toxicol. Appl. Pharmacol.*, 1996, **141**, 138.
120. D. Steinritz, A. Elischer and F. Balszuweit, *et al.*, Sulphur mustard induces time- and concentration-dependent regulation of NO-synthesizing enzymes, *Toxicol. Lett.*, 2009, **188**, 263.
121. H. C. O'Neill, D. J. Orlicky, T. B. Hendry-Hofer, J. E. Loader, B. J. Day and C. W. White, Role of reactive oxygen and nitrogen species in olfactory epithelial injury by the sulfur mustard analogue 2-chloroethyl ethyl sulfide, *Am. J. Respir. Cell Mol. Biol.*, 2011, **45**, 323.
122. D. Steinritz, A. Schmidt and T. Simons, *et al.*, Chlorambucil (nitrogen mustard) induced impairment of early vascular endothelial cell migration – Effects of α-linolenic acid and N-acetylcysteine, *Chem.-Biol. Interact.*, 2014, **219C**, 143.
123. N. Tewari-Singh, S. Inturi and A. K. Jain, *et al.*, Catalytic antioxidant AEOL 10150 treatment ameliorates sulfur mustard analog 2-chloroethyl ethyl sulfide-associated cutaneous toxic effects, *Free Radicals Biol. Med.*, 2014, **72**, 285.
124. T. McGovern, B. J. Day, C. W. White, W. S. Powell and J. G. Martin, AEOL10150: a novel therapeutic for rescue treatment after toxic gas lung injury, *Free Radicals Biol. Med.*, 2011, **50**, 602.
125. H. C. O'Neill, C. W. White and L. A. Veress, *et al.*, Treatment with the catalytic metalloporphyrin AEOL 10150 reduces inflammation and oxidative stress due to inhalation of the sulfur mustard analog 2-chloroethyl ethyl sulfide, *Free Radicals Biol. Med.*, 2010, **48**, 1188.
126. M. Ghanei, K. Abolmaali and J. Aslani, Efficacy of concomitant administration of clarithromycin and acetylcysteine in bronchiolitis obliterans in seventeen sulfur mustard—exposed patients: an open-label study, *Curr. Ther. Res.*, 2004, **65**, 495.
127. B. Jugg, S. Fairhall and A. Smith, *et al.*, N-acetyl-L-cysteine protects against inhaled sulfur mustard poisoning in the large swine, *Clin. Toxicol.*, 2013, **51**, 216.
128. S. Mukhopadhyay, S. Mukherjee, W. L. Stone, M. Smith and S. K. Das, Role of MAPK/AP-1 signaling pathway in the protection of CEES-induced lung injury by antioxidant liposome, *Toxicology*, 2009, **261**, 143.
129. S. Mukhopadhyay, S. Mukherjee, B. K. Ray, A. Ray, W. L. Stone and S. K. Das, Antioxidant liposomes protect against CEES-induced lung injury by decreasing SAF-1/MAZ-mediated inflammation in the guinea pig lung, *J. Biochem. Mol. Toxicol.*, 2010, **24**, 187.
130. N. Tewari-Singh, C. Agarwal, J. Huang, B. J. Day, C. W. White and R. Agarwal, Efficacy of glutathione in ameliorating sulfur mustard analog-induced toxicity in cultured skin epidermal cells and in SKH-1 mouse skin in vivo, *J. Pharmacol. Exp. Ther.*, 2011, **336**, 450.

131. D. Steinritz, B. Bölck and J. Schwarz, *et al.*, Effect of N-acetyl cysteine and alpha-linolenic acid on sulfur mustard caused impairment of in vitro endothelial tube formation, *Toxicol. Sci.*, 2010, **118**, 521.
132. T. Anand, R. Vijayaraghavan, P. V. L. Rao, I. Bansal and B. K. Bhattacharya, Attenuation of sulfur mustard toxicity by S-2(2-aminoethylamino) ethyl phenyl sulfide (DRDE-07) in mouse liver, *Toxicol. Mech. Methods*, 2011, **21**, 596.
133. V. Lomash, S. E. Jadhav, F. Ahmed, R. Vijayaraghavan and S. C. Pant, Evaluation of wound-healing formulation against sulphur mustard-induced skin injury in mice, *Hum. Exp. Toxicol.*, 2012, **31**, 588.
134. M. Pohanka, J. Sobotka, M. Jilkova and R. Stetina, Oxidative stress after sulfur mustard intoxication and its reduction by melatonin: efficacy of antioxidant therapy during serious intoxication, *Drug Chem. Toxicol.*, 2011, **34**, 85.
135. H. Ishida, R. Ray, J. Amnuaysirikul, K. Ishida and P. Ray, Nitric oxide synthase gene transfer overcomes the inhibition of wound healing by sulfur mustard in a human keratinocyte in vitro model, *ISRN Toxicol.*, 2012, **2012**, 190429.
136. X. Gao, R. Ray, Y. Xiao, P. E. Barker and P. Ray, Inhibition of sulfur mustard-induced cytotoxicity and inflammation by the macrolide antibiotic roxithromycin in human respiratory epithelial cells, *BMC Cell Biol.*, 2007, **8**, 17.
137. X. Gao, R. Ray, Y. Xiao and P. Ray, Suppression of inducible nitric oxide synthase expression and nitric oxide production by macrolide antibiotics in sulfur mustard-exposed airway epithelial cells, *Basic Clin. Pharmacol. Toxicol.*, 2008, **103**, 255.
138. X. Gao, R. Ray, Y. Xiao, K. Ishida and P. Ray, Macrolide antibiotics improve chemotactic and phagocytic capacity as well as reduce inflammation in sulfur mustard-exposed monocytes, *Pulm. Pharmacol. Ther.*, 2009, **23**, 97.
139. X. Gao, D. R. Anderson and A. W. Brown, *et al.*, Pathological studies on the protective effect of a macrolide antibiotic, roxithromycin, against sulfur mustard inhalation toxicity in a rat model, *Toxicol. Pathol.*, 2011, **39**, 1056.
140. A. A. Zarin, M. Behmanesh, M. Tavallaei, M. Shohrati and M. Ghanei, Overexpression of transforming growth factor (TGF)-beta1 and TGF-beta3 genes in lung of toxic-inhaled patients, *Exp. Lung Res.*, 2010, **36**, 284.
141. F. Balszuweit, H. John, A. Schmidt, K. Kehe, H. Thiermann and D. Steinritz, Silibinin as a potential therapeutic for sulfur mustard injuries, *Chem.-Biol. Interact.*, 2013, **206**, 496.
142. A. Tekiner, O. Yucel and A. K. Sargin, *et al.*, The effect of nitrogen mustard on the rat brain and the therapeutic value of proanthocyanidin, *Turk. Neurosurg.*, 2009, **19**, 360.
143. A. Tekiner, D. Yucel, M. A. Bayar, O. Yucel, Y. Erdem and J. Karakaya, The effect of Nitrogen Mustard on the enzymatic antioxidant defense of rat brain tissue and the therapeutic value of proanthocyanidin, *Turk. Neurosurg.*, 2011, **21**, 461.

144. M. Pohanka, J. Sobotka and R. Stetina, Sulfur mustard induced oxidative stress and its alteration by epigallocatechin gallate, *Toxicol. Lett.*, 2011, **201**, 105.
145. M. H. Boskabady, N. Vahedi, S. Amery and M. R. Khakzad, The effect of Nigella sativa alone, and in combination with dexamethasone, on tracheal muscle responsiveness and lung inflammation in sulfur mustard exposed guinea pigs, *J. Ethnopharmacol.*, 2011, **137**, 1028.
146. M. H. Boskabady, A. Tabatabayee, S. Amiri and N. Vahedi, The effect of vitamin E on pathological changes in kidney and liver of sulphur mustard-exposed guinea pigs, *Toxicol. Ind. Health*, 2012, **28**, 216.
147. Y. Panahi, A. Sahebkar and M. Amiri, *et al.*, Improvement of sulphur mustard-induced chronic pruritus, quality of life and antioxidant status by curcumin: results of a randomised, double-blind, placebo-controlled trial, *Br. J. Nutr.*, 2012, **108**, 1272.
148. Y. Panahi, A. Sahebkar, S. Parvin and A. Saadat, A randomized controlled trial on the anti-inflammatory effects of curcumin in patients with chronic sulphur mustard-induced cutaneous complications, *Ann. Clin. Biochem.*, 2012, **49**, 580.
149. A. Sahebkar, Baicalin as a potentially promising drug for the management of sulfur mustard induced cutaneous complications: a review of molecular mechanisms, *Cutaneous Ocul. Toxicol.*, 2012, **31**, 226.
150. T. Kadar, A. Amir and L. Cohen, *et al.*, Anti-VEGF therapy (bevacizumab) for sulfur mustard-induced corneal neovascularization associated with delayed limbal stem cell deficiency in rabbits, *Curr. Eye Res.*, 2014, **39**, 439.
151. M. A. Javadi, M. R. Jafarinasab, S. Feizi, F. Karimian and K. Negahban, Management of mustard gas-induced limbal stem cell deficiency and keratitis, *Ophthalmology*, 2011, **118**, 1272.
152. S. Dachir, M. Cohen and R. Sahar, *et al.*, Beneficial effects of activated macrophages on sulfur mustard-induced cutaneous burns, an in vivo experience, *Cutaneous Ocul. Toxicol.*, 2014, 1.
153. A. Schmidt, M. Scherer, H. Thiermann and D. Steinritz, Mesenchymal stem cells are highly resistant to sulfur mustard, *Chem.-Biol. Interact.*, 2013, **206**, 505.

CHAPTER 5

Clinical and Laboratory Diagnosis of Chemical Warfare Agent Exposure

FRANZ WOREK*[a], HORST THIERMANN[a], AND TIMO WILLE[a]

[a]Bundeswehr Institute of Pharmacology and Toxicology, Neuherbergstraße 11, 80937 Munich, Germany
*E-mail: franzworek@bundeswehr.org

5.1 Introduction

Highly toxic organophosphorus based (OP) nerve agents have been developed by different countries for use as chemical warfare agents (CWAs) since the 1930s.[1] Nerve agents have been repeatedly used during military conflicts,[2] against civilian populations[3] and by terrorists.[4] In the meantime, the production, storage and use of CWAs have been banned by the international community and compliance with the regulations of the Chemical Weapons Convention is controlled by the Organisation for the Prohibition of Chemical Weapons. However, the nerve agent sarin was repeatedly used against civilians in Syria in 2013,[5,6] emphasizing the continuing threat CWAs pose.

Exposure to nerve agents can result in life threatening toxic effects and requires rapid diagnosis and treatment. Typical signs of poisoning enable clinical diagnosis in cases of nerve agent exposure with rapid onset of toxic signs; however, these may be delayed in scenarios with low level and

Issues in Toxicology No. 27
Chemical Warfare Toxicology, Volume 2: Management of Poisoning
Edited by Franz Worek, John Jenner, and Horst Thiermann

Published by the Royal Society of Chemistry, www.rsc.org

percutaneous exposure to nerve agents. This demands the development and availability of laboratory tools for supporting the clinical diagnosis of nerve agent exposure and to provide decisive information for the initiation and optimization of specific antidotal treatment.

This chapter on clinical and laboratory diagnosis of CWA exposure will focus on the diagnosis of nerve agent exposure and will put an emphasis on differences in clinical signs of poisoning after inhalation and percutaneous exposure, and on novel developments in the field of laboratory diagnosis. The toxicology, clinical and laboratory diagnoses of exposure to vesicants, lung damaging agents and opioids are presented in Chapters 2 and 4 in Volume 1 and Chapters 4 and 8 in this book.

5.2 Structure and Mechanism

Highly toxic OP nerve agents are a heterogeneous group of phosphonates, phosphoramidates and phosphonothionates (Figure 5.1), and have been developed by different countries for use as CWAs since the 1930s.[1] The most relevant nerve agents are tabun (GA), sarin (GB), soman (GD), cyclosarin (GF), VX and Russian VX (VR; Figure 5.1). Modification of the phosphorus bound residues R1 and R2 allows the design of numerous derivatives with modified physicochemical properties and, in particular, even higher toxicities.[7–12] In addition, there are close structural and biochemical similarities between OP nerve agents and pesticides (Figure 5.1).[13–15]

OP nerve agents and pesticides interact with a variety of proteins[16] and are highly reactive with serine esterases, primarily acetylcholinesterase (AChE; EC 3.1.1.7), butyrylcholinesterase (BChE; EC 3.1.1.8) and carboxylesterase (CaE; EC 3.1.1.1).[14,17–20] The acute toxicity of nerve agents is due to covalent binding to a serine residue of the catalytic triad at the base of a narrow gorge of AChE (Figure 5.2).[21,22] Nerve agent induced AChE inhibition impairs its physiological function, *i.e.* hydrolysis of the neurotransmitter acetylcholine.[23] This leads to accumulation of acetylcholine at cholinergic synapses throughout the body and overstimulation of muscarinic and nicotinic receptors.[24–26]

Nerve agent inhibited AChE underlies the post-inhibitory reactions that may affect the course of poisoning, the persistence of clinical signs and that are important for the therapeutic efficacy of specific antidotes, *i.e.* oximes (Figure 5.2).[18] Spontaneous hydrolysis of nerve agent–AChE conjugates results in spontaneous regeneration of the enzyme's activity and cessation of the toxic signs if no residual agent is present in the body. This reaction does not occur with human AChE inhibited by tabun, sarin, soman or cyclosarin, and is slow with VX and VR inhibited AChE, with a half-time ($t_{1/2}$) of 33 and 18 h, respectively.[27] Spontaneous dealkylation ('aging') of a nerve agent–AChE conjugate is exceptionally fast with soman inhibited human AChE ($t_{1/2} \approx 2$ min), but substantially slower with other nerve agents ($t_{1/2} = 3$ to >100 h).[28] This reaction does not influence the clinical course of poisoning but affects the ability of nucleophiles to remove the OP moiety from the enzyme.[29]

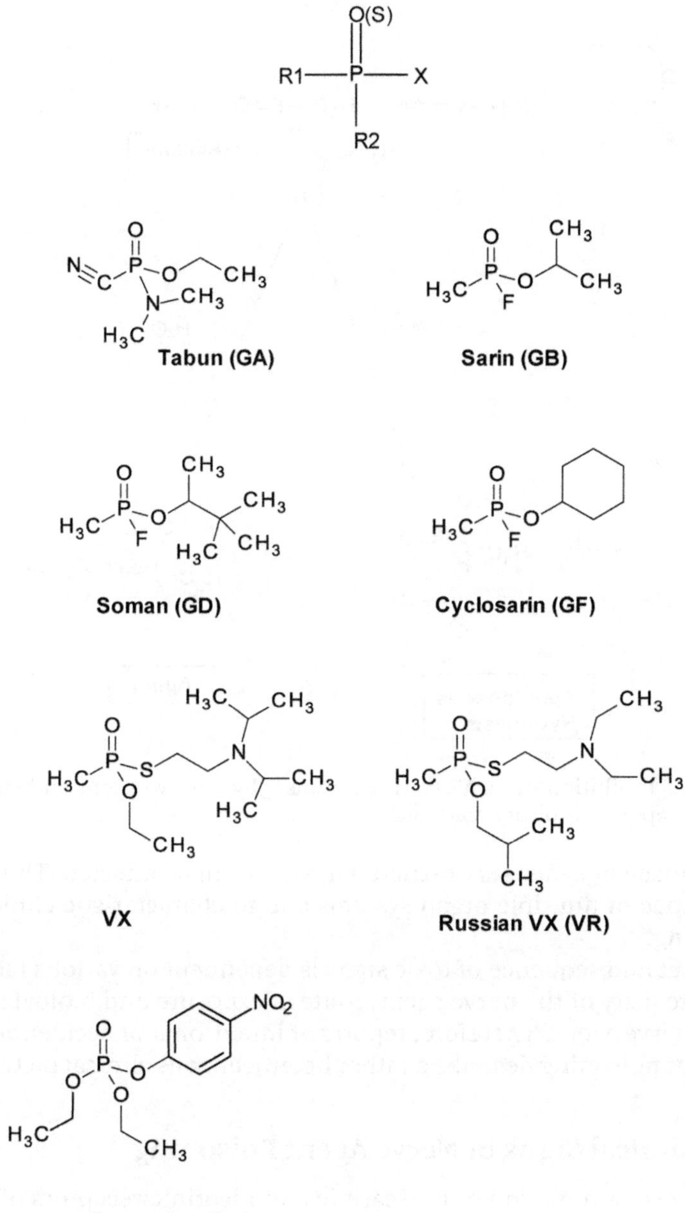

Figure 5.1 Generic structure of OP compounds and chemical structure of nerve agents and a model pesticide (paraoxon-ethyl).

5.3 Clinical Diagnosis

Inhibition of AChE by nerve agents is followed by an impairment of neurotransmission in the central and peripheral cholinergic system.[1] In consequence, neurotransmission in the central and autonomous system, as well as

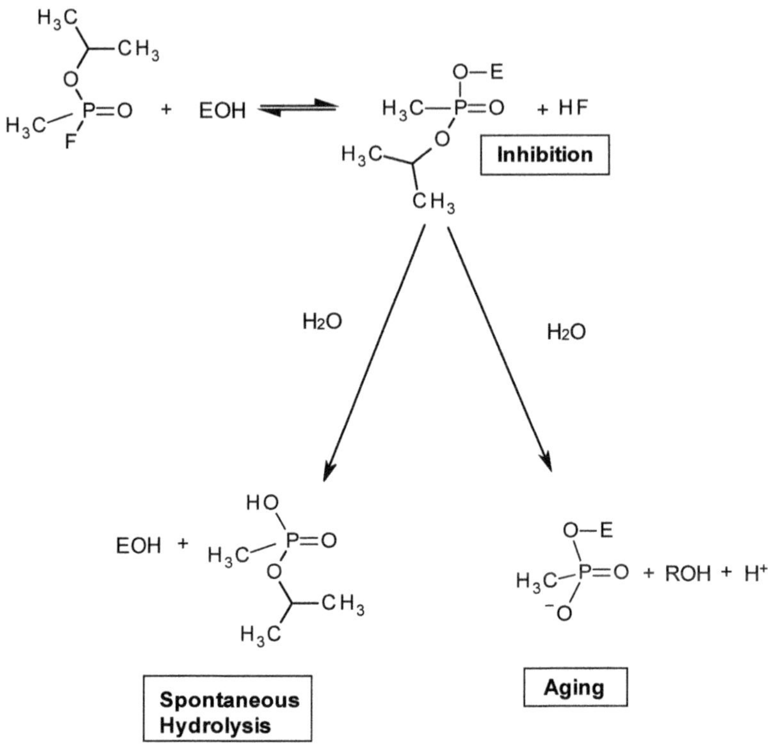

Figure 5.2 Inhibition of AChE (serine esterase) by a nerve agent and subsequent post-inhibitory reactions.

at neuromuscular synapses of striated muscles will be affected. This leads to a disturbance of multiple organ systems and to characteristic clinical signs of poisoning.

The onset and sequence of toxic signs is dependent on various factors, *i.e.* dose and toxicity of the nerve agent, route of exposure and biological stability of the nerve agent. Therefore, reports of intentional or accidental human nerve agent poisoning describe a rather heterogeneous clinical picture.[24,30–34]

5.3.1 Clinical Signs of Nerve Agent Poisoning

The acute overstimulation of muscarinic and nicotinic receptors of the central and peripheral cholinergic system induces increased activity of different parts of the central nervous system, of pre- and post-ganglionic synapses of parasympathetic nerves, of preganglionic synapses of sympathetic nerves and of neuromuscular synapses of striated muscles, including respiratory muscles (Table 5.1).

Figure 5.3 gives an overview of the most important clinical signs of nerve agent poisoning in relation to the severity of intoxication. Depending on the exposure route and nerve agent dose, the manifestation of certain signs may

Table 5.1 Toxic nerve agent effects in relation to cholinergic receptor subtypes.

Cholinergic receptor	Target organ	Clinical signs
Muscarinic	Glands	Rhinorrhea, lachrymation, salivation, sweating, bronchorrhea
	Smooth muscle	Miosis, accommodation disorder, intestinal cramps, involuntary defecation and micturition, bradycardia, arrhythmia
Nicotinic	Skeletal muscle	Fasciculation, cramps, weakness
	Autonomic ganglia	Tachycardia, hypertension, pallor
Muscarinic/nicotinic	Central nervous system	Dizziness, restlessness, anxiety, confusion, tremor, convulsions, respiratory depression

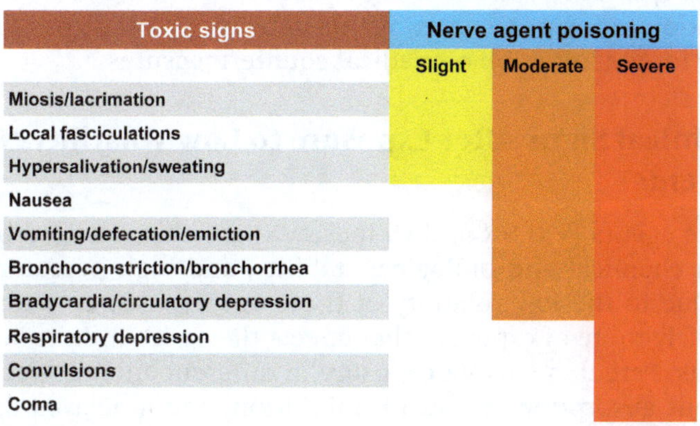

Figure 5.3 Toxic signs of nerve agent poisoning in relation to severity of intoxication.

vary and in the course of poisoning signs may aggravate, *i.e.* an initially mild poisoning may develop into a severe and life threatening state, especially in the case of percutaneous exposure.

5.3.2 Clinical Signs After Exposure to Volatile Nerve Agents

The exposure of unprotected individuals to volatile nerve agents, *e.g.* sarin, soman and cyclosarin, will result in local effects at accessible mucous membranes (eye, nasopharynx, trachea and bronchi) and, after absorption of the agent into the systemic circulation, in widespread systemic effects.[24,30,31,33,34] Reports on human volunteer studies, accidental exposures and nerve agent attacks consistently showed a rapid onset of signs, *i.e.* within minutes. The most common sign in casualties of the Tokyo subway sarin attack was miosis (80–99%), mostly connected with eye pain, visual darkness, conjunctival injection and rhinorrhea, which was obviously a local effect of the sarin vapor.[4,34,35] Other frequent signs, *e.g.* dyspnea, cough, chest oppression and fasciculations, may have been primarily local, while other signs, *e.g.* nausea, vomiting, weakness, decreased consciousness and agitation, must be attributed to the systemic effects of absorbed sarin. From these reports, miosis must be considered as an early and extremely sensitive indicator of exposure to a volatile nerve agent.

This assumption is supported by reports on the secondary exposure of medical staff to sarin vapor from casualties of the Tokyo subway sarin attack.[36] Symptomatic patients were transferred into the treatment facility without prior decontamination and the evaporation of sarin from hair, skin and clothes resulted in contamination of 13 out of 15 medical doctors. Miosis and dim vision were the most frequent signs (11 out of 15) followed by rhinorrhea (8 out of 15), six doctors required atropine to counteract the signs of sarin poisoning.

Finally, a rapid onset of cholinergic overstimulation can be anticipated after inhalation exposure to nerve agents and the typical signs of poisoning are decisive for the initiation of medical countermeasures.

5.3.3 Clinical Signs After Exposure to Low Volatility Nerve Agents

V-type nerve agents (VX, VR and Chinese VX) are characterized by low volatility, high chemical and biological stability, and high percutaneous toxicity.[7,37,38] Due to the low volatility of these agents, skin contamination is the most likely route of exposure that affects the onset and the sequence of clinical signs. Percutaneous VX exposure in different animal species results in slow agent absorption and AChE inhibition, and a delayed appearance of unbound VX in the systemic circulation.[39–43] Figure 5.4 exemplifies the different toxicokinetics of inhaled sarin and percutaneous VX exposure. Sarin inhalation results in a rapid increase of the agent in the systemic circulation followed by fast degradation by endogenous detoxification mechanisms.[44,45] In contrast, percutaneous exposure to VX results in a delayed and slow increase in agent concentration in the systemic circulation followed by a steady-state phase over a prolonged time period.[40,46] This toxicokinetic behavior induces a delayed onset of clinical signs; depending on the model this can take up to several hours.[39,42,47,48] Hereby, animal data indicate that the time period between the onset of first clinical signs and the manifestation of severe, life threatening signs, *e.g.* apnea, may be short.[39] The sequence of signs may be dependent on the animal species. In guinea pigs, chewing was followed by shivering, salivation, tremor and finally respiratory distress, while in anesthetized swine the sequence was mastication, miosis, salivation and then respiratory distress.

A larger number of human volunteer studies with percutaneous VX exposure have been performed in the past, but only a few results have been published in the open literature.[49] In these trials, sub-lethal VX doses were applied to different body regions and a common feature was a long delay until a decrease in cholinesterase activity could be recorded. Moderate

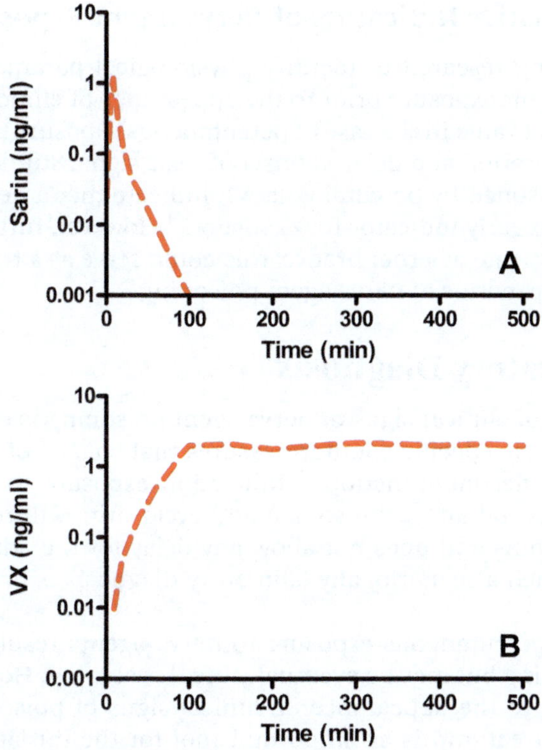

Figure 5.4 Simulated nerve agent concentrations after inhaled sarin (A) and percutaneous VX exposure (B). Data were taken from studies in guinea pigs (sarin) and swine (VX).[44,46]

clinical signs appeared after several hours and were correlated to the level of AChE inhibition.

Only a limited amount of data on homicidal human VX exposure is available in the open literature. One individual was exposed percutaneously on the back to an unknown amount of VX and experienced seizures, coma, sweating, fasciculations and cyanosis but no miosis.[50] A second individual was poisoned with a hypodermic VX injection to the neck.[51] The man suffered from cardiorespiratory arrest, miosis, sweating, fasciculations, diarrhea and hypothermia. In both cases, the time between exposure and the onset of clinical signs was not reported; however, these cases indicate that in percutaneous human VX poisoning local fasciculations at the exposure site may be an early indicator for exposure to VX.

The slow absorption of V-agents after percutaneous exposure leads to a delayed distribution of the agents in the systemic circulation and target tissues, and to a substantial retardation in the onset of clinical signs. Hence, early indicators are needed to initiate rapid decontamination and administration of specific antidotes prior to the manifestation of life threatening signs of poisoning.[52,53]

5.3.4 Alternative Indicators of Nerve Agent Exposure

There is ongoing research to identify physiological parameters for recognizing nerve agent exposure prior to the appearance of clinical signs, which would be of great value in the case of percutaneous exposure to V-agents with slow agent absorption and delayed onset of toxic signs. Studies in conscious guinea pigs poisoned by percutaneous VX indicate that a decrease of heart rate could be an early indicator for exposure.[54] However, further studies are needed to investigate whether bradycardia could serve as a trigger to treat in more realistic scenarios of nerve agent poisoning.

5.4 Laboratory Diagnosis

The evaluation of clinical signs of nerve agent poisoning is essential for the decision to initiate specific countermeasures that consist of antidotal treatment and skin decontamination.[55] Inhalation exposure to volatile G-type nerve agents, *e.g.* tabun, sarin, soman and cyclosarin, will result in a rapid onset of symptoms and does not allow any delay for the administration of antidotes. In such a scenario, any laboratory diagnosis is only of confirmatory value.

In contrast, percutaneous exposure to nerve agents results in a delayed onset of poisoning but may be eventually life threatening. Here, a laboratory diagnosis prior to the appearance of clinical signs of poisoning can serve as a trigger to treat and is an important tool for the initiation of medical countermeasures.

At present, only the analysis of blood samples is a meaningful tool for the diagnosis of nerve agent exposure as well as for the definitive verification of exposure to these CWAs.[56,57] Different parameters were investigated for this purpose:

- Determination of AChE activity in whole blood and BChE activity in plasma;[58]
- Identification and quantification of unbound nerve agent in plasma or whole blood;[59]
- Identification of nerve agent metabolites in plasma and urine;[60,61]
- Fluoride induced reactivation of inhibited AChE or BChE isolated from whole blood or plasma;[62,63]
- Digestion of nerve agent inhibited BChE or albumin followed by analysis of phosphyl–protein adducts.[64–66]

Hereby, the analysis of unbound nerve agents, nerve agent metabolites and protein adducts is laborious, time consuming and requires sophisticated laboratory equipment and well trained personnel. In view of these drawbacks these parameters are inadequate for diagnostic purposes but essential tools for the retrospective verification of nerve agent exposure, and will be discussed in detail in Chapter 6.

5.4.1 Cholinesterases as Diagnostic Markers

Cholinesterases are the primary target of nerve agents, and AChE and BChE activities in blood samples are essential parameters for supporting the clinical diagnosis of nerve agent exposure and can provide decisive information for the initiation and optimization of specific antidotal treatment.[58,67] At present, determination of cholinesterase activity is the only method for rapid and onsite laboratory diagnosis.

Numerous human volunteer studies, as well as accidental and homicidal exposure to nerve agents provide convincing evidence that erythrocyte AChE and plasma BChE activities are sensitive parameters for the diagnosis of nerve agent exposure.[24,30–33,49,68–70] Ongoing inhibition of AChE and BChE activities closely reflects the increase of nerve agent concentration in the blood, which is of importance in the case of slow transfer of agents from the skin into the systemic circulation.

Synaptic AChE is not obtainable for direct measurement, but erythrocyte AChE can be analyzed easily in small blood samples. In humans, AChE is encoded by a single gene,[23] and numerous experimental and clinical studies have provided convincing data that erythrocyte AChE is highly comparable to synaptic AChE and therefore may serve as a surrogate parameter for diagnostic purposes.[71–74] In contrast, marked structural and kinetic differences between human AChE and BChE have to be considered.[75,76] These differences are primarily related to aging and oxime reactivation kinetics of nerve agent inhibited AChE and BChE, and are less relevant for the inhibition by nerve agents. Hence, determination of the activity of human erythrocyte AChE and plasma BChE may be considered as a suitable parameter for the diagnosis of nerve agent exposure, while only AChE activity is considered as a valuable tool for monitoring the efficacy of oxime therapy.[76]

Numerous assays for the analysis of human AChE and BChE activity in blood and plasma have been developed in the past decades and their suitability has been reviewed extensively.[58,77–80] At present, the spectrophotometric Ellman assay[81] is widely used and various modifications of the original procedure have been proposed.[58]

The Ellman assay allows simple, rapid and cheap determination of cholinesterase activity in blood and plasma. Figure 5.5 shows the principle of this assay, which is based on the hydrolysis of the substrate acetylthiocholine (ATCh) or butyrylthiocholine (BTCh) by AChE or BChE, followed by reaction of thiocholine with the chromogen 5,5′-dithio-bis-2-nitrobenzoic acid (DTNB) and formation of yellow thionitrobenzoate (TNB^-), which can be analyzed photometrically. Hereby, BChE activity can be determined selectively with BTCh in plasma and whole blood samples, while ATCh allows the analysis of AChE and BChE activity in whole blood samples. Selective determination of AChE activity in whole blood requires the addition of a selective BChE inhibitor.[58]

The original Ellman assay is accompanied by a number of drawbacks.[82] Analysis of AChE activity in whole blood samples at the wavelength originally

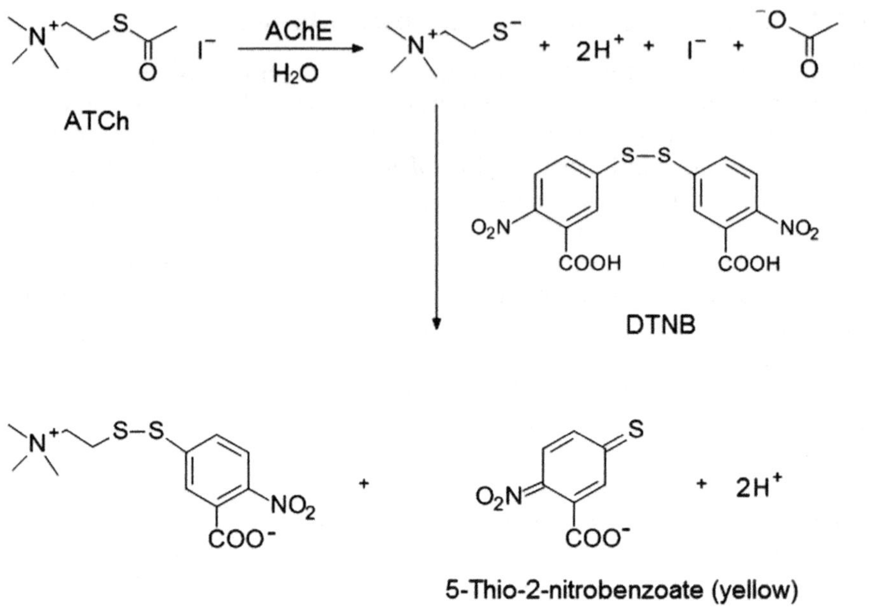

Figure 5.5 Schematic of the reactions of the spectrophotometric Ellman assay for the determination of AChE activity.

used by Ellman, 412 nm, results in an annoying disturbance caused by hemoglobin absorbance, and the BChE inhibitor quinidine lacks specificity. This led to modifications of the Ellman assay in order to increase its sensitivity and specificity. Use of a different wavelength, *i.e.* 436–470 nm, markedly improves the TNB^- : hemoglobin ratio, and replacement of quinidine with ethopropazine enables a more selective and sensitive determination of AChE activity in whole blood samples.[82,83]

5.4.2 Onsite Determination of Cholinesterase Activity

In the meantime, multiple applications of the Ellman assay were developed and implemented on microplate based and fully automated robot assisted liquid handling systems for high throughput analysis of multiple blood samples.[84,85] A major disadvantage of laboratory based systems for the analysis of AChE and BChE activity in nerve agent exposure scenarios is the need to handle and to transport blood samples adequately to minimize *ex vivo* reactions between cholinesterases and nerve agents, and to minimize the time delay between blood sampling and analysis.

This called for the development of technologies for the immediate onsite analysis of AChE and BChE activities.[67] Some 30 years ago, a simple ready to use kit, based on the Ellman assay, was developed and is marketed by EQM Research Inc. (Cincinnati, OH, USA). This mobile kit has been successfully tested in human OP pesticide poisoning.[86]

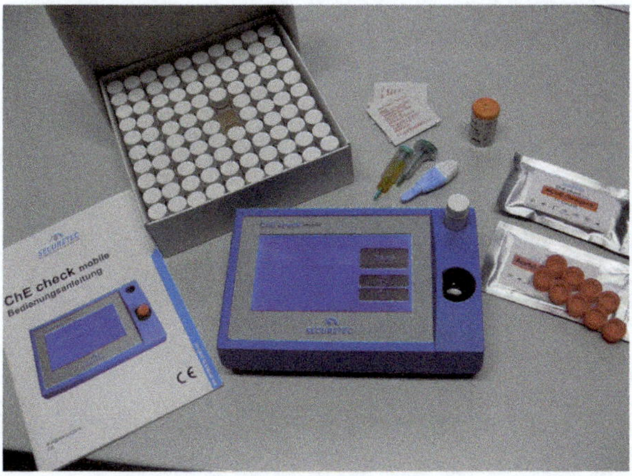

Figure 5.6 Components of the mobile assay kit for the onsite determination of AChE and BChE activity in whole blood (ChE check mobile).

Recently, a novel mobile kit was developed by Securetec Detektions-Systeme AG (Brunnthal, Germany; http://www.securetec.net) in cooperation with the German Armed Forces. The ChE check mobile test-kit (Figure 5.6) includes a number of advanced features and allows the selective, sensitive and reproducible determination of AChE or BChE activity in a 10 µl capillary or venous blood sample within 4 min. The test-kit includes two components, one is a reagent kit for the determination of AChE or BChE activity consisting of vials with 2 ml of buffer and a white transport cap and reagent caps for AChE (red) or BChE (yellow), as well as capillaries for EDTA blood (10 µl). The red AChE reagent caps contain lyophilized DTNB, the substrate ATCh and the selective BChE inhibitor AS1397 (Figure 5.7). For the determination of BChE activity the yellow reagent caps are stocked with DTNB and the substrate BTCh.

The second component is a small photometer with an LED set at 470 nm. A large touchscreen allows patient data input, menu control and display of instructions, results and explanations. Power supply is achieved *via* (rechargeable) batteries or a power outlet. The results are stored and can be exported *via* a USB hub. Enzyme activities can be determined at ambient temperature (10–50 °C) and are normalized to 37 °C. In addition, AChE activity refers to the hemoglobin content of the blood dilution, which minimizes potential dilution errors.

The ChE check is an easy to use assay kit that can be executed with minimal training. The whole assay procedure consists of a few steps:

- Blank measurement
- Blood collection and hemoglobin measurement
- Replacement of the white transport cap with red AChE cap or yellow BChE cap
- Measurement of AChE or BChE activity

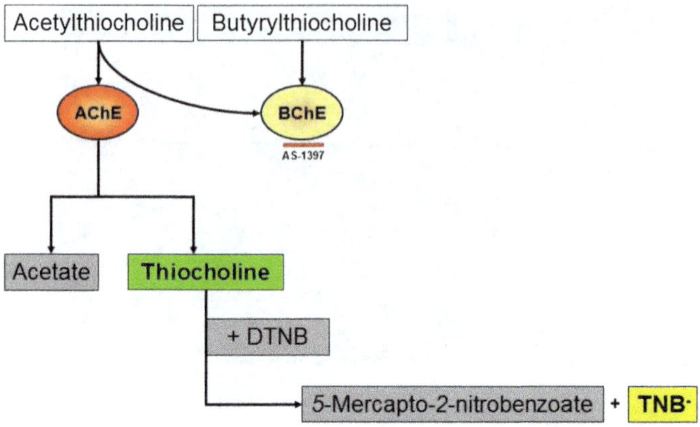

Figure 5.7 Schematic of the reactions of the modified Ellman assay for the determination of AChE and BChE activity with the mobile assay kit (ChE check mobile).

Enzyme activities are given as U gHb^{-1} and U l^{-1} for AChE and BChE, respectively, and information is shown on the display regarding whether the determined value is in the normal range or depressed. Additional advice for the evaluation of the test result can be retrieved, a valuable feature for users with little knowledge on nerve agent poisoning.

The activity of human erythrocyte AChE and plasma BChE underlies large inter-individual variations with a wide range of normal values.[87–89] Intra-individual variations of human erythrocyte AChE activity are low over a prolonged time period, while activity of human BChE activity shows larger variations.[90,91] Hence, knowledge of baseline erythrocyte AChE activity values enables the evaluation of partial enzyme inhibition and the immediate diagnosis of low level nerve agent exposure or slow onset of nerve agent poisoning, *e.g.* after percutaneous VX contamination.

In conclusion, determination of AChE or BChE activity in blood is at present the only laboratory parameter to give an indication of exposure to nerve agents and to support the clinical diagnosis of nerve agent poisoning.[58] Repetitive analysis of AChE activity can give information on the effectiveness of oximes in reactivating nerve agent inhibited enzymes, but cannot provide a definitive explanation if treatment with an oxime fails to reactivate AChE.[57] Reasons for an insufficient oxime effect may be rapid aging of the inhibited AChE, a specific problem of soman poisoning,[92] the inability of an administered oxime to reactivate AChE inhibited by a certain nerve agent, *e.g.* HI-6 in the case of tabun poisoning,[27] or poisoning with a high nerve agent dose resulting in a re-inhibition of reactivated AChE by excess nerve agent.[93]

5.4.3 Therapeutic Monitoring: The Cholinesterase Status

The investigation of clinical courses of OP pesticide poisoning revealed that, besides determination of AChE and BChE activity, additional laboratory parameters are needed to enable a proper evaluation of the effectiveness of

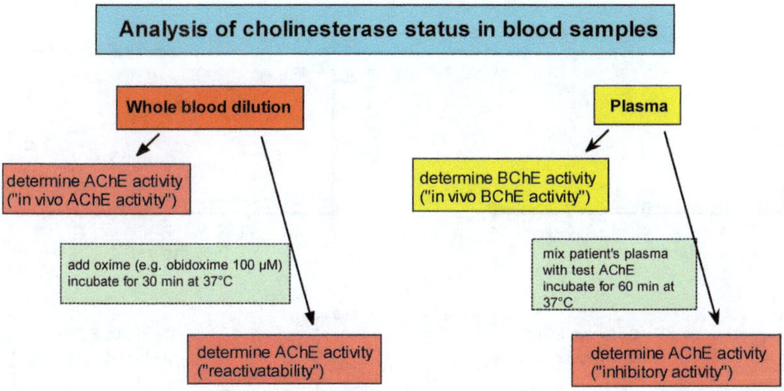

Figure 5.8 Schematic of the reactions of the cholinesterase status assay for the analysis of AChE and BChE activity, reactivatability and inhibitory activity in patient blood samples.

oxime therapy.[93–95] This led to the development and clinical validation of a set of laboratory parameters, the cholinesterase status.[58,96,97] This test battery consists of four independent assays (Figure 5.8):

- Determination of erythrocyte AChE activity in a patient blood sample or blood dilution (*in vivo* AChE activity);
- Determination of plasma BChE activity in a patient plasma sample (*in vivo* BChE activity);
- Determination of maximum reactivatability of AChE by incubation of a patient blood dilution with a specified oxime concentration for a defined time period followed by determination of AChE activity (reactivatability);
- Determination of inhibitory activity by incubation of a patient plasma sample with test AChE for a defined time period followed by determination of AChE activity (inhibitory activity).

Determination of the *in vivo* AChE and BChE activities gives information on their actual levels in the patient's blood. Dilution of a patient's blood sample results in a substantial decrease in nerve agent concentration and incubation with a supratherapeutic oxime concentration, *e.g.* 100 µM obidoxime, provides information on the maximum reactivation that could be achieved by an administered oxime. Finally, the incubation of patient plasma with test AChE and subsequent determination of AChE activity indicates the presence of the nerve agent in the blood. Repetitive determination of the cholinesterase status provides essential information on the changes in AChE and BChE activities over time and allows a rational assessment as to whether oxime therapy should be maintained or discontinued. Figure 5.9 presents the cholinesterase status of simulated soman (Figure 5.9A and B) and VX intoxications (Figure 5.9C and D) with oxime treatment. In both examples, the determination of AChE and BChE activities would result in

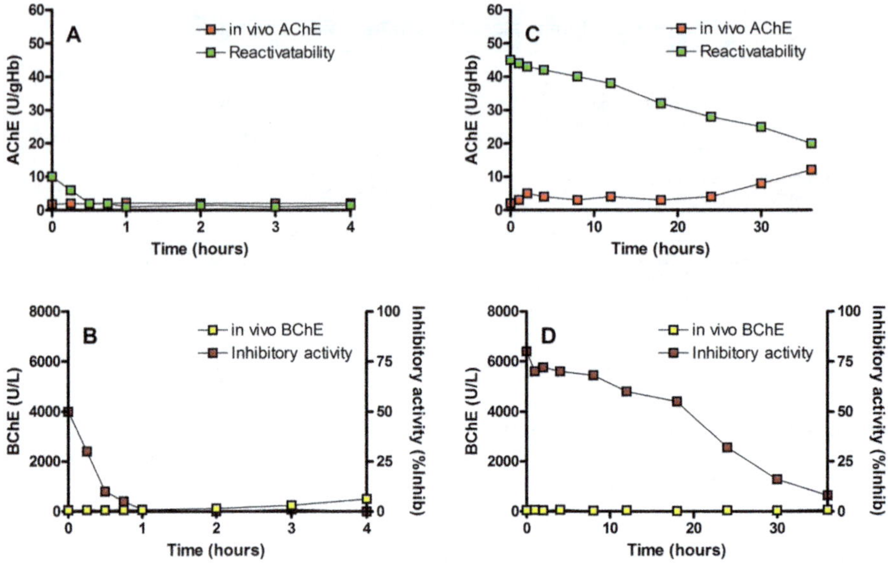

Figure 5.9 Simulated cholinesterase status in soman (A and B) and VX poisoning (C and D) with oxime therapy.

almost completely inhibited enzyme and would indicate that the continuously administered oxime is ineffective. However, only the additional determination of reactivatability and inhibitory activity provides an explanation for the lack of oxime effect. In the case of soman poisoning the rapid aging of AChE prevents reactivation by an oxime (Figure 5.9A). The rapid decrease of inhibitory activity demonstrates that no excess inhibitor is present after 1 h and that continuation of oxime therapy should not have any benefit for the patient (Figure 5.9B). In contrast, the simulated VX poisoning shows that the administered oxime should be able to reactivate inhibited AChE (Figure 5.9C; reactivatability), but the prolonged presence of inhibitory activity initially prevents net reactivation of AChE (Figure 5.9C). A decrease of the inhibitory activity, *i.e.* decrease of VX concentration (Figure 5.9D), results in a moderate increase of *in vivo* AChE activity at a later stage. Due to the slow aging $t_{1/2}$ of VX inhibited AChE, the ongoing administration of oxime should prevent aging of at least some of the synaptic AChE and should result in a relevant reactivation of the enzyme after clearance of the nerve agent.

The cholinesterase status was originally developed for use with spectrophotometers and robot assisted microplate readers.[98] In order to provide an application of the cholinesterase status for onsite use, the ChE check mobile system was modified and is now available as a ChE status monitor assay kit (Securetec Detektions-Systeme AG) for the determination of the cholinesterase status (Figure 5.10). This handy device needs minimal infrastructure, *i.e.* a centrifuge for plasma preparation, pipet and power supply, and is intended for use in the field or rural hospitals. The kit consists of a photometer with an incorporated temperature controlled (37 °C) incubation unit, vials, reagent

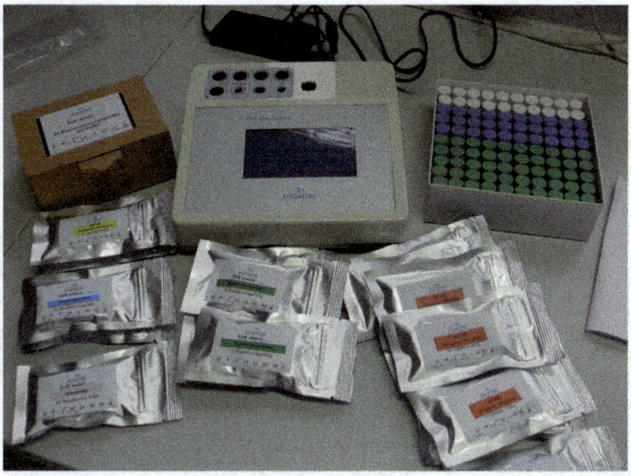

Figure 5.10 Components of the assay kit for onsite determination of the cholinesterase status in whole blood and plasma (ChE status monitor).

caps for AChE and BChE activity determination, and reagent cups with lyophilized oxime and test AChE for the determination of reactivatability and inhibitory activity, respectively. Again, the assay procedure is menu driven and can be performed with minimal training. The kit enables the monitoring of two intoxicated patients over a prolonged time period and allows the therapeutic monitoring of oxime treated nerve agent poisoned patients in the field.

5.5 Summary and Outlook

Exposure to nerve agents leads to specific clinical signs of cholinergic overstimulation. The time to onset and the sequence of clinical signs is dependent on the nerve agent dose and exposure route. In the case of exposure to nerve agent vapor, the rapid onset of signs is decisive for the initiation of medical countermeasures. In contrast, the delayed onset of signs after percutaneous exposure to nerve agents calls for alternative indicators as the trigger to treat parameters.

At present, the determination of AChE and BChE activity is the only feasible laboratory tool for the confirmation of a clinical diagnosis of nerve agent exposure, but is an invaluable tool for the pre-symptomatic diagnosis of percutaneous nerve agent exposure.

The determination of the cholinesterase status is an easy to use tool for therapeutic monitoring in nerve agent poisoning requiring oxime therapy, and can provide essential information for a decision on the duration of oxime administration.

In the meantime, ready to use kits for the onsite diagnostic determination of AChE and BChE activities in human blood and for bedside therapeutic monitoring utilizing the cholinesterase status have been developed and implemented.

The need for early indicators as a trigger to treat in percutaneous nerve agent exposure calls for the development of novel devices for the individualized and repetitive determination of AChE activity.

References

1. T. C. Marrs, Toxicology of organophosphate nerve agents, in *Chemical warfare agents: Toxicology and treatment*, ed. T. C. Marrs, R. L. Maynard and F. R. Sidell, John Wiley & Sons Ltd., Chichester, 2007, pp. 191–221.
2. R. M. Black, R. J. Clarke, R. W. Read and M. T. J. Reid, Application of gas chromatography-mass spectrometry and gas chromatography-tandem mass spectrometry to the analysis of chemical warfare samples, found to contain residues of the nerve agent sarin, sulphur mustard and their degradation products, *J. Chromatogr. A*, 1994, **662**, 301–321.
3. C. MacIlwain, Study proves Iraq used nerve gas, *Nature*, 1993, **363**, 3.
4. T. Okumura, T. Nomura, T. Suzuki, M. Sugita, Y. Takeuchi and T. Naito, *et al.* The dark morning: the experiences and lessons learned from the Tokyo subway sarin attack, in *Chemical warfare agents: Toxicology and treatment*, ed. T. C. Marrs, R. L. Maynard and F. R. Sidell, John Wiley & Sons Ltd., Chichester, 2007, pp. 277–285.
5. R. Pita and J. Domingo, The use of chemical weapons in the Syrian conflict, *Toxics*, 2014, **2**, 391–402.
6. A. Eisenkraft, D. Gilburd, M. Kassirer and Y. Kreiss, What can we learn on medical preparedness from the use of chemical agents against civilians in Syria?, *Am. J. Emerg. Med.*, 2014, **32**, 186.
7. R. M. Black and J. M. Harrison, The chemistry of organophosphorus chemical warfare agents, in *The chemistry of organophosphorus compounds*, ed. F. R. Hartley, John Wiley & Sons, Chichester, 1996, pp. 781–840.
8. M. I. Kabachnik, A. P. Brestkin, N. N. Godovikov, M. J. Michelson, E. V. Rozengart and V. I. Rozengart, Hydrophobic areas on the active surface of cholinesterases, *Pharmacol. Rev.*, 1970, **22**, 355–388.
9. N. Aurbek, N. M. Herkert, M. Koller, H. Thiermann and F. Worek, Kinetic analysis of interactions of different sarin and tabun analogues with human acetylcholinesterase and oximes: Is there a structure–activity relationship?, *Chem.–Biol. Interact.*, 2010, **187**, 215–219.
10. F. Worek, N. M. Herkert, M. Koller, N. Aurbek and H. Thiermann, Interaction of pentylsarin analogues with human acetylcholinesterase: A kinetic study, *Toxicol. Lett.*, 2009, **187**, 119–123.
11. A. Bartling, F. Worek, L. Szinicz and H. Thiermann, Enzyme-kinetic investigation of different sarin analogues reacting with human acetylcholinesterase and butyrylcholinesterase, *Toxicology*, 2007, **233**, 166–172.
12. S. N. Moralev and E. V. Rozengart, *Comparative enzymology of cholinesterases*, International University Line, La Jolla, 2007.
13. G. Schrader, Die Entwicklung neuer Insektizide auf Grundlage organischer Fluor- und Phosphor-Verbindungen, *Monogr. Angew. Chem.*, 1951, **62**, 1–62.

14. B. Holmstedt, Pharmacology of organophosphorus cholinesterase inhibitors, *Pharmacol. Rev.*, 1959, **11**, 567–688.
15. M. Eto, *Organophosphorus pesticides: organic and biological chemistry*, CRC Press, Cleveland, 1974.
16. B. J. Jandorf, H. O. Michel, N. K. Schaffer, R. Egan and W. H. Summerson, The mechanism of reaction between esterases and phosphorus-containing anti-esterases, *Discuss. Faraday Soc.*, 1955, **20**, 134–142.
17. D. R. Davies, Cholinesterases and the mode of action of some anticholinesterases, *J. Pharm. Pharmacol.*, 1954, **6**, 1–26.
18. W. N. Aldridge and E. Reiner, *Enzyme inhibitors as substrates – interactions of esterases with esters of organophosphorus and carbamic acids*, North-Holland Publishing Company, Amsterdam, London, 1972.
19. D. M. Maxwell and D. E. Lenz, Structure-activity relationships and anticholinesterase activity, in *Clinical and experimental toxicoloy of organophosphates and carbamates*, ed. B. Ballantyne and T. C. Marrs, Butterworth & Heinemann, Oxford, 1992, pp. 47–58.
20. D. M. Maxwell, The specificity of carboxylesterase protection against the toxicity of organophosphorus compounds, *Toxicol. Appl. Pharmacol.*, 1992, **114**, 306–312.
21. P. Taylor, Z. Radic, N. A. Hosca, S. Camp, P. Marchot and H. A. Berman, Structural basis for the specificity of cholinesterase catalysis and inhibition, *Toxicol. Lett.*, 1995, **82–83**, 453–458.
22. V. Tougu, Acetylcholinesterase: Mechanism of catalysis and inhibition, *Curr. Med. Chem.*, 2001, **1**, 155–170.
23. J. Massoulie, L. Pezzementi, S. Bon, E. Krejci and F. M. Vallette, Molecular and cellular biology of cholinesterases, *Prog. Neurobiol.*, 1993, **41**, 31–91.
24. D. Grob, The manifestations and treatment of poisoning due to nerve gas and other organic phosphate anticholinesterase compounds, *Arch. Intern. Med.*, 1956, **98**, 221–239.
25. E. C. Lee, Clinical manifestations of sarin nerve gas exposure, *J. Am. Med. Assoc.*, 2003, **290**, 659–662.
26. Y. Rosman, A. Eisenkraft, N. Milk, A. Shiyovich, N. Ophir, S. Shrot, Y. Kreiss and M. Kassirer, Lessons learned from the Syrian sarin attack: Evaluation of a clinical syndrome through social media, *Ann. Intern. Med.*, 2014, **160**, 644–648.
27. F. Worek, H. Thiermann, L. Szinicz and P. Eyer, Kinetic analysis of interactions between human acetylcholinesterase, structurally different organophosphorus compounds and oximes, *Biochem. Pharmacol.*, 2004, **68**, 2237–2248.
28. F. Worek and H. Thiermann, The value of novel oximes for treatment of poisoning by organophosphorus compounds, *Pharmacol. Ther.*, 2013, **139**, 249–259.
29. P. Eyer and F. Worek, Oximes, in *Chemical warfare agents: Toxicology and treatment*, ed. T. C. Marrs, R. L. Maynard and F. R. Sidell, John Wiley & Sons Ltd., Chichester, 2007, pp. 305–329.

30. D. Grob and A. M. Harvey, The effects and treatment of nerve gas poisoning, *Am. J. Med.*, 1953, **14**, 52–63.
31. D. Grob and J. C. Harvey, Effects in man of the anticholinesterase compound sarin (isopropyl methyl phosphonofluoridate), *J. Clin. Invest.*, 1958, **37**, 350–368.
32. F. R. Sidell and W. A. Groff, The reactivatibility of cholinesterase inhibited by VX and sarin in man, *Toxicol. Appl. Pharmacol.*, 1974, **27**, 241–252.
33. F. R. Sidell, Soman and sarin: clinical manifestations and treatment of accidental poisoning by organophosphates, *Clin. Toxicol.*, 1974, **7**, 1–17.
34. T. Okumura, N. Takasu, S. Ishimatsu, S. Miyanoki, A. Mitsuhashi, K. Kumuda, K. Tanaka and S. Hinohara, Report of 640 victims of the Tokyo subway sarin attack, *Ann. Emerg. Med.*, 1996, **28**, 129–135.
35. T. Kato and T. Hamanaka, Ocular signs and symptoms caused by exposure to sarin gas, *Am. J. Ophthalmol.*, 1996, **121**, 209–210.
36. H. Nozaki, S. Hori, Y. Shinozawa, S. Fujishima, K. Takuma, M. Sagoh, H. Kimura, T. Ohki, M. Suzuki and N. Aikawa, Secondary exposure of medical staff to sarin vapor in the emergency room, *Intensive Care Med.*, 1995, **21**, 1032–1035.
37. H. P. Benschop and L. P. A. de Jong, Toxicokinetics of nerve agents, in *Chemical warfare agents: toxicity at low levels*, ed. S. M. Somani and J. A. Romano, CRC Press, Boca Raton, 2001, pp. 25–81.
38. F. R. Sidell, Nerve agents, in *Medical aspects of chemical and biological warfare*, ed. F. R. Sidell, E. T. Takafuji and D. R. Franz, Borden Institute, Washington, D.C., 1997, pp. 129–179.
39. R. P. Chilcott, C. H. Dalton, I. Hill, C. M. Davidson, K. L. Blohm and M. G. Hamilton, Clinical manifestations of VX poisoning following percutaneous exposure in the domestic white pig, *Hum. Exp. Toxicol.*, 2003, **22**, 255–261.
40. M. J. van der Schans, B. J. Lander, H. van der Wiel, J. P. Langenberg and H. P. Benschop, Toxicokinetics of the nerve agent (±)-VX in anesthetized and atropinized hairless guinea pigs and marmosets after intravenous and percutaneous administration, *Toxicol. Appl. Pharmacol.*, 2003, **191**, 48–62.
41. J. R. Wetherell, S. J. Armstrong, R. W. Read and G. F. Clough, VX penetration following percutaneous poisoning: A dermal microdialysis study in the guinea pig, *Toxicol. Mech. Methods*, 2008, **18**, 313–321.
42. M. J. A. Joosen, M. J. van der Schans and H. P. M. Van Helden, Percutaneous exposure to the nerve agent VX: Efficacy of combined atropine, obidoxime and diazepam treatment, *Chem.-Biol. Interact.*, 2010, **188**, 255–263.
43. T. W. Sawyer, J. Mikler, F. Worek, G. Reiter, H. Thiermann, C. Tenn, K. Weatherby and S. Bohnert, The therapeutic use of localized cooling in the treatment of VX poisoning, *Toxicol. Lett.*, 2011, **204**, 52–56.
44. H. E. T. Spruit, J. P. Langenberg, H. C. Trap, H. J. Van Der Wiel, R. B. Helmich, H. P. M. Van Helden and H. P. Benschop, Intravenous and inhalation toxicokinetics of sarin stereoisomers in atropinized guinea pigs, *Toxicol. Appl. Pharmacol.*, 2000, **169**, 249–254.

45. M. Jokanovic, Current understanding of the mechanisms involved in metabolic detoxification of warfare nerve agents, *Toxicol. Lett.*, 2009, **188**, 1–10.
46. G. Reiter, J. Mikler, I. Hill, K. Weatherby, H. Thiermann and F. Worek, Chromatographic resolution, characterisation and quantification of VX enantiomers in hemolysed swine blood samples, *J. Chromatogr. B*, 2008, **873**, 86–94.
47. H. Mumford, M. E. Price, D. M. Cerasoli, W. Teschner, H. Ehrlich, H. P. Schwarz and D. E. Lenz, Efficacy and physiological effects of human butyrylcholinesterase as a post-exposure therapy against percutaneous poisoning by VX in the guinea-pig, *Chem.-Biol. Interact.*, 2010, **187**, 304–308.
48. H. Mumford, M. E. Price, D. E. Lenz and D. M. Cerasoli, Post-exposure therapy with human butyrylcholinesterase following percutaneous VX challenge in guinea pigs, *Clin. Toxicol.*, 2011, **49**, 287–297.
49. F. R. Sidell, A history of human studies with nerve agents by the UK and USA, in *Chemical warfare agents: Toxicology and treatment*, ed. T. C. Marrs, R. L. Maynard and F. R. Sidell, John Wiley & Sons Ltd., Chichester, 2007, pp. 223–239.
50. H. Nozaki, N. Aikawa, S. Fujishima, M. Suzuki, Y. Shinozawa, S. Hori and S. Nogawa, A case of VX poisoning and the difference from sarin, *Lancet*, 1995, **346**, 698–699.
51. F. Morimoto, T. Shimazu and T. Yoshioka, Intoxication of VX in humans, *Am. J. Emerg. Med.*, 1999, **17**, 493–494.
52. M. G. Hamilton, I. Hill, J. Conley, T. W. Sawyer, D. C. Caneva and P. M. Lundy, Clinical aspects of percutaneous poisoning by the chemical warfare agent VX: Effects of application site and decontamination, *Mil. Med.*, 2004, **169**, 856–862.
53. M. J. A. Joosen, M. J. van der Schans, W. C. Kuijpers, H. P. M. Van Helden and D. Noort, Timing of decontamination and treatment in case of percutaneous VX poisoning: A mini review, *Chem.-Biol. Interact.*, 2013, **203**, 149–153.
54. H. Mumford, M. E. Price and J. R. Wetherell, A novel approach to assessing percutaneous VX poisoning in the conscious guinea-pig, *J. Appl. Toxicol.*, 2008, **28**, 694–702.
55. C. P. Holstege, M. Kirk and F. R. Sidell, Chemical warfare – nerve agent poisoning, *Crit. Care Clin.*, 1997, **13**, 923–942.
56. D. Noort, H. P. Benschop and R. M. Black, Biomonitoring of exposure to chemical warfare agents: A review, *Toxicol. Appl. Pharmacol.*, 2002, **184**, 116–126.
57. F. Worek, M. Koller, H. Thiermann and L. Szinicz, Diagnostic aspects of organophosphate poisoning, *Toxicology*, 2005, **214**, 182–189.
58. P. Eyer and F. Worek, Cholinesterase, in *Clinical toxicological analysis*, ed. W.-R. Külpmann, Wiley-VCH, Weinheim, 2009, pp. 755–774.
59. R. M. Black and R. W. Read, Biological markers of exposure to organophosphorus nerve agents, *Arch. Toxicol.*, 2013, **87**, 421–437.
60. D. Noort, A. G. Hulst, H. J. M. Platenburg, M. Polhuijs and H. P. Benschop, Quantitative analysis of O-isopropyl methylphosphonic acid in

serum samples of Japanese citizens allegedly exposed to sarin: estimation of internal dosage, *Arch. Toxicol.*, 1998, **72**, 671–675.

61. J. R. Barr, W. J. Driskell, L. S. Aston and R. A. Martinez, Quantitation of metabolites of the nerve agents sarin, soman, cyclohexylsarin, VX, and Russian VX in human urine using isotope-dilution gas chromatography-tandem mass spectrometry, *J. Anal. Toxicol.*, 2004, **28**, 372–378.
62. M. Polhuijs, J. P. Langenberg and H. P. Benschop, New method for retrospective detection of exposure to organophosphorus anticholinesterases: application to alleged sarin victims of Japanese terrorists, *Toxicol. Appl. Pharmacol.*, 1997, **146**, 156–161.
63. M. J. van der Schans, M. Polhuijs, C. van Dijk, C. E. A. M. Degenhardt, K. Pleijsier, J. P. Langenberg and H. P. Benschop, Retrospective detection of exposure to nerve agents: analysis of phosphofluoridates originating from fluoride-induced reactivation of phosphylated BuChE, *Arch. Toxicol.*, 2004, **78**, 508–524.
64. A. Fidder, A. G. Hulst, D. Noort, R. de Ruiter, M. J. van der Schans, H. P. Benschop and J. P. Langenberg, Retrospective detection of exposure to organophosphorus anti-cholinesterases: mass spectrometric analysis of phosphylated human butyrylcholinesterase, *Chem. Res. Toxicol.*, 2002, **15**, 582–590.
65. D. Noort, A. Fidder, M. J. van der Schans and A. G. Hulst, Verification of exposure to organophosphates: Generic mass spectrometric method for detection of human butyrylcholinesterase adducts, *Anal. Chem.*, 2006, **78**, 6640–6644.
66. H. John, F. Breyer, J. O. Thumfart, H. Höchstätter and H. Thiermann, Matrix-assisted laser desorption/ionization time-of-flight mass spectrometry (MALDI-TOF MS) for detection and identification of albumin phosphylation by organophosphorus pesticides and G- and V-type nerve agents, *Anal. Bioanal. Chem.*, 2010, **398**, 2677–2691.
67. S. Chowdhary, R. Bhattacharyya and D. Banerjee, Acute organophosphorus poisoning, *Clin. Chim. Acta*, 2014, **431**, 66–76.
68. J. Suzuki, T. Kohno, M. Tsukagosi, T. Furuhata and K. Yamazaki, Eighteen cases exposed to sarin in Matsumoto, Japan, *Intern. Med.*, 1997, **36**, 466–470.
69. H. Morita, N. Yanagisawa, T. Nakajima, M. Shimizu, H. Hirabayashi, H. Okudera, M. Nohara, Y. Midorikawa and S. Mimura, Sarin poisoning in Matsumoto, Japan, *Lancet*, 1995, **346**, 290–293.
70. F. R. Sidell, G. K. Aghajanian and W. A. Groff, The reversal of anticholinergic intoxication in man with the cholinesterase inhibitor VX, *Exp. Biol. Med.*, 1973, **144**, 725–730.
71. H. Thiermann, T. Seeger, S. Gonder, N. Herkert, B. Antkowiak, T. Zilker, F. Eyer and F. Worek, Assessment of neuromuscular dysfunction during poisoning by organophosphorus compounds, *Chem.–Biol. Interact.*, 2010, **187**, 265–269.
72. H. Thiermann, T. Zilker, F. Eyer, K. Felgenhauer, P. Eyer and F. Worek, Monitoring of neuromuscular transmission in organophosphate pesticide-poisoned patients, *Toxicol. Lett.*, 2009, **191**, 297–304.

73. S. Eckert, P. Eyer, N. Herkert, R. Bumm, G. Weber, H. Thiermann and F. Worek, Comparison of the oxime-induced reactivation of erythrocyte and muscle acetylcholinesterase following inhibition by sarin and paraoxon, using a perfusion model for the real-time determination of membrane-bound acetylcholinesterase activity, *Biochem. Pharmacol.*, 2008, **75**, 698–703.
74. N. M. Herkert, G. Freude, U. Kunz, H. Thiermann and F. Worek, Comparative kinetics of organophosphates and oximes with erythrocyte, muscle and brain acetylcholinesterase, *Toxicol. Lett.*, 2012, **209**, 173–178.
75. P. Masson, E. Carletti and F. Nachon, Structure, activities and biomedical applications of human butyrylcholinesterase, *Protein Pept. Lett.*, 2009, **16**, 1215–1224.
76. N. Aurbek, H. Thiermann, F. Eyer, P. Eyer and F. Worek, Suitability of human butyrylcholinesterase as therapeutic marker and pseudo catalytic scavenger in organophosphate poisoning: A kinetic analysis, *Toxicology*, 2009, **259**, 133–139.
77. R. F. Witter, Measurement of blood cholinesterase, *Arch. Environ. Health*, 1963, **6**, 537–563.
78. J. H. Wills and K. P. DuBois, The measurement and significance of changes in the cholinesterase activities of erythrocytes and plasma in man and animals, *Crit. Rev. Toxicol.*, 1972, **1**, 153–202.
79. B. W. Wilson and J. D. Henderson, Blood esterase determinations as markers of exposure, *Rev. Environ. Contam. Toxicol.*, 1992, **128**, 55–69.
80. V. E. V. St. Omer and G. E. Rottinghaus, Biochemical determination of cholinesterase activity in biological fluids and tissues, in *Clinical and experimental toxicology of organophosphates and carbamates*, ed. B. Ballantyne and T. C. Marrs, Butterworth & Heinemann, Oxford, 1992, pp. 15–27.
81. G. L. Ellman, K. D. Courtney, V. Anders and R. M. Featherstone, A new and rapid colorimetric determination of acetylcholinesterase activity, *Biochem. Pharmacol.*, 1961, **7**, 88–95.
82. F. Worek, P. Eyer and H. Thiermann, Determination of acetylcholinesterase activity by the Ellman assay: A versatile tool for in vitro research on medical countermeasures against organophosphate poisoning, *Drug Test. Anal.*, 2012, **4**, 282–291.
83. F. Worek, U. Mast, D. Kiderlen, C. Diepold and P. Eyer, Improved determination of acetylcholinesterase activity in human whole blood, *Clin. Chim. Acta*, 1999, **288**, 73–90.
84. B. P. Doctor, L. Toker, E. Roth and I. Silman, Microtiter assay for acetylcholinesterase, *Anal. Biochem.*, 1987, **166**, 399–403.
85. T. Wille, H. Thiermann and F. Worek, Development of a high-throughput screening for nerve agent detoxifying materials using a fully-automated robot-assisted biological assay, *Toxicol. In Vitro*, 2010, **24**, 1026–1031.
86. B. N. Rajapakse, H. Thiermann, P. Eyer, F. Worek, S. J. Bowe, A. H. Dawson and N. A. Buckley, Evaluation of the Test-mate ChE (cholinesterase) field kit in acute organophosphorus poisoning, *Ann. Emerg. Med.*, 2011, **58**, 559–564.

87. K. B. Augustinsson, The normal variation of human blood cholinesterase activity, *Acta Physiol. Scand.*, 1955, **35**, 40–52.
88. J. A. Rider, J. L. Hodges, J. Swader and A. D. Wiggins, Plasma and red cell cholinesterase in 800 "healthy" blood donors, *J. Lab. Clin. Med.*, 1957, **50**, 376–383.
89. D. E. Arrieta, S. A. McCurdy, J. D. Henderson, L. J. Lefkowitz, R. Reitstetter and B. W. Wilson, Normal range of human red blood cell acetylcholinesterase activity, *Drug Chem. Toxicol.*, 2009, **32**, 182–185.
90. F. R. Sidell and A. Kaminskis, Temporal intrapersonal physiological variability of cholinesterase activity in human plasma and erythrocytes, *Clin. Chem.*, 1975, **21**, 1961–1963.
91. L. J. Lefkowitz, J. M. Kupina, N. L. Hirth, R. M. Henry, G. Y. Noland, J. Y. Barbee, J. Y. Zhou and C. B. Weese, Intraindividual stability of human erythrocyte cholinesterase activity, *Clin. Chem.*, 2007, **53**, 1358–1363.
92. W. K. Berry and D. R. Davies, Factors influencing the rate of 'aging' in a series of alkyl methylphosphonyl-acetylcholinesterases, *Biochem. J.*, 1966, **100**, 572–576.
93. P. Eyer, The role of oximes in the management of organophosphorus pesticide poisoning, *Toxicol. Rev.*, 2003, **22**, 165–190.
94. H. Thiermann, U. Mast, R. Klimmek, P. Eyer, A. Hibler, R. Pfab, N. Felgenhauer and T. Zilker, Cholinesterase status, pharmacokinetics and laboratory findings during obidoxime therapy in organophosphate poisoned patients, *Hum. Exp. Toxicol.*, 1997, **16**, 473–480.
95. H. Thiermann, L. Szinicz, F. Eyer, F. Worek, P. Eyer, N. Felgenhauer and T. Zilker, Modern strategies in therapy of organophosphate poisoning, *Toxicol. Lett.*, 1999, **107**, 233–239.
96. M. Eddleston, P. Eyer, F. Worek, F. Mohamed, L. Senarathna, L. von Meyer, E. Juszczak, A. Hittarage, S. Azhar, W. Dissanayake, M. H. R. Sheriff, L. Szinicz, A. H. Dawson and N. A. Buckley, Differences between organophosphorus insecticides in human self-poisoning: a prospective cohort study, *Lancet*, 2005, **366**, 1452–1459.
97. M. Eddleston, F. Worek, P. Eyer, H. Thiermann, L. von Meyer, K. Jeganathan, M. H. R. Sheriff, A. H. Dawson and N. A. Buckley, Poisoning with the S-alkyl organophosphorus insecticides profenofos and prothiofos, *Q. J. Med.*, 2009, **102**, 785–792.
98. H. Thiermann, K. Kehe, D. Steinritz, J. Mikler, I. Hill, T. Zilker, P. Eyer and F. Worek, Red blood cell acetylcholinesterase and plasma butyrylcholinesterase status: important indicators of the treatment of patients poisoned by organophosphorus compounds, *Arh. Hig. Rada Toksikol.*, 2007, **58**, 359–366.

CHAPTER 6

Verification of Exposure to Chemical Warfare Agents

ROBERT W. READ[a]

[a]Defence Science and Technology Laboratory, Porton Down, Salisbury, Wiltshire SP4 0JQ, UK

6.1 Introduction

Although prohibited by international treaties since the Hague Declaration of 1899 and the Hague Convention of 1907, chemical warfare (CW) agents have been used in a number of conflicts during the 20th century. The best known large scale uses were by both sides during World War 1. Significant quantities were also used, for example, by Imperial Japan in Manchuria and by Italy in Abyssinia (Ethiopia), both in the 1930s. These and other uses are well documented.[1] The entry into force of the Chemical Weapons Convention (CWC)[2] in 1997 gave impetus to the elimination of chemical weapons, but possible possession by the few countries that have not signed the CWC and terrorist organisations remains of concern. Recent confirmed uses of the organophosphorus nerve agent sarin in Syria demonstrated the importance of maintaining the capability for verification of exposure to CW agents for diagnostic and forensic purposes.[3] Analysis of environmental samples, such as soil, water and munition fragments, for detection of CW agents and their degradation products is well established.[4] In conflict zones it is often not possible to collect suitable environmental samples and in such cases the collection of biomedical samples, usually blood and urine, from escaped

Issues in Toxicology No. 27
Chemical Warfare Toxicology, Volume 2: Management of Poisoning
Edited by Franz Worek, John Jenner, and Horst Thiermann

Published by the Royal Society of Chemistry, www.rsc.org

or evacuated casualties is of great importance. The Organisation for the Prohibition of Chemical Weapons (OPCW), which administers the CWC, is in the process of setting up a system of designated laboratories for analysis of biomedical samples. Confidence building exercises held as part of this process have already resulted in significant capability increases in laboratories worldwide. These laboratories will complement the existing designated laboratories for the analysis of environmental samples.

Historically, evidence for the presence of a CW agent was provided by its physiological effects on casualties and by use of a variety of methods ranging from the human sense of smell to devices that relied on detection based on chemical and physicochemical properties. Development of equipment for sensitive detection in the field continues to this day, however unequivocal identification to forensic standards always requires laboratory analysis. The first recorded scientific investigations were those following allegations that trichothecene mycotoxins had been used as a CW agent, known as 'Yellow Rain', in southeast Asia in the late 1970s and early 1980s. These allegations have been thoroughly documented elsewhere.[1,5] Despite the controversies surrounding those investigations, they provided the first real experiences of the associated analyses and demonstrated the importance of analytical quality control. These experiences were put to good use in later investigations. As confirmation of the use of a CW agent may result in a political or military response the quality of analytical results is critical.

Alleged use of CW agents by both sides in the Iran–Iraq conflict and against the Kurdish population in Iraq in the 1980s demonstrated the need for analytical methods for unequivocal confirmation of such use. In many cases, analysis of environmental samples collected from the battlefield provided evidence. However, the treatment of Iranian and Kurdish casualties in hospitals in Belgium, The Netherlands and the United Kingdom allowed collection of biomedical samples from humans exposed to sulphur mustard. It was recognised that analysis of such samples required significantly more sensitive and selective methods than existing ones for environmental samples. Although the physiological effects of exposure, predominantly severe blistering and severe eye and lung effects, were well known, there was little knowledge of the chemical action of sulphur mustard in the body or of its metabolism. Lengthy investigations into these aspects, and consequent analytical method development, were undertaken.

The terrorist use of sarin by the Japanese Aum Shinrikyo cult in two incidents in Matsumoto City and Tokyo in 1994 and 1995, together with an assassination with another nerve agent, VX, in Osaka in 1994, showed that analytical methods for verification of exposure to nerve agents were also required.

6.2 Biomarkers of Exposure

A biomarker of exposure may be defined as a chemical, metabolite or reaction product with a target molecule in the human body that is measured to verify or quantitate exposure. Owing to their reactivity, intact CW agents are unlikely to be suitable as biomarkers. The principal biomarkers of interest for verification of exposure to CW agents are urinary metabolites and reaction products, or adducts, with proteins and DNA.[6,7] Differing analytical approaches are required. Urinary metabolites are generally small, polar molecules and soon after exposure may be present at relatively high concentrations. During the first few days following a moderate to high exposure their detection does not require particularly sensitive or sophisticated instrumentation, although such instrumentation should provide higher confidence results. However, the concentration of metabolites declines rapidly and detection at later times post-exposure, or in the case of a low level exposure, requires much higher sensitivity. It is unlikely that the majority of metabolites would be detectable more than about 2 weeks post-exposure.

Adducts with proteins, usually the blood proteins haemoglobin and albumin, and the enzymes acetylcholinesterase (AChE) and butyrylcholinesterase (BuChE) in the case of nerve agents, are normally present at significantly lower concentrations than urinary metabolites. Their lifetime in the body may be up to the lifetime of the native protein, *e.g.* 100–120 days for human haemoglobin and 20–25 days for albumin, so detection is possible over longer timescales provided that analytical sensitivity is sufficiently high. In cases where it is impossible to collect samples from casualties until several days post-exposure, this long term detectability becomes more important. Detection of an adduct with an intact protein in the presence of a much larger quantity of native protein would be extremely difficult, if not impossible. Proteins are therefore broken down into small peptides or individual amino acids by enzymatic digestion or acid hydrolysis prior to analysis. The resulting digests or hydrolysates are complex mixtures, and selective sample preparation and sophisticated instrumentation are prerequisites for their analysis. Consequently, these methods are more technically demanding than those for urinary metabolites. Methods that release a small molecule related to the CW agent from adducted proteins are applicable in some cases. Owing to repair mechanisms, adducts with DNA would be expected to have shorter lifetimes than those with proteins. Degradation products of these adducts are excreted in the urine and analytical methods are similar to those for urinary metabolites.

Although efforts are made to extend the time for which biomarkers may be detected after exposure to a CW agent, an aspect that has received little attention is the earliest time following an exposure that detection is possible. This would depend on the agent and route of exposure. Correct timing of sample collection would be required in order to verify exposure. The majority of metabolism studies in animals use samples collected over 12 or 24 h periods and, therefore, information on levels of metabolites or adducts in the first few hours following exposure is absent. A study with inhaled sulphur mustard in pigs showed that urinary metabolites were not detected until 2 h post-exposure.[8] In some cases of human exposure, samples have been collected at intervals to follow the concentrations of metabolites or adducts over time.

6.2.1 Analytical Methods and Instrumentation

Past investigations into alleged use of CW agents have involved the analysis of relatively small numbers of samples from individuals believed to have been exposed, mainly in a military context. The Tokyo subway incident, in which there were more than five thousand casualties but only twelve fatalities, resulted in analysis of tens of samples, the exact number being uncertain. These small sample numbers were easily handled by manual procedures. More recently, increased concerns regarding possible terrorist use of CW agents on un-protected civilian populations encouraged interest in automated, high throughput analytical methods. In such an event, a large number of samples, including those from the 'worried well', may be expected, and rapid results required for diagnosis and to guide medical treatment.

Developed analytical methods fall into three main categories: those with applications in toxicological investigations only, *e.g.* methods for chiral analysis of organophosphorus nerve agents; those applied to animal studies that may also be applicable to human samples; and those that have been applied to human samples. Many methods have been developed for the detection of urinary metabolites[6] and adducts with proteins and DNA[7] as biomarkers of exposure. A few methods for detection of intact agents have been developed but positive results for samples from exposed individuals are unlikely unless obtained very soon after a high level exposure. These methods have some applications in animal studies, for example in toxicokinetic investigations. The greatest efforts have been applied to the development of methods for agents deemed to pose the greatest threat, namely sulphur mustard and nerve agents.

Whichever biomarker is considered, analytical methods must demonstrate sufficient selectivity and sensitivity, and avoid false positive results. For these reasons most analytical protocols pay great attention to optimisation of instrumental conditions to achieve low, usually sub-ng ml^{-1}, limits of detection (LOD) and lower limits of quantitation (LLOQ), and to both positive and negative quality control samples.

The majority of modern analytical methods for biomarkers of CW agents are based on the combination of a gas chromatography (GC) or liquid chromatography (LC) separation with detection by mass spectrometry (MS; GC-MS, LC-MS), although some other analytical techniques have been investigated. OPCW requirements for the analysis of biomedical samples are primarily focused on chromatographic and mass spectrometric techniques providing unequivocal identification of biomarkers. As highly sensitive and selective analyses are required, preferred methods use GC-MS/MS or LC-MS/MS. Most GC-MS and GC-MS/MS methods utilise positive or negative ion chemical ionisation (CI), although electron ionisation (EI) has some applications. Use of electrospray ionisation (ESI) in LC-MS and LC-MS/MS methods is now almost universal; atmospheric pressure chemical ionisation (APCI) has been used in some methods. The most commonly used mass spectrometers are triple quadrupole and ion-trap types operated in selected reaction monitoring (SRM) MS/MS mode; use of magnetic sector instruments is now rare. However, with the increasing availability of high resolution, accurate mass instruments such as time of flight (TOF) and Orbitrap™ in many laboratories their use in biomarker analysis is becoming more common. Single quadrupole instruments operated in the selected ion monitoring (SIM) mode are still used in many laboratories involved in the analysis of biomarkers, however the additional selectivity and confidence provided by SRM methods is generally preferred.

Suitable sample preparation procedures prior to GC or LC separation are critical. The majority of published methods use more-or-less selective solid phase extraction (SPE) for isolation and clean up of analytes. Automated SPE and 96 well plate technology may be utilised to provide high throughput, rapid sample preparation. These technologies have been incorporated into some analytical methods that previously were performed manually. It should be noted that some high throughput methods using immunomagnetic beads for sample extraction rely on the availability of often very expensive antibodies and binding of these to the beads is not a trivial process. The effort required and cost of implementation of this type of method, and high throughput methods in general, should be balanced against the likelihood that a laboratory might receive large numbers of samples.

Accurate quantitation requires the use of suitable internal standards (IS). Stable isotopically labelled, usually deuterium or carbon-13, forms of analytes are preferred for methods using MS detection, although some methods use non-labelled, structurally similar compounds. Isotopically pure, labelled IS for quantitation of urinary metabolites may be synthesised and some are commercially available. Production of IS for quantitation of blood protein adducts is more difficult. Ideally, the IS should be added to an aliquot of the original sample and taken through the complete analytical procedure. In the case of blood protein or cholinesterase (ChE) adducts this requires an IS to be prepared from a well characterised incubate of the appropriate blood fraction with the labelled CW agent. Aliquots of incubate containing labelled adduct are added to samples to be quantitated. Alternatively, labelled amino acid or peptide adducts may be synthesised, the latter being particularly complex. These are then added after the digestion step in the sample preparation procedure. Even if accurate quantitation is not required, the use of a suitable IS provides confidence in the success of sample preparation and that analytical sensitivity is maintained.

Several reviews incorporating details of analytical methods have been published in recent years.[6,7,9–12] The majority of methods have been developed for the detection of biomarkers of a single CW agent or series of similar agents. There have, however, been some developments in the detection of protein adducts that are designed to be more generally applicable.[13] LC methods increasingly have been utilised, mainly because the amount of sample preparation required is often less and derivatisation reactions are not usually necessary, resulting in greater sample throughput. However, the high resolution separation and sensitivity of many GC-MS and GC-MS/MS methods should not be overlooked.

As samples from human casualties are relatively rare, when they do become available it is usually the case that multiple methods are applied for their analysis. The main emphasis of the following sections is on methods for detection of biomarkers of exposure that have been applied to human samples. Although some methods described have not been applied to samples from casualties, a number have been applied to the analysis of samples from non-exposed individuals to demonstrate the absence of background levels of metabolites or adducts. Wherever possible, biomarkers should be unique to the CW agent and not capable of being produced from other sources. If other sources are available, then background levels in non-exposed individuals may be significant and alternative biomarkers should be sought.

The reader will find many additional references to the underlying basic research and details of alternative methods in the majority of publications cited both in this and other chapters in this volume.

6.3 Sulphur Mustard

The chemistry and metabolism of sulphur mustard, bis(2-chloroethyl) sulphide, $S(CH_2CH_2Cl)_2$, is complex and dominated by reactions with nucleophiles; the sulphur atom may also be oxidised.[6,7] Metabolism studies were performed in the early 1990s in response to alleged uses in the Iran–Iraq conflict. Three urinary metabolites derived from hydrolysis and oxidation, and a further seven derived from initial alkylation of the relatively abundant tripeptide glutathione were identified.[6] Metabolites were identified by desorption chemical ionisation MS/MS following isolation from urine of exposed rats by repetitive LC. It is likely that more could be identified using modern LC-MS techniques.

Initial investigations into reactions of sulphur mustard in the blood concentrated on red cell haemoglobin, specifically its protein component globin. Globin consists of two peptide chains, α and β, and the protein of normal haemoglobin consists of identical pairs of each. Studies into alkylation of globin by sulphur mustard *in vitro* showed reaction products with amino, carboxyl, hydroxyl and sulphhydryl groups in amino acid side chains, and the *N*-terminal amino groups. Alkylated amino acids detected in globin digested with the enzyme pronase E were valine at the *N*-terminals of both α and β chains, as well as histidine, cysteine, aspartic acid, glutamic acid, lysine and tryptophan.[1,7] All of these amino acids were modified with a 2-hydroxyethylthioethyl (HETE) group formed by reaction with sulphur mustard and hydrolysis of the remaining free chlorine. The positions of the alkylated amino acids in globin were determined by sequencing of alkylated peptides resulting from digestion with the enzyme trypsin.[1,7]

Albumin, the major protein in blood plasma, was also found to be alkylated by sulphur mustard. Analysis of trypsin digests of human serum albumin treated *in vitro* with sulphur mustard showed that the only free cysteine residue in the molecule, Cys-34, was a major site of alkylation, along with histidine and glutamic and/or aspartic acids.[14] The cysteine adduct was the most amenable to sensitive detection by LC-MS/MS.

A urinary excretion product isolated from plasma and urine of dermally exposed pigs, assumed to be derived from reaction with a protein histidine residue, was also reported.[15]

As one of the major effects of exposure to sulphur mustard is blistering of the skin, reaction with the abundant skin protein keratin was investigated. Strong evidence was obtained for the majority of alkylation involving aspartic and glutamic acid residues.[16]

Investigations into adducts with DNA showed the primary site of alkylation to be the N^7 position of deoxyguanosine.[7] An adduct with guanine from the breakdown of alkylated DNA was detected in the urine of exposed guinea pigs.[17] A recent study in rats has shown the presence of adducts with the N^7 position of guanine, the O^6 position of guanine and the N^3 position of adenine in DNA isolated from the skin of exposed animals. An adduct crosslinking the N^7 positions of two guanine molecules was also detected.[18]

During and following these studies, a number of methods for detection of urinary metabolites and adducts with blood and skin proteins and DNA were applied to human samples and published. The first methods were developments of those used for the investigations into metabolism and reaction with proteins. Later developments have been directed at improving performance and applicability. A number of methods have been applied to the analysis of human samples and these are detailed in the following section.

6.3.1 Application to Human Samples

Samples from military casualties were obtained from incidents during the Iran–Iraq conflict, and the al-Anfal campaign by Iraq against its Kurdish population in 1988. A few samples originated from accidental exposures to sulphur mustard. The majority of analyses were performed in The Netherlands, the United Kingdom and the United States of America. Significant later developments and improvements made to methods that have been applied to human samples are included in this section.

6.3.1.1 Intact Agent and Metabolites

One of the earliest analyses of samples from a human exposed to sulphur mustard was performed in Germany in 1986.[19] Tissues and body fluids from an Iranian soldier, deceased 7 days after exposure, were analysed for intact agent after storage at −20 °C for 12 months. Positive identification was obtained by electron ionisation GC-MS analysis of extracts of abdominal fat. Quantitation in a number of tissues, blood, urine and cerebrospinal fluid was performed by detection of a complex with gold using electrothermal atomic absorption spectroscopy. Concentrations of agent determined were in the range 1.1–15.1 mg kg^{-1}. The quoted LOD was in the region of 0.1 mg kg^{-1}. The methods used were mainly applicable to the analysis of *post-mortem* tissue samples and, as mentioned previously, detection of intact agent should be considered unusual.

At around the same time, urine samples from Iranian casualties were analysed in The Netherlands. The hydrolysis product, thiodiglycol, bis(2-hydroxyethyl) sulphide, $S(CH_2CH_2OH)_2$, in urine was converted back to sulphur mustard by reaction with concentrated hydrochloric acid and collected from the reaction headspace on Tenax® adsorption tubes.[20] The trapped sulphur mustard was detected by GC-MS. Using a 10 ml urine sample the LOD was reported to be a few ng ml^{-1} and thiodiglycol in casualty samples was in the range 3–140 ng ml^{-1}. However, thiodiglycol was detected at concentrations up to 55 ng ml^{-1} in control samples, thus making unambiguous verification of exposure impossible. Later modifications to the method, including use of a deuterated thiodiglycol IS, allowed greater confidence in quantitation.[21] Concentrations in casualty samples were in the range 10–100 ng ml^{-1} with the exception of one sample at 330 ng ml^{-1}. Control samples contained less than 20 ng ml^{-1} thiodiglycol and 80% of casualty samples had concentrations above the 95% confidence level calculated from controls. If performed today, these analyses would not be considered to give acceptable proof of exposure owing to the presence of thiodiglycol in the negative controls.

Developments in sample preparation techniques provided the possibility of extraction of thiodiglycol from urine and blood.[22] Samples were prepared using the technique now known as solid supported liquid–liquid extraction (SSLLE). Urine, plasma or whole blood absorbed on Clin-Elut diatomaceous earth columns, were extracted with ethyl acetate and the extracts partially purified on C18 (for blood and plasma) or Florisil® (for urine) SPE cartridges. After evaporation to dryness the extract residues were derivatised with pentafluorobenzoyl chloride in pyridine and analysed by GC-MS with negative ion SIM. Deuterated thiodiglycol IS was used for quantitation. A LOD of 1 ng ml^{-1} was achieved with 1 ml samples. Importantly, concentrations of thiodiglycol in a set of eight control human urine samples were all less than 1 ng ml^{-1}. A set of eight control blood samples, from the same subjects as the control urine, gave concentrations in the range 6–16 ng ml^{-1} with two additional samples less than 1 ng ml^{-1}.

A similar method for analysis of thiodiglycol sulphoxide, bis(2-hydroxyethyl) sulphoxide, $OS(CH_2CH_2OH)_2$, in urine, either with or without prior treatment with acidic titanium trichloride, and with deuterated IS, gave a LOD of 1 ng ml^{-1} in a 0.5 ml sample.[23] Treatment with titanium trichloride reduces thiodiglycol sulphoxide to thiodiglycol, allowing combined analysis of thiodiglycol, thiodiglycol sulphoxide and any acid labile esters present in urine. Using this method, it was found that the concentration of thiodiglycol sulphoxide in a set of five control human samples was in the range 2–8 ng ml^{-1}, however a sixth sample contained 36 ng ml^{-1}. The source of the background level of thiodiglycol sulphoxide is assumed to be dietary but much larger reference range studies would be needed to define a 'normal' background. The source of the thiodiglycol detected in the blood and, using more sensitive methods, the urine, may be presumed to be the same. Again, the presence of a variable natural background degrades the usefulness of these methods for verification of exposure.

In contrast to the above methods, those developed for analysis of the two metabolites 1,1′-sulphonylbis[2-(methylsulphinyl)ethane] (SBMSE) and 1-methylsulphinyl-2-[2-(methylthio)ethylsulphonyl]ethane (MSMTESE), derived from the initial reaction with glutathione and further action of the enzyme β-lyase, have shown no natural background. These β-lyase metabolites are considered to be unequivocal biomarkers of sulphur mustard exposure. Before the general availability of sensitive LC-MS instruments, these metabolites were detected by GC-MS following reduction to a single analyte, 1,1′-sulphonylbis[2-(methylthio)ethane] (SBMTE), by titanium trichloride (see Scheme 6.1).[24] After reduction, SBMTE was extracted using either Clin-Elut columns or C8 SPE cartridges. Ammonia chemical ionisation GC-MS analysis with SIM provided a LOD of 2 ng ml^{-1} in a 1 ml sample. Deuterated ISs were used for quantitation.

Improvements in detection methods for thiodiglycol, thiodiglycol sulphoxide and β-lyase metabolites using GC-MS/MS SRM allowed lower LODs to be achieved.[25] The LOD for the reduced β-lyase metabolites was decreased to 0.1 ng ml^{-1} in a 1 ml sample. The true LODs for thiodiglycol and thiodiglycol sulphoxide in urine could not be determined owing to the background present in normal urine, however chromatographic background peaks were significantly reduced. When applied to urine samples from five Iranian and two Kurdish casualties, combined analysis of thiodiglycol and sulphoxide showed concentrations in the range 11–72 ng ml^{-1} in five of the samples, and not detectable in the remaining two. A negative control sample also showed a concentration of 11 ng ml^{-1}. Concentrations of β-lyase metabolites as SBMTE were in the range 0.1–5 ng ml^{-1} for six of the samples, and one at the very high concentration of 220 ng ml^{-1}. No SBMTE was detected in a negative control. The casualty showing the highest concentrations in both sets of analyses later died. The two Kurdish casualties were from the well known attack on the town of Halabja on 17 March 1988. Chromatograms for β-lyase metabolites detected as SBMTE from analysis of the urine from two casualties are shown in Figure 6.1.

The same methods were applied to urine samples from two casualties suffering extensive blistering from accidental exposure to the contents of a World War 1 munition.[26] Analyses were performed in duplicate or triplicate for thiodiglycol, thiodiglycol sulphoxide, combined thiodiglycol plus sulphoxide, β-lyase metabolites, and an additional bis-conjugate metabolite derived from reaction with glutathione, 1,1′-sulphonylbis[2-*S*-(*N*-acetylcysteinyl)ethane]

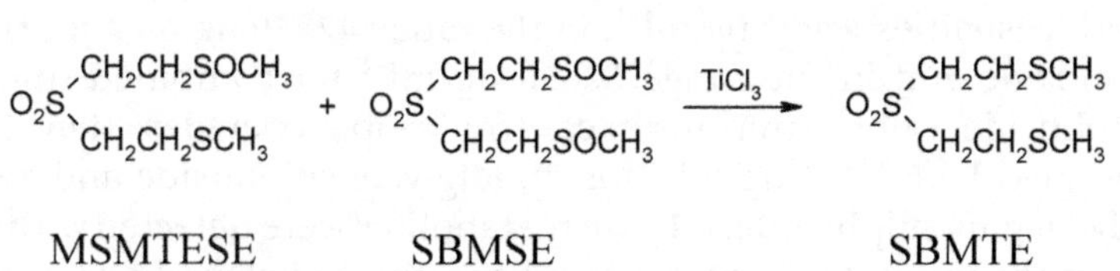

Scheme 6.1 Structures of β-lyase metabolites of sulphur mustard and their reduction product.

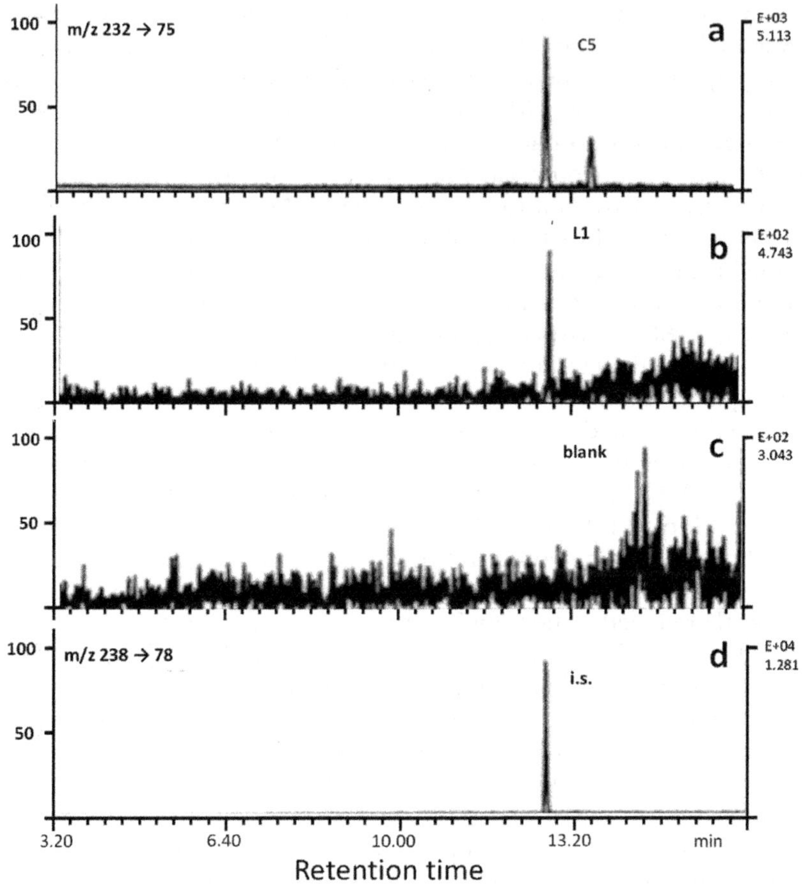

Figure 6.1 SRM chromatograms showing detection of β-lyase metabolites of sulphur mustard as SBMTE. Urine from (a) Iranian casualty C5 (1 ng ml^{-1}) and (b) Kurdish casualty L1 (0.1 ng ml^{-1}); (c) glassware blank for L1; and (d) D_6 IS (5 ng ml^{-1}). Analysis was performed using GC-MS/MS with ammonia CI. Reprinted from R. M. Black and R. W. Read, Improved methodology for the detection and quantitation of urinary metabolites of sulphur mustard using gas chromatography-tandem mass spectrometry, *J. Chromatogr. B: Biomed. Sci. Appl.*, 1995, **665**, 97–105, Copyright (1995), with permission from Elsevier.[25]

(SBSNAE; see Scheme 6.2). The concentration of thiodiglycol in samples from both casualties was 2 ng ml^{-1}, in the range 42–70 ng ml^{-1} for thiodiglycol sulphoxide and in the range 52–80 ng ml^{-1} for combined thiodiglycol plus sulphoxide. Concentrations in control samples were less than 1 ng ml^{-1} for thiodiglycol, and 4–5 ng ml^{-1} for thiodiglycol sulphoxide and combined thiodiglycol plus sulphoxide. β-Lyase metabolites were detected with concentrations in the range 42–57 ng ml^{-1} and controls at below the LOD of 0.1 ng ml^{-1}. The bis-conjugate was analysed by LC-MS with thermospray ionisation, however the LOD of 25 ng ml^{-1} did not allow detection in the samples.

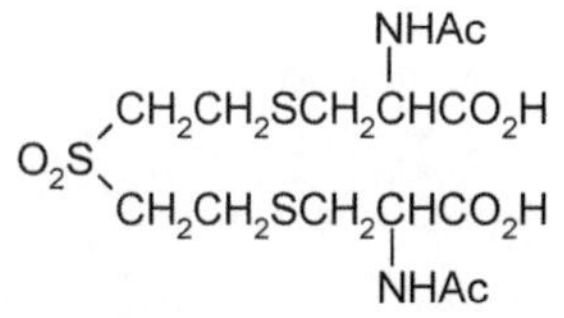

Scheme 6.2 Structure of the SBSNAE metabolite of sulphur mustard.

Following the development of sensitive ESI LC-MS/MS methods for β-lyase and bis-conjugate metabolites of sulphur mustard, these methods were applied to analyse samples from the Kurdish and accidental casualties.[27,28] The individual β-lyase metabolites, MSMTESE and SBMSE, were both detected in samples from the Kurdish casualties at close to the LOD of 0.1 ng ml^{-1}, and at much higher concentrations in samples from the accidental casualties. The bis-conjugate, SBSNAE, was detected by negative ion ESI at very low concentrations close to the LOD of 0.5 ng ml^{-1} in samples from the accidental casualties. The bis-conjugate is a major metabolite in the rat,[6] but based on these results, is much less abundant in humans. Chromatograms from the analysis of the urine from one of the accidental casualties are shown in Figure 6.2.

Following an accidental laboratory exposure to sulphur mustard aerosol and vapour, urine samples collected up to 14 days post-exposure were analysed for the presence of thiodiglycol.[29] Thiodiglycol was detected as its bis-heptafluorobutyryl ester derivative by GC-MS with EI and SIM, and an excretion profile was constructed from the results of analysis of daily samples. A maximum level of excretion was reached on day 4 with positive results obtained up to day 13. The half-life of elimination was estimated as 1.18 days and the total percutaneous dose calculated as 49 mg or greater. Further samples collected up to 6 months post-exposure showed no further elimination of thiodiglycol. Analysis of fluid from a blister showed evidence of a sulphur mustard related compound but it could not be identified unambiguously. Although thiodiglycol is not considered an unequivocal biomarker for confirmation of sulphur mustard exposure, this example shows that its detection can provide very useful data in the case of a known exposure.

Another accidental exposure, to the contents of an old munition during a disposal operation, provided the opportunity to apply a suite of methods to samples from two casualties.[30] One casualty suffered blistering to 6.5% of their body surface area and the other had one small blister. Urine samples were collected up to 41 days post-exposure. Both urinary metabolites and blood protein adducts (see Section 6.3.1.2) were detected. The urinary metabolites, thiodiglycol, thiodiglycol plus thiodiglycol sulphoxide, and β-lyase metabolites (as SBMTE) were detected by GC-MS/MS, and SBSNAE by LC-MS/MS. Thiodiglycol, thiodiglycol plus thiodiglycol sulphoxide, and SBMTE were all detected for up to 11 days and elimination profiles were constructed for the first casualty. Positive results were reported for the second casualty up to 7 days. SBSNAE was detected only in the initial sample taken

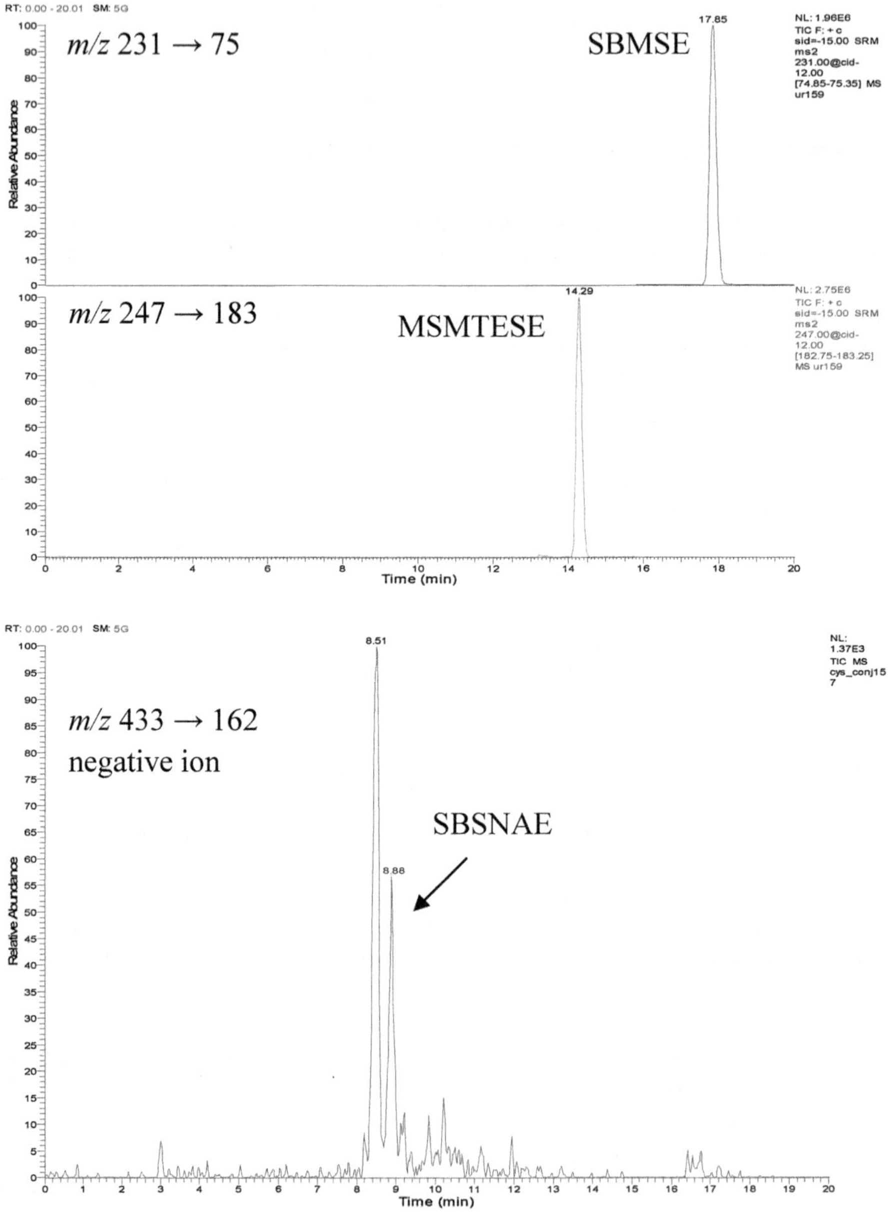

Figure 6.2 SRM chromatograms showing the detection of β-lyase (upper) and SBSNAE (lower) metabolites of sulphur mustard in urine from an accidentally exposed casualty. Analysis was performed using LC-MS/MS with ESI. Concentrations of metabolites were 30 ng ml^{-1} SBMSE, 15 ng ml^{-1} MSMTESE and ~1 ng ml^{-1} SBSNAE.

2 days post-exposure from the first casualty. As in the analyses described above, SBSNAE was detected at a very low concentration, adding to the evidence that it is not a major metabolite in humans. The β-lyase metabolites were shown to be the best indicators of exposure, with confirmation obtained for the casualty showing minimal symptoms by analysis of a urine sample taken 7 days after exposure.

A variety of methods for the analysis of sulphur mustard metabolites by LC-MS/MS have been published in recent years. These have mainly concentrated on the β-lyase metabolites, either individually[31] or reduced to SBMTE.[32,33] An additional method has been published for analysis of the bis-conjugate SBSNAE.[34] A method for simultaneous analysis of seven metabolites, including the oxidation product of sulphur mustard, bis(2-chloroethyl) sulphoxide or mustard sulphoxide, in plasma has also been published.[35] None of these have been applied to human samples.

6.3.1.2 *Protein and DNA Adducts*

Samples of blood from Iranian casualties of sulphur mustard exposure were analysed in the United Kingdom and The Netherlands. Samples were collected in 1986 (United Kingdom) and 1988 (The Netherlands), but owing to the lengthy investigations and method development described above, the first analyses were not reported until 1997. Adducts with *N*-terminal valine and histidine residues of globin were detected along with a DNA adduct.

The *N*-terminal valine adduct was detected by GC-MS with negative ion CI and SIM following cleavage from globin.[36] Globin was isolated from blood using a precipitation procedure and the *N*-terminal valine residue selectively cleaved by modified Edman degradation with pentafluorophenyl isothiocyanate (PFPITC). The resulting thiohydantoin product was derivatised with heptafluorobutyric anhydride (HFBA; see Scheme 6.3). This method allowed detection of adduct in samples collected 22 and 26 days post-exposure from two Iranian casualties.[37] The method used globin from human blood incubated with D_8-labelled sulphur mustard as IS. A second set of samples collected between 5 and 10 days post-exposure from a further four Iranian casualties, and within 48 h from one accidental casualty, were analysed by a similar method using a magnetic sector mass spectrometer at a mass resolution of 8000 (10% valley definition).[38] Adduct was detected in all samples. These samples were received as lysed whole blood, so the isolated globin was impure, containing some plasma proteins; globin is normally prepared from

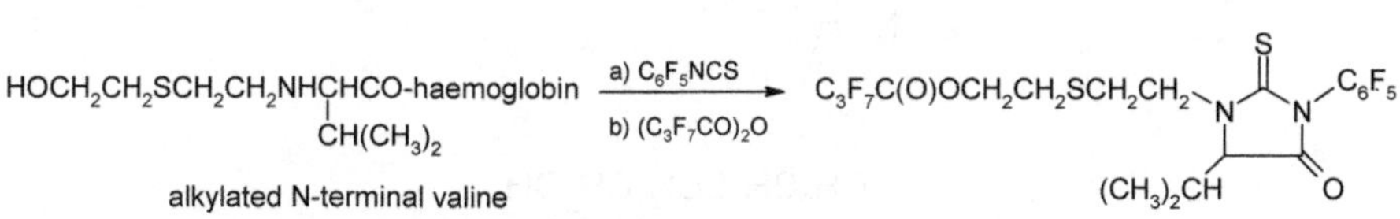

Scheme 6.3 Cleavage by modified Edman degradation and derivatisation of the *N*-terminal valine adduct of sulphur mustard.

washed red cells. However, chromatograms were very clean showing only a single peak for the adduct.

A complete procedure for the analysis of the *N*-terminal valine adduct and its use in simple bench-top GC-MS instruments in field laboratory conditions has been published.[39] The minimum detectable exposure level of the method was 100 nM. A later, improved method, using an optimised SPE procedure for purification of the thiohydantoin product prior to derivatisation, claims a minimum detectable exposure level of 20 nM.[40] A rapid and sensitive method for analysis of *N*-terminal valine adducts by LC-MS/MS has also been developed.[41] The method has not been evaluated for the adduct with sulphur mustard but is suitable for automation and applicable to whole blood.

The human casualty samples were also analysed by an immunochemical method for the N^7 adduct of 2′-deoxyguanosine from DNA, and by LC-MS/MS for a histidine adduct, N^1-(2-hydroxyethylthioethyl)histidine, from globin (see Scheme 6.4).[37,38] Both analyses gave positive results for all casualty samples. Although rather abundant and useful for confirmation of exposure, detection of the histidine adduct requires considerable sample preparation, involving overnight vacuum hydrolysis with 6 M hydrochloric acid, evaporation to dryness, SPE and derivatisation with fluorenylmethoxycarbonyl chloride (FmocCl). As far as is known, this method has not been applied to human samples elsewhere.

A method for detection of an adduct with cysteine in human serum albumin was successfully applied for the analysis of samples from nine Iranian casualties.[14] Following digestion of isolated albumin with the enzyme pronase, the adduct was detected as the modified tripeptide HETE-Cys-Pro-Phe by LC-MS/MS in samples collected 8–9 days post-exposure. The method allowed detection at an exposure level of 10 nM. A later improved method isolated albumin using a Cibacron Blue F3GA affinity column (Hi-Trap™ Blue HP) in place of the original precipitation procedure.[42] The minimum detectable exposure level was estimated at 1.5 nM. Although no samples from casualties were analysed, a small reference range study using 80 samples from non-exposed subjects showed no detectable background.

A recent modification of the method to a 96 well plate format reduced the analysis time by a factor of three, however the sensitivity (50 nM) was not as good as previously.[43] Loss of sensitivity was attributed to less efficient production of adducted tripeptide by the pronase enzyme preparation used in comparison with previous preparations. Possible differences in enzyme

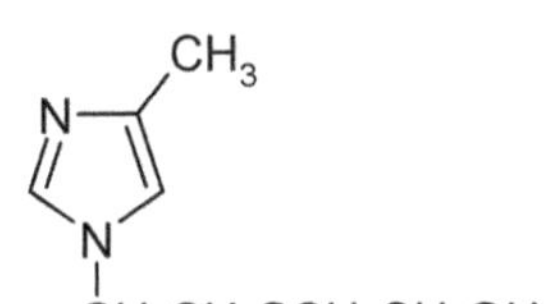

Scheme 6.4 Structure of the sulphur mustard adduct N^1-(2-hydroxyethylthioethyl)histidine.

activity are a consideration in all analyses requiring digestion steps. Again, no human casualty samples were analysed but a set of 124 plasma samples from non-exposed subjects demonstrated the absence of background.

Samples obtained from two individuals exposed to sulphur mustard during disposal of an old munitions (see Section 6.3.1.1) provided an opportunity to apply two methods for detection of adducts with blood proteins in parallel.[44] Plasma samples were obtained over a 42 day period from the severely exposed first casualty and over a 6 day period from the much less exposed second. Analyses were performed for the sulphur mustard cysteine adduct, using the affinity column isolation method and LC-MS/MS as described above,[42] and for thiodiglycol cleaved by alkaline hydrolysis from ester adducts with aspartic and glutamic acid residues in precipitated, dried plasma proteins.[45] Thiodiglycol was detected as its pentafluorobenzoyl derivative by GC-MS with negative ion CI and SIM. All analyses for the adducted tripeptide and thiodiglycol were positive for the most severely exposed casualty. As for urinary metabolites, elimination profiles for both adduct types were constructed for this casualty. For the casualty showing only minor exposure, adducted tripeptide was detected in all samples, however no cleaved thiodiglycol was detected. Improvements in sensitivity made to allow detection of thiodiglycol in later samples from the first casualty were not applied to samples from the second casualty owing to lack of sample volume. The LLOQ of the method was later reduced from 25 nM to 1.56 nM sulphur mustard in human plasma (*in vitro*) by inclusion of a concentration step, neutralisation of excess derivatisation reagent and optimisation of conditions.[46] Unlike the methods for detection of free thiodiglycol in the blood, this method appears to be free from background in negative controls. The analyses performed on samples from these casualties clearly demonstrate the advantages of blood protein adducts over urinary metabolites as biomarkers of exposure for extended periods post-exposure.

6.3.1.3 Recent Human Exposures to Sulphur Mustard

During the preparation of this chapter, results were reported for analyses of samples from four Chinese casualties of exposure to abandoned sulphur mustard, dating from World War 2 and presumably of Imperial Japanese forces origin.[47] A comprehensive series of analyses were performed on urine, blood and blister exudate samples collected from 3 days post-exposure onwards. Results demonstrate the timescales over which the various biomarkers may be applicable for verification of exposure. Analyses performed were: GC-MS for thiodiglycol and thiodiglycol plus thiodiglycol sulphoxide in urine; GC-MS/MS for β-lyase metabolites in urine; LC-MS/MS for thiodiglycol, thiodiglycol sulphoxide, bis(2-chloroethyl) sulphoxide (mustard sulphoxide) and β-lyase metabolites in urine, blood and blister exudate; LC-MS/MS for DNA adducts, N^7-[2-[(2-hydroxyethyl)thio]ethyl]-guanine, O^6-[2-[(2-hydroxyethyl)thio]ethyl]-guanine, N^3-[2-[(2-hydroxyethyl)thio]ethyl]-adenine and bis[2-(guanin-7-yl)ethyl] sulphide, in urine and blood; and GC-MS for

N-terminal valine globin adduct in blood. All methods used were previously published.

Blister exudate samples were found to contain thiodiglycol, thiodiglycol sulphoxide, mustard sulphoxide and β-lyase metabolites, all detected for up to 6 days post-exposure. Amounts of exudate after this time were too small to provide useable samples. Urine contained thiodiglycol and thiodiglycol sulphoxide detected for up to 7 days post-exposure, at which time concentrations were at or below previously published background levels.[22,23] β-Lyase metabolites were detected for up to 10 days and DNA adducts up to 32 days post-exposure. Blood contained mustard sulphoxide, detected but below the LLOQ, low levels of β-lyase metabolites were detected up to 6 days post-exposure, and DNA adducts were detected up to 14 days post-exposure. Significantly, the *N*-terminal valine adduct was detected above the LLOQ at 95 days post-exposure for three of the casualties, and at 60 days post-exposure for the less exposed fourth casualty, illustrating the utility of blood protein adducts as long-term biomarkers of exposure.

As sampling did not commence until day 3, the maximum concentrations of the majority of analytes, particularly in the urine, are likely to have been missed. However, concentrations determined for all metabolites and adducts showed good correlation with the severity of symptoms exhibited by the casualties. Timescales for detection appear to be broadly consistent with previous reports.

6.4 Nerve Agents

In contrast to sulphur mustard, the chemistry and metabolism of organophosphorus nerve agents are less complex, and were well known before any human samples were collected. The classical nerve agents comprise two main classes: G-agents and V-agents (see Scheme 6.5). The G-agents are *O*-alkyl alkylphosphonofluoridates, such as sarin, soman and cyclosarin, and *O*-alkyl *N*,*N*-dialkylphosphoramidocyanidates, such as tabun. The V-agents are *O*-alkyl *S*-(2-dialkylaminoethyl) alkylphosphonothiolates, such as VX. The chemistry of these agents has been documented extensively.[48] Metabolism is dominated by hydrolysis to alkyl alkylphosphonic acids and alkylphosphonic acids.[6,49] Reactions with proteins are more complex, but much less

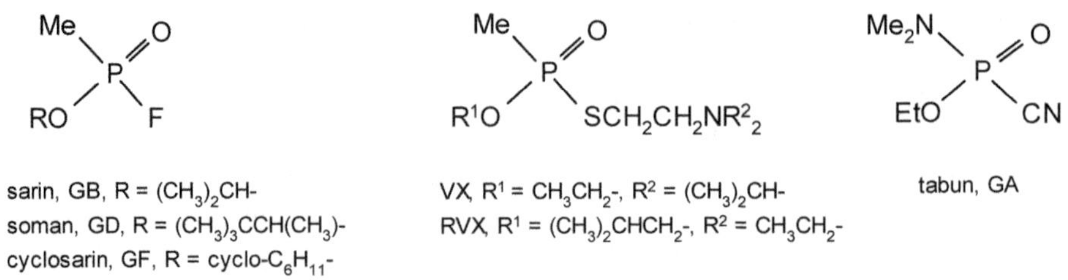

Scheme 6.5 Structures of organophosphorus nerve agents.

so than for sulphur mustard. The agents react rapidly with a serine hydroxyl group in the active site of AChE, the enzyme that catalyses the hydrolysis of the neurotransmitter acetylcholine in neuromuscular junctions and the central nervous system, thus inhibiting its action. From the point of view of verification of exposure, reactions with AChE present in red blood cell (erythrocyte) membranes and with BuChE, which is present in plasma but has no known physiological function, are more important.[7,49] Reactions with amino acid residues in other proteins also occur. Adducts with a tyrosine residue in albumin have some advantages as biomarkers of exposure in some circumstances as described below.[49]

As for sulphur mustard, a large number of methods for the analysis of biomarkers of nerve agent exposure have been reviewed.[6,7,9–12,49–51]

The simplest method for monitoring exposure to nerve agents uses the measurement of active AChE in erythrocytes or BuChE in plasma.[52,53] Inhibition of the enzyme is determined by a corresponding reduction in activity. The colourimetric Ellman method and its modifications monitor release of thiocholine from acetyl- or butyryl-thiocholine using the reagent 5,5′-dithio-bis-nitrobenzoic acid. A major disadvantage of this method is that ChE activities are rather variable between individuals and, as a reduction in activity is measured, baseline measurements are required prior to any possible exposure. As well as nerve agents, other organophosphorus compounds, such as many pesticides, and carbamates also inhibit ChE. This method is therefore not suitable for verification of exposure to nerve agents but is widely used in health monitoring, including in some devices proposed for point of care use.[50]

Intact nerve agent is unlikely to be detectable except in the most severe cases of exposure, and owing to the high toxicity of the agents, samples from casualties of such exposures are likely to be *post-mortem*. Methods for detection of intact agents have been limited to toxicological studies in animals where the dose is carefully controlled and medical countermeasures may be administered.

Urinary metabolites of nerve agents provide accessible biomarkers of exposure. The initial alkyl alkylphosphonic acid metabolites are extractable relatively easily from urine and may be analysed either by GC-MS[54,55] or GC-MS/MS[55–60] following suitable derivatisation, or directly by LC-MS[61] or LC-MS/MS.[62–66] The same metabolites may also be detected in plasma or serum.[67,68] Hydrophilic interaction LC (HILIC) is now often used in place of reverse-phase separations. The high organic content mobile phases used in HILIC are very compatible with ESI and high sensitivity is usually achievable. An example of detection of alkyl methylphosphonic acids in spiked human urine using HILIC conditions and detection by ESI with negative ion SRM is shown in Figure 6.3. The final alkylphosphonic acid metabolites are very polar and thus difficult to extract. The loss of the *O*-alkyl group also reduces the amount of information regarding the original agent and these metabolites are rarely included in analytical methods. Detection of metabolites of tabun presents additional problems. The initial hydrolysis products, ethyl *N,N*-dimethylphosphoramidic acid and ethyl phosphorocyanidic acid, hydrolyse further to ethyl phosphoric acid.[48,49] This is also a metabolite of some pesticides and plasticisers and thus not suitable as a biomarker for verification of exposure to tabun. A method including detection of the ethyl *N,N*-dimethylphosphoramidic acid metabolite has been published, however it is unstable and its occurrence *in vivo* has not been established.[56,57]

Adducts of nerve agents with ChEs may be determined using differing approaches. The experimentally simplest method uses displacement of the adducted phosphyl (phosphonyl or phosphoryl) group from the inhibited enzyme by an excess of fluoride ion.[69] The displaced phosphyl group, as the corresponding fluoridate, is extracted by SPE and detected by GC-MS or GC-MS/MS. Several variations of this approach have been published.[70–73] Although most often applied to detection of adduct with BuChE in plasma, the method has also been applied to detection of adduct with AChE in red blood cells[74,75] and tissues.[76] A disadvantage of the method is that all adducts are detected as fluoridates, thus the same phosphyl group originating from

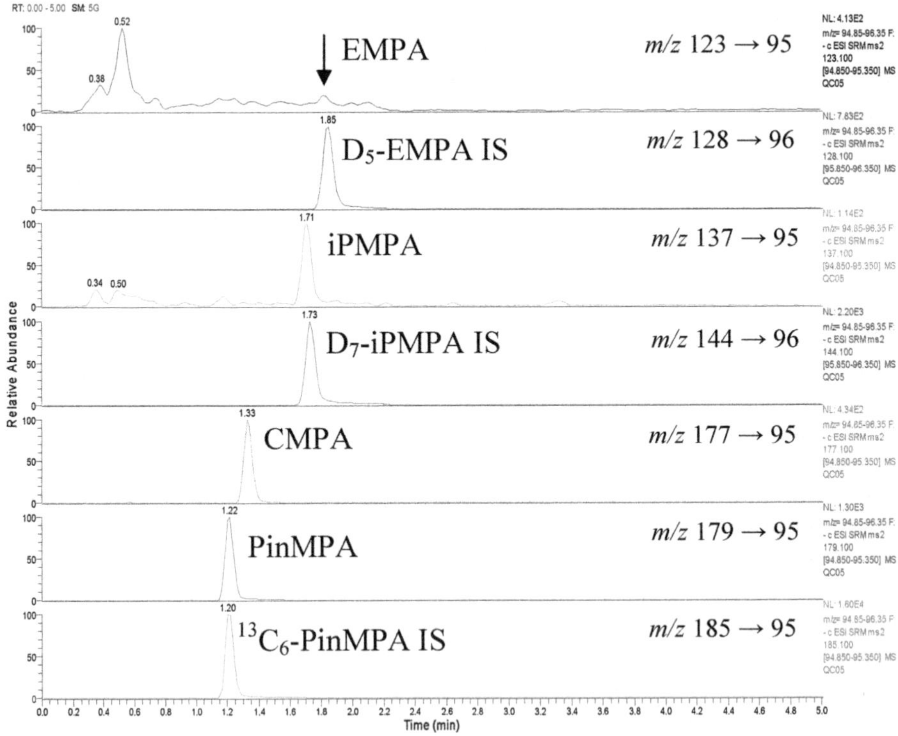

Figure 6.3 SRM chromatograms for alkyl methylphosphonic acids (1 ng ml^{-1}) and IS (10 ng ml^{-1}) from an extract of spiked human urine. Analysis was performed using HILIC conditions and LC-MS/MS with negative ion ESI. EMPA: ethyl methylphosphonic acid, iPMPA: isopropyl methylphosphonic acid, CMPA: cyclohexyl methylphosphonic acid, PinMPA: pinacolyl methylphosphonic acid.

a G-agent (fluoridate) or a V-agent (phosphonothiolate) cannot be distinguished. For example, the fluoridate resulting from displacement of the VX adduct could also originate from *O*-ethyl methylphosphonofluoridate (ethyl sarin) and is detected as such. Tabun is detected as its analogue, fluoro tabun. Figure 6.4 shows an example of GC-MS/MS detection of sarin regenerated from an incubate of human plasma with 1 nM sarin.

A second approach detects an adduct as a nonapeptide containing the phosphylated active site serine residue (Ser-203 in human AChE, Ser-198 in human BuChE). The method is usually applied to BuChE, which is much more abundant than AChE (BuChE 40–80 nM in plasma, AChE ~3 nM in erythrocytes). BuChE is isolated from plasma or serum and digested with the enzyme pepsin to give the phosphylated nonapeptide Phe-Gly-Glu-Ser*-Ala-Gly-Ala-Ala-Ser (where Ser* is the phosphylated Ser-198 residue), which is detected by LC-MS/MS.[77] Again, variations and improvements have been published,[78–80] including a method for detection of a common amine tagged nonapeptide derived from BuChE phosphylated by any nerve agent or organophosphorus pesticide.[80] Most recently, the emphasis has been on

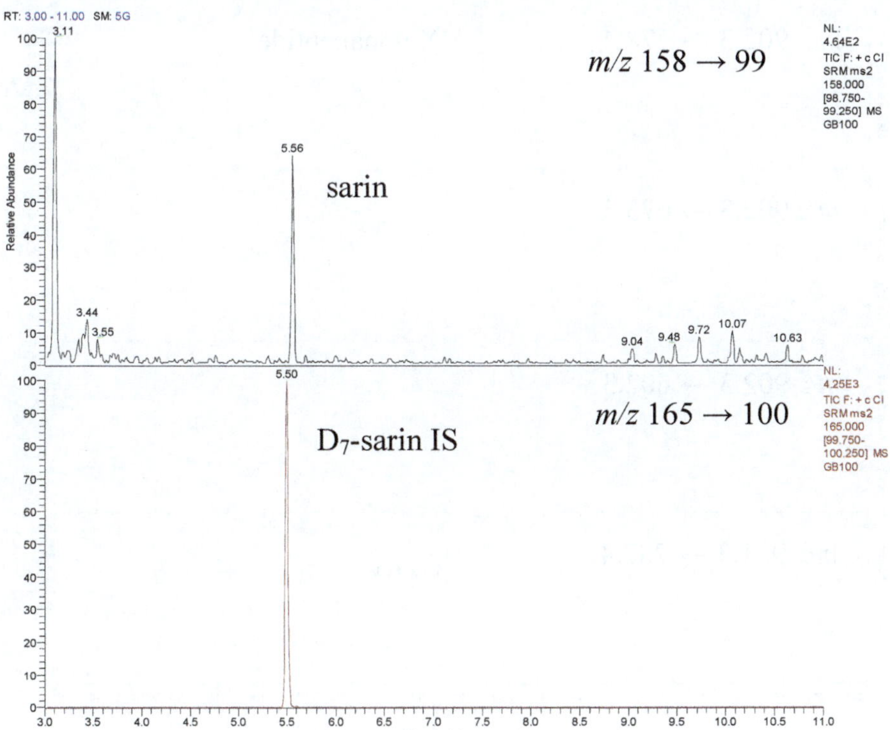

Figure 6.4 SRM chromatograms for sarin regenerated from an incubate of human plasma with 1 nM (140 pg ml^{-1}) sarin. IS was added following fluoride regeneration and prior to SPE. Analysis was performed using GC-MS/MS with ammonia CI.

the use of immunomagnetic isolation of BuChE and high throughput 96 well plate technology.[81–83] This technology has also been used to develop a method for simultaneous quantitation of adducted BuChE, non-adducted BuChE and free agent.[84] An example of detection of the ethyl methylphosphonyl adduct from VX in a plasma sample analysed during an OPCW biomedical sample analysis exercise is shown in Figure 6.5. The method used was based on that of Fidder *et al.*[77] with a carbon-13 labelled IS added before drying the final filtrate.

A significant problem with any method for detection of AChE and BuChE adducts is the phenomenon known as 'ageing'. The ageing process cleaves the *O*-alkyl moiety from the phosphylated serine in the active site of the enzyme. Ageing occurs at varying rates for the majority of nerve agents and is most rapid with soman, the *O*-pinacolyl moiety being removed within a few minutes. This renders the phosphyl group resistant to displacement by fluoride ion, and therapeutic oximes, and the resultant residue on the nonapeptide can only be identified as an alkylphosphonate.[49] Therefore the level of information obtained regarding the agent is much reduced. Nevertheless,

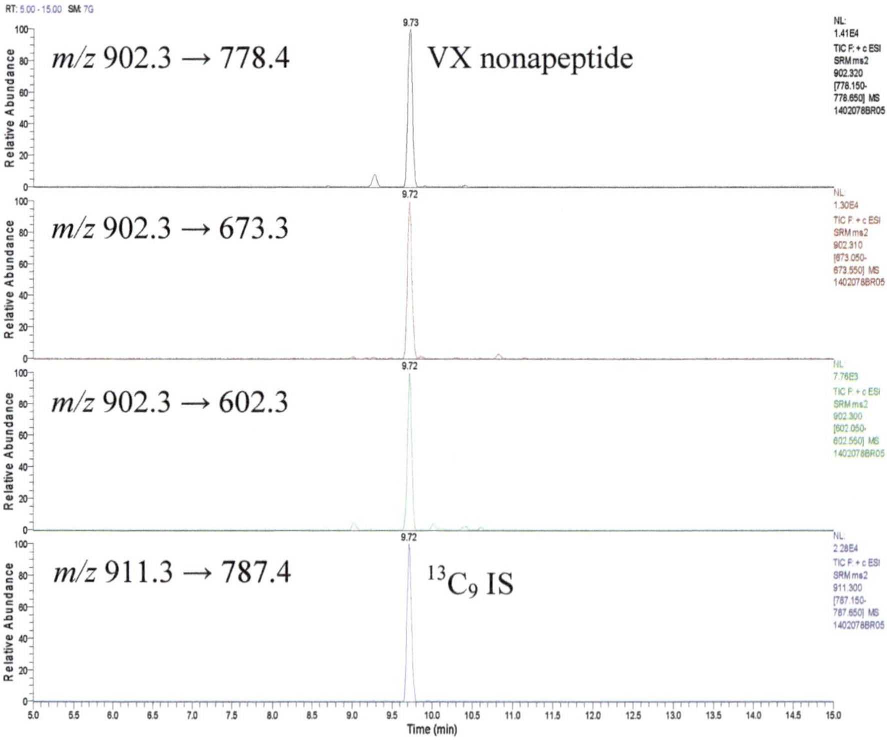

Figure 6.5 SRM chromatograms for VX adducted nonapeptide [Phe-Gly-Glu-Ser(EMP)-Ala-Gly-Ala-Ala-Ser] isolated from a sample of human plasma incubated with 30 nM (8 ng ml^{-1}) VX, analysed during an OPCW biomedical sample analysis exercise. Analysis was performed using LC-MS/MS with ESI. IS: $^{13}C_9$-Phe-Gly-Glu-Ser(EMP)-Ala-Gly-Ala-Ala-Ser.

detection of an aged residue would indicate that an exposure to a nerve agent had indeed occurred. A method for quantitation of methylphosphonate adducted BuChE by LC-MS/MS following immunomagnetic isolation and pepsin digestion has been published.[85] An alternative method for detection of aged adducts used binding to titanium oxide to enrich peptides produced by pepsin digestion of BuChE that had been treated with nerve agents [soman, sarin, cyclosarin, VX and *O*-isobutyl *S*-(2-diethylaminoethyl) methylphosphonothiolate (VR or RVX)] and stored at room temperature for 6 years.[86] Aged adducts were detected by matrix-assisted laser desorption/ionisation (MALDI) MS. Although application to real samples would still require isolation of BuChE, and preferably detection by LC-MS/MS, a large improvement in sensitivity was achieved by titanium oxide enrichment. An additional important finding was that adducts of VR showed no sign of ageing even after such a long period at room temperature. By using such methods, it is now possible to perform a complete analysis of native BuChE, and both non-aged and aged BuChE adducts in a sample, together with quantitation of any free agent.

An alternative adduct with a tyrosine residue in albumin (Tyr-411 in human albumin) is not subject to ageing and the complete structure of the phosphyl adduct is retained.[49,87–89] Example structures of the adducts are shown in Scheme 6.6. The adduct is extracted by SPE from plasma digested with the enzymes pronase or protease type XIV, and detected by ESI LC-MS/MS. Unlike non-aged adducts with BuChE, the adduct is also resistant to displacement by therapeutic oximes.[90] The adducts were formed in *in vitro* incubates with realistically low concentrations of the G-agents soman, sarin, cyclosarin and tabun; the adduct of VX was formed only in very high concentration incubates. Adducts containing the intact phosphyl group were detected for all of the G-agents in samples from exposed animals.[89,90] An example of the detection of the adduct with a low concentration of sarin in a human plasma incubate is shown in Figure 6.6. Using a method that includes affinity isolation of albumin from rat plasma prior to enzyme digestion, the detection of the VX–tyrosine adduct has been demonstrated.[91] This method also showed an improved signal to noise ratio compared with previous methods. Tyrosine adducts are only expected to be detected at levels of exposure higher than those detectable by analysis of BuChE adducts. However, in cases of exposure where therapeutic oximes have been administered, and possibly with delayed collection of samples, analysis of tyrosine adducts may be more appropriate.

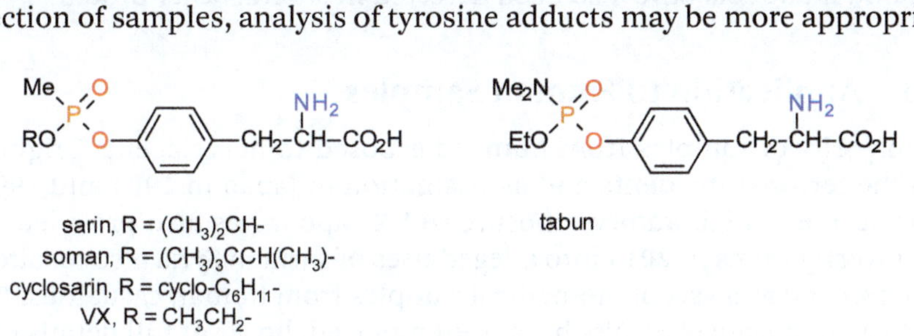

Scheme 6.6 Structures of adducts of nerve agents with tyrosine.

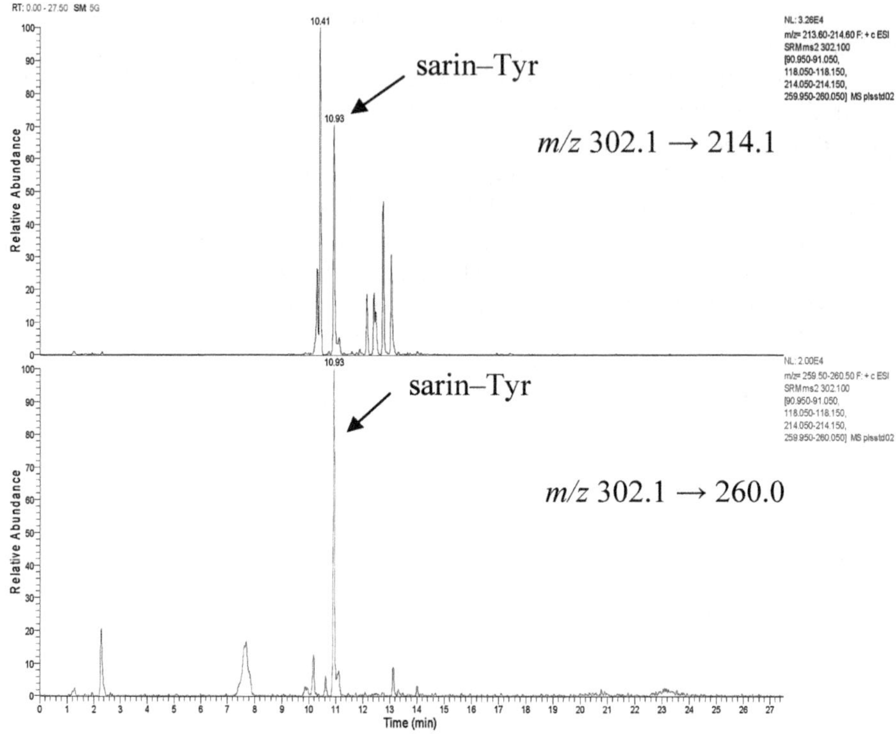

Figure 6.6 SRM chromatograms for sarin adduct with tyrosine from an incubate of 1 nM (140 pg ml^{-1}) sarin in human plasma. Analysis was performed using LC-MS/MS with ESI.

Similarly to enrichment of peptides derived from BuChE, enrichment of peptides from pepsin digests of albumin on iron affinity (PHOS-Select™) gel beads has been demonstrated.[92] Again, detection of peptides was by MALDI-TOF MS, but the enrichment procedure has potential application to samples from nerve agent exposures. Adducts of VX with two tyrosine residues in keratins in the human skin have been identified in pronase and trypsin digests of skin exposed to the agent.[93] The adducts were detected by LC-MS/MS. Similar adducts have also been detected in several other proteins.[94]

6.4.1 Application to Human Samples

The majority of samples from humans exposed to nerve agents originated from the terrorist incidents and assassination in Japan in 1994 and 1995. A single accidental laboratory exposure to VX vapour has also provided samples. Investigations in 2013 into alleged uses of sarin in Syria also resulted in collection and analysis of biomedical samples from human casualties. Basic 'positive' or 'negative' results have been reported, however full details of the analyses are yet to be published.[3]

6.4.1.1 Samples from Japanese Casualties of Sarin Exposure

Although among the best available at the time, the methods used for the initial analyses of samples from Japanese casualties would no longer be considered appropriate for verification of exposure. Rather non-selective silyl derivatisation reagents were used for GC with phosphorus flame photometric detection (FPD) of urinary metabolites.[95,96]

Urine samples from casualties of the Tokyo subway incident were partially cleaned up by passage through a column containing layers of cation exchange resin in the silver, barium and hydrogen forms.[95] The flow through was adjusted to pH 3.65–3.75 and lyophilised prior to derivatisation with *N*,*O*-bis(trimethylsilyl)trifluoroacetamide plus trimethylchlorosilane (BSTFA + TMCS) 10 : 1. The resulting trimethylsilyl (TMS) derivatives were detected by GC-FPD with LODs of 0.025 μg ml^{-1} for ethyl methylphosphonic acid (EMPA) and isopropyl methylphosphonic acid (iPMPA), and 0.625 μM for methylphosphonic acid (MPA). Ethyl phosphonic acid (EPA) was added to samples as IS for quantitation. Despite the selective nature of the FPD a considerable number of background peaks were present. Even in chromatograms from the most seriously intoxicated casualty these peaks were of significant intensity. The method was used to follow the excretion of isopropyl MPA in two casualties over a period of 8 days, the maximum concentration being observed within 12 h.

A similar method was used to analyse a single urine sample from a casualty of the Matsumoto City incident.[96] In this case urine was diluted with an equal volume of water and passed through a C18 cartridge and a hydrogen form cation exchange column prior to concentration to a small volume under reduced pressure. The concentrate, together with a tetrahydrofuran (THF) wash of the flask in which it was prepared, was then concentrated to dryness under nitrogen. The residue was dissolved in THF and derivatised with *N*-methyl-*N*-(*tert*-butyldimethylsilyl)trifluoroacetamide (MTBSTFA). After addition of 5% sodium chloride solution, the resulting *tert*-butyldimethylsilyl (TBDMS) derivatives were extracted into *n*-hexane containing 3-cyanophenyl dimethylphosphorothiolate [*O*,*O*-dimethyl *S*-(3-cyanophenyl)phosphorothiolate] as IS. The extract was dried with anhydrous sodium sulphate. Analysis by GC-FPD gave remarkably clean chromatograms with only small background peaks present. Both iPMPA and MPA were detected in urine samples collected on days 1 and 3 post-exposure. Only iPMPA was detected in a sample collected on day 7. Concentrations of MPA determined were 0.14 μg ml^{-1} on day 1 and 0.02 μg ml^{-1} on day 3. Owing to the lack of an authentic standard of iPMPA, its concentrations were estimated at 0.76, 0.08 and 0.01 μg ml^{-1} on days 1, 3 and 7, respectively.

TMS derivatives, this time with detection by GC-MS, were also used to confirm the presence of sarin adducts with erythrocyte AChE in four casualties from Tokyo.[97] Two of the casualties were fatalities. Red blood cell ghosts (erythrocyte membranes) were prepared and AChE extracted by a solubilisation and ultra-centrifugation procedure. AChE as well as other proteins contained in the extract were digested with trypsin, and bound sarin hydrolysis products were released by further digestion with alkaline phosphatase. High molecular weight impurities were removed by ultrafiltration and hydrolysis products derivatised with BSTFA plus 1% TMCS. The resulting TMS derivatives were analysed by GC-MS with EI and methane CI. Chromatograms were complex, however spectra were obtained that were consistent with TMS derivatives of iPMPA and MPA in samples from all four casualties.

A similar procedure, with the addition of an immunoaffinity purification of AChE, was used to detect MPA in brain tissue from four Tokyo casualties.[98] Tissue (cerebellums) had been preserved in formalin and stored for about 2 years before analysis. As above, GC-MS EI chromatograms were very complex, but peaks consistent with the TMS derivative of MPA were present. No iPMPA was detected, probably because of hydrolysis during storage.

Although deemed fit for the purpose of confirmation of exposure in the cases described, the above methods have some disadvantages. They lack the selectivity and sensitivity required to verify low level exposures and, in some instances, the positive identification of the nerve agent involved lacks certainty. The lengthy sample preparation procedures are also of concern when analysis of large numbers of samples may be required. The now most often used methods for verification of nerve agent exposure were developed to overcome these problems. They were applied to samples from casualties of both the Matsumoto and Tokyo subway incidents.

The first method to be developed in response to the incidents in Japan was that for fluoride regeneration of sarin.[69] Serum samples were diluted with three volumes of pH 3.5 sodium acetate buffer and incubated with 2 M potassium fluoride at 25 °C for 2 min. Incubates were then loaded onto C18 SPE cartridges and regenerated sarin was eluted with ethyl acetate. Ethyl acetate was separated from the residual aqueous phase by freezing with a dry ice/acetone mixture. Extracts were analysed by GC with alkaline flame nitrogen/phosphorus detection or high resolution MS (resolution 5000) with EI and SIM. The extract from one serum sample was also analysed by GC-high resolution MS in EI full scan mode. Sample introduction was *via* a thermal desorber autosampler that allowed a volume of 300 µl of ethyl acetate solution to be injected. Regenerated sarin was detected in serum from 10 out of 11 Tokyo casualties and 2 out of 7 Matsumoto casualties. Sarin concentrations were in the range 0.2–4.1 ng ml^{-1}. The extract analysed by full scan GC-MS gave a chromatographic peak containing characteristic fragment ions at *m*/*z* 81, 99 and 125, and could thus be identified as sarin. The method provided proof that casualties had been exposed to an agent with the structure i-PrO(CH_3)P(O)X, where it was assumed that X = F, *i.e.* sarin.

The second method developed was that for detection of adducts with BuChE as a phosphylated nonapeptide.[77] BuChE was isolated from serum using a procainamide affinity gel column. The column was eluted with 20 mM phosphate buffer containing 1 mM EDTA and 600 mM sodium chloride. Eluates were heated at 95 °C for 15 min and precipitated proteins removed by centrifugation. Following concentration by molecular weight cut off filtration, digestion with pepsin was performed. The digest was concentrated under vacuum prior to analysis by LC-MS/MS with ESI on a quadrupole-TOF (Q-TOF) instrument. Samples from two casualties of the Tokyo subway incident were analysed. Both had been analysed previously using the fluoride regeneration method described above. Nonapeptide with serine modified with an isopropyl methylphosphonyl group was detected in both samples. A full product ion spectrum of the *m*/*z* 916.4 protonated molecule precursor ion was obtained for one of the samples. The concentration of inhibited BuChE detected was estimated at 10–20 pmol ml^{-1}. Fluoride regeneration analysis of the same samples had detected sarin at approximately 14 pmol ml^{-1}. The utility of the method for detection of exposure to other agents and pesticides was also demonstrated.

As described above, several variations of these methods have since been published, including extension to other nerve agents. Some of these methods will be more broadly applicable to other ChE inhibitors.

6.4.1.2 Sample from a Japanese Casualty of VX Exposure

Serum collected from the male victim of an assassination with VX was analysed approximately 6 months after death, which occurred 10 days post-exposure.[99] The serum was collected approximately 1 h post-exposure but the use of VX was suspected only after testimony was obtained from the suspects. Serum was initially extracted with dichloromethane, the extract dried with anhydrous sodium sulphate and evaporated under nitrogen. The residue was redissolved in dichloromethane. The remaining aqueous fraction was deproteinised by the addition of acetonitrile. Oxalate buffer and sodium chloride were added to the supernatant and extracted with acetonitrile. The extract was evaporated to dryness under nitrogen and the residue derivatised with MTBSTFA plus *tert*-butyldimethylchlorosilane (TBDMCS). Analyses were performed by GC-MS and GC-MS/MS with EI and isobutane CI in full scan mode. EI and SIM were used for quantitation.

Analysis of the acetonitrile extract showed the presence of the TBDMS derivative of EMPA. Both EI and CI spectra, and CI product ion spectra, were consistent with those from an authentic standard. A very high concentration of 1.25 µg ml^{-1} of EMPA was determined. Analysis of the dichloromethane extract showed the presence of a small peak with a prominent fragment ion at *m*/*z* 114. Other ions present were *m*/*z* 72, 75 and 128. These ions were indicative of a compound related to the *N*,*N*-diisopropylaminoethylthio side-chain of VX. The CI spectrum contained an intense protonated ion at *m*/*z* 176, indicating a molecular mass of 175, and a product ion spectrum showed *m*/*z* 75 as its major fragment. The unknown compound was identified as 2-(*N*,*N*-diisopropylaminoethyl)methylsulphide. Identification was confirmed by comparison with an authentic standard and its concentration was determined as 143 ng ml^{-1}. This finding was important as detection of a compound derived from the VX side chain, together with EMPA, allowed the exposure to be differentiated from one to ethyl sarin.

6.4.1.3 Samples from an Accidental VX Exposure

Blood collected from a laboratory worker who accidentally inhaled VX vapour was analysed for the presence of ChE adducts using fluoride regeneration methods. Analyses were performed on both plasma and red cell fractions.[75,100] The casualty had received treatment including administration of atropine and the oxime pralidoxime. No significant reduction in blood ChE activity was reported and all symptoms of exposure disappeared within 24 h. Blood samples were collected on days 1, 6, 8, 13, 20 and 27; urine was collected on days 1 and 6.

Analysis of plasma followed a previously published method.[72,100] Plasma was incubated with 5.25 M potassium fluoride in pH 3.5 sodium acetate buffer at 40 °C for 1 h. A deuterated (CD_3) VX fluoridate analogue (*O*-ethyl D_3-methylphosphonofluoridate) was added as IS. Samples were loaded onto preconditioned polymeric SPE cartridges and dried by applying suction for 30 min. Regenerated agent was eluted with chloroform. Ethyl acetate was added to the eluate and concentrated to small volume under nitrogen. Residual ethyl acetate solutions were analysed by GC with high resolution EI and SIM. The regenerated fluoridate analogue of VX, *O*-ethyl methylphosphonofluoridate, was detected in all samples. Concentrations ranged from 81.2 pg ml^{-1} on day 1 to 6.9 pg ml^{-1} on day 27. The LOD was determined as 5.5 pg ml^{-1}. The measured concentrations were fitted to an exponential decay curve and the half-life of the VX–BuChE adduct estimated at 7.5 days. Analysis of urine samples failed to detect any EMPA metabolite of VX.

Analysis of red blood cells also followed a previously published method.[74,75] Acetate buffer, 6 M potassium fluoride solution and a deuterated IS were added to red cells, vortexed and centrifuged. Supernatant was added to a preconditioned C18 SPE cartridge. Further portions of acetate buffer and potassium fluoride solution were added to the residual red blood cells, vortexed, centrifuged and the supernatant added to the SPE cartridge. The combined supernatants were allowed to drain through the cartridge under gentle suction. Regenerated agent was eluted with ethyl acetate and the eluate dried over anhydrous sodium sulphate. Following filtration, the ethyl acetate solution was concentrated under nitrogen prior to analysis by GC-MS/MS with ammonia CI and SRM. Again, the fluoridate analogue of VX was detected in all samples with concentrations ranging from 219.9 pg ml^{-1} on day 1 to 96.9 pg ml^{-1} on day 27. Triplicate analyses gave results with rather large variability, however the half-life of the adduct in red blood cells was calculated as 24.5 days. No red blood cell sample corresponding to the day 13 plasma was analysed. The higher concentrations found in red blood cells supported the finding that VX preferentially inhibits red blood cell ChE. Results also demonstrated that detection in red blood cells should be possible for longer post-exposure compared with in plasma.

Both methods demonstrated the high sensitivity achievable and allowed detection of ChE adducts even in a casualty showing only minor symptoms of exposure and receiving therapy. Large numbers of such casualties and worried well would be expected in a terrorist use scenario, heavily outnumbering any fatalities, as was the case in the Tokyo subway.

6.5 Other Agents

In contrast to sulphur mustard and nerve agents, much less attention has been paid to the development of methods for verification of exposure to other CW agents. Such agents include analogues of sulphur mustard, nitrogen mustards, the arsenical vesicant lewisite, the hallucinogen quinuclidinyl benzilate (BZ), phosgene and hydrogen cyanide. Only brief details of selected methods for detection of biomarkers of exposure are provided here. No known human exposures have occurred in which biomedical samples have been analysed, the exception being the nitrogen mustard bis(2-chloroethyl) methylamine (HN-2), which has been used in cancer therapy and in this context some metabolism studies have been performed.

6.5.1 Analogues of Sulphur Mustard

The analogues of sulphur mustard of greatest interest are those that may be present in weaponised agents as by-products of synthesis or as freezing point depressants. Urine from a casualty of exposure to such an agent would be expected to contain metabolites of these materials as well as of sulphur mustard. A method for detection of seven hydrolysis product metabolites of these analogues by LC-MS/MS with detection by negative ion APCI has been published.[101] Titanium trichloride was used to reduce sulphoxide metabolites. The lowest reportable concentration was 1 ng ml^{-1}, and in contrast to thiodiglycol and its sulphoxide, no background was found in a set of 100 urine samples from non-exposed individuals.

6.5.2 Nitrogen Mustards

The nitrogen mustards, bis(2-chloroethyl)ethylamine (HN-1), HN-2 and tris(2-chloroethyl)amine (HN-3), are potent vesicants and are less volatile than sulphur mustard. Methods for detection of their hydrolysis product urinary metabolites and their adducts with a cysteine residue in albumin have been published. The urinary metabolites *N*-ethyldiethanolamine (from HN-1), *N*-methyldiethanolamine (HN-2) and triethanolamine (HN-3) may be detected by LC-MS/MS following automated strong cation exchange SPE.[102] Although no background of *N*-ethyldiethanolamine or *N*-methyldiethanolamine was detected in a set of 120 urine samples, 47% contained background of triethanolamine at concentrations between the LOD of 3 ng ml^{-1} and approximately 6500 ng ml^{-1}.

A high throughput automated method used 96 well plate, mixed mode, C8/strong cation exchange SPE and detection by LC-MS/MS with ESI and SRM.[103] A LOQ of 1 ng ml^{-1} was achieved for *N*-ethyldiethanolamine and

N-methyldiethanolamine in 300 µl aliquots of urine. The metabolite of HN-3 was not included in this method.

Like sulphur mustard, nitrogen mustards form adducts with the Cys-34 residue in albumin.[104] The modified Cys-Pro-Phe tripeptide may be detected by LC-MS/MS following pronase digestion in the same way as for the sulphur mustard adduct. A method combining detection of the tripeptide from sulphur mustard and nitrogen mustard adducts has been published, although the sensitivity was only moderate.[105] LODs in incubates with whole blood were 50 nM for sulphur mustard, 100 nM for HN-2, and 200 nM for HN-1 and HN-3.

6.5.3 Lewisite

Because the arsenical vesicant lewisite has been weaponised in the past, either separately or in mixtures with sulphur mustard, biomarkers of exposure have been the subject of some interest. Weaponised lewisite is a mixture of three compounds, all predominantly as trans isomers: ~90% lewisite 1, $ClCH{=}CHAsCl_2$; up to ~10% lewisite 2, $(ClCH{=}CH)_2AsCl$; and <1% lewisite 3, $(ClCH{=}CH)_3As$. Method development for biomarker detection has focused on metabolites and adducts of the most abundant lewisite 1.

2-Chlorovinylarsonous acid (CVAA), the urinary metabolite of lewisite 1, has been detected as a derivative formed by the reaction of CVAA in urine with an alkanedithiol, such as ethanedithiol or 1,3-propanedithiol.[106–108] Derivatives may readily be extracted from the reaction headspace by solid phase microextraction (SPME).[106,107] SPME combined with GC-MS with EI and SIM achieved LODs as low as 7.4 pg ml^{-1} in 1 ml urine samples.[106] The method was also applied for the analysis of plasma and red blood cells.[107] An alternative method used dispersive derivatisation liquid–liquid microextraction.[108] Ethanedithiol in a mixture of methanol (dispersive solvent) and chloroform (extraction solvent) was added rapidly to urine samples. Following vigorous shaking and standing for 1 min, the sample was centrifuged and the chloroform layer removed for analysis by GC-MS with EI and SIM. This relatively simple method achieved a LOD of 0.015 ng ml^{-1}.

Urinary metabolites have also been detected by LC with inductively coupled plasma MS (ICP-MS)[109] and LC-MS/MS.[110] An advantage of LC-based methods is the ability to detect both CVAA and its oxidation product, 2-chlorovinylarsonic acid (CVAOA). The disadvantage of ICP-MS methods is that confirmation of identity is based solely on retention time and the presence of arsenic. Simple dilution of urine samples with sodium arsonoacetate IS in mobile phase buffer followed by an isocratic LC separation and ICP-MS allowed a high throughput of 12 samples per hour to be achieved. LODs were 1.3 ng ml^{-1} for CVAA and 1.4 ng ml^{-1} for CVAOA.[109] Analysis by LC-MS/MS achieved LODs of 0.5 ng ml^{-1} for CVAA and 3 ng ml^{-1} for CVAOA. Urine samples were basified (pH 9) with ammonia and partially cleaned up by passage through a mixed mode C8/strong cation exchange SPE cartridge. Samples were analysed by LC-MS/MS with negative ion ESI and SRM.[110]

Lewisite has been shown to bind to human haemoglobin, with crosslinking of cysteine residues 93 and 112 of the globin β-chain identified as one binding site.[111] Bound CVAA was displaced from red blood cells by reaction with 2,3-dimercapto-1-propanol (BAL; British Anti-Lewisite) in acetonitrile and the product extracted by SPE on C18 cartridges. The BAL derivative was eluted with dichloromethane, concentrated to dryness and derivatised with heptafluorobutyrylimidazole in toluene. After washing with water and drying with magnesium sulphate, samples were analysed by GC-MS with EI and negative ion CI and SIM. The LOD for *in vitro* exposed human blood was 1 nM. The same method was applied to isolation of CVAA from human urine with a LOD of 10 nM.

6.5.4 Quinuclidinyl Benzilate

Methods have been developed for the detection of the hallucinogen quinuclidinyl benzilate (BZ) and its hydrolysis product metabolites, benzilic acid and 3-quinuclidinol, in urine.[112] BZ and benzilic acid were isolated by SPE on C18 cartridges and 3-quinuclidinol on Florisil® cartridges. TMS derivatives were prepared and analysed by GC-MS with EI in SIM mode. LODs were 0.5 ng ml^{-1} for BZ and 5 ng ml^{-1} for the metabolites, but large, 20 ml, urine volumes were required.

6.5.5 Phosgene and Hydrogen Cyanide

Both phosgene and hydrogen cyanide are common industrial chemicals that were used as CW agents during World War 1. The use of toxic industrial chemicals for terrorist purposes is still of concern. The presence of biomarkers of exposure to phosgene and hydrogen cyanide may result from industrial occupational exposure, exposure to smoke from fires and, in the case of hydrogen cyanide, cigarettes. Biomarkers are therefore not unique to their use as CW agents.

Phosgene has been shown to form adducts *in vitro* with albumin and haemoglobin.[113] An adduct with globin was identified as a crosslink between *N*-terminal valine and the adjacent leucine residues of the α-chain. A similar adduct was detected in control samples, possibly from reaction with carbon dioxide, rendering this adduct unsuitable as a biomarker of exposure to phosgene.[7] An adduct with albumin was identified as a crosslink between lysine residues 195 and 199. Methods for detection of these adducts have not been applied to human or animal samples.

In a recent method for determination of exposure to hydrogen cyanide, and cyanides in general, plasma proteins were precipitated and adducted thiocyanate extracted by hydrolysis with a pH 10 carbonate buffer.[114] Following derivatisation with pentafluorobenzyl bromide, analysis was performed by GC-MS with EI and SIM. The LOD was estimated as 2.5 ng ml^{-1} of thiocyanate in the extraction matrix.

6.6 Further Developments

Developments in analytical methods for verification of exposure to CW agents are mainly aimed at improvements in sensitivity and sample throughput. Owing to the large variations in properties of analytes it is likely that methods will still need to be targeted at single or small numbers of analytes. The use of high resolution, scanning mass spectrometric methods is showing great promise for the detection of multiple analytes in a single analysis. The use of such a method for detection of nerve agent metabolites has been demonstrated.[115] The major advantage of the technique is that full scan data can be used for detection of analytes that would be missed by targeted methods such as SRM, the proviso being that sample preparation methods must allow such detection to be achieved.

Simple, rapid methods for screening samples prior to analysis by more complex methods may have wider applications. Point of care devices have been proposed for such purposes and there is no reason why the same devices could not be used in the laboratory.[50] It remains to be seen whether such devices will have the required sensitivity and selectivity to avoid significant numbers of false positives or negatives. An alternative screening approach is to use selective mass spectrometric detection with minimal sample preparation and no chromatographic separation. Detection of nerve agent metabolites in synthetic urine has been demonstrated using such an approach.[116] Alkyl methylphosphonic acids thermally desorbed from an atmospheric solids analysis probe were ionised in an APCI source and detected by high resolution MS in an Orbitrap™ instrument. The acids were all detected in samples spiked at 1 ng ml^{-1}, except for EMPA, which was detected at 100 ng ml^{-1}. This method approaches the sensitivity and selectivity required to be useful for the screening of real samples. It should be noted that all screening methods developed to date have been applied to nerve agents. Extension of rapid screening methods to other agents, with widely differing properties, will be complex and it remains to be seen whether simple solutions to the problems involved are possible. Application to urinary metabolites is probably less demanding than to blood protein and ChE adducts, although attempts have been made in the latter context.[13]

Developments in instrumentation continue and mass spectrometers are becoming ever more powerful. Modern instruments are extremely sensitive, robust and much more user friendly than in the past. Together with improved sample preparation and separation techniques these developments will lead to further advances in the detection of biomarkers for the verification of exposure.

References

1. R. W. Read, Applications of mass spectrometry in investigations of alleged use of chemical warfare agents, in *Detection of Biological Agents for the Prevention of Bioterrorism, NATO Science for Peace and Security Series A – Chemistry and Biology*, ed. J. Banoub, Springer, Heidelberg, 2011, pp. 201–219.

2. OPCW, *Convention on the prohibition of the development, production, stockpiling and use of chemical weapons and on their destruction*, Organisation for the Prohibition of Chemical Weapons, The Hague, 1994.
3. UN, *United Nations mission to investigate allegations of the use of chemical weapons in the Syrian Arab Republic, Final report*, United Nations, New York, 2013.
4. R. M. Black and R. W. Read, Environmental and biomedical sample analysis in support of allegations of use of chemical warfare agents, *Toxin Rev.*, 2007, **26**, 275–298.
5. J. B. Tucker, The 'Yellow Rain' controversy: Lessons for arms control compliance, *Nonproliferation Rev.*, 2001, **8**, 25–42.
6. R. M. Black, R. W. Read and D. Noort, Methods for the retrospective detection of exposure to toxic scheduled chemicals: Analysis of free metabolites, in *Encyclopedia of Analytical Chemistry, Online*, ed. R. A. Meyers, John Wiley and Sons Ltd, Chichester, UK, 2012.
7. D. Noort and R. M. Black, Methods for retrospective detection of exposure to toxic scheduled chemicals. Part B: Mass spectrometric and immunochemical analysis of covalent adducts to proteins and DNA, in *Encyclopedia of Analytical Chemistry, Online*, ed. R. A. Meyers, John Wiley and Sons Ltd, Chichester, UK, 2012.
8. S. J. Fairhall, B. J. A. Jugg, R. W. Read, S. J. Stubbs, S. J. Rutter, A. J. Smith, T. M. Mann, J. Jenner and A. M. Sciuto, Exposure-response effects of inhaled sulfur mustard in a large porcine model: a 6-h study, *Inhalation Toxicol.*, 2010, **22**, 1135–1143.
9. R. M. Black, An overview of biological markers of exposure to chemical warfare agents, *J. Anal. Toxicol.*, 2008, **32**, 2–9.
10. R. M. Black, History and perspectives of bioanalytical methods for chemical warfare agent detection, *J. Chromatogr. B*, 2010, **878**, 1207–1215.
11. B. R. Capacio, J. R. Smith, R. K. Gordon, J. R. Haigh, J. R. Barr and B. J. Lukey, Clinical detection of exposure to chemical warfare agents, in *Chemical Warfare Agents. Chemistry, Pharmacology, Toxicology, and Therapeutics*, ed. J. A. Romano Jr, B. J. Lukey and H. Salem, CRC Press, Boca Raton, Florida, 2nd edn, 2008, ch. 19, pp. 501–548.
12. K. Tsuge and Y. Seto, Mass spectrometric identification of chemical warfare agent adducts with biological macromolecule for verification of their exposure, *J. Health Sci.*, 2009, **55**, 879–886.
13. J. Carol-Visser, M. van der Schans, A. Fidder, A. G. Hulst, B. L. M. van Baar, H. Irth and D. Noort, Development of an automated on-line pepsin digestion-liquid chromatography-tandem mass spectrometry configuration for the rapid analysis of protein adducts of chemical warfare agents, *J. Chromatogr. B*, 2008, **870**, 91–97.
14. D. Noort, A. G. Hulst, L. P. A. De Jong and H. P. Benschop, Alkylation of human serum albumin by sulfur mustard in vitro and in vivo: Mass spectrometric analysis of a cysteine adduct as a sensitive biomarker of exposure, *Chem. Res. Toxicol.*, 1999, **12**, 715–721.
15. I. Sandelowsky, G. A. Simon, P. Bel, R. Barak and A. Vincze, N^1-(2-hydroxyethylthioethyl)-4-methylimidazole (4-met-1-imid-thiodiglycol)

in plasma and urine: a novel metabolite following dermal exposure to sulphur mustard, *Arch. Toxicol.*, 1992, **66**, 296–297.

16. G. P. van der Schans, D. Noort, R. H. Mars-Groenendijk, A. Fidder, L. F. Chau, L. P. A. De Jong and H. P. Benschop, Immunochemical detection of sulfur mustard adducts with keratins in the stratum corneum of human skin, *Chem. Res. Toxicol.*, 2003, **15**, 21–25.
17. A. Fidder, D. Noort, L. P. A. de Jong, H. P. Benschop and A. G. Hulst, N7-(2-hydroxyethylthioethyl)-guanine: a novel urinary metabolite following exposure to sulphur mustard, *Arch. Toxicol.*, 1996, **70**, 854–855.
18. L. Yue, Y. Wei, J. Chen, H. Shi, Q. Liu, Y. Zhang, J. He, L. Guo, T. Zhang, J. Xie and S. Peng, Abundance of four sulfur mustard-DNA adducts ex vivo and in vivo revealed by simultaneous quantification in stable isotope dilution-ultrahigh performance liquid chromatography-tandem mass spectrometry, *Chem. Res. Toxicol.*, 2014, **27**, 490–500.
19. G. Drasch, E. Kretschmer, G. Kauert and L. Von Meyer, Concentrations of mustard gas [bis(2-chloroethyl)sulfide] in the tissues of a victim of vesicant exposure, *J. Forensic Sci.*, 1987, **32**, 1788–1793.
20. E. R. J. Wils, A. G. Hulst, A. L. de Jong, A. Verweij and H. L. Boter, Analysis of thiodiglycol in urine of victims of an alleged attack with mustard gas, *J. Anal. Toxicol.*, 1985, **9**, 254–257.
21. E. R. J. Wils, A. G. Hulst and J. van Laar, Analysis of thiodiglycol in urine of victims of an alleged attack with mustard gas, Part II, *J. Anal. Toxicol.*, 1988, **12**, 15–19.
22. R. M. Black and R. W. Read, Detection of trace levels of thiodiglycol in blood, plasma and urine using gas chromatography – electron-capture negative-ion chemical ionisation mass spectrometry, *J. Chromatogr.*, 1988, **449**, 261–270.
23. R. M. Black and R. W. Read, Methods for the analysis of thiodiglycol sulphoxide, a metabolite of sulphur mustard, in urine using gas chromatography-mass spectrometry, *J. Chromatogr.*, 1991, **558**, 393–404.
24. R. M. Black, R. J. Clarke and R. W. Read, Analysis of 1,1′-sulphonylbis[2-(methylsulphinyl)ethane]and 1-methylsulphinyl-2-[2-(methylthio) ethylsulphonyl]ethane, metabolites of sulphur mustard, in urine using gas chromatography-mass spectrometry, *J. Chromatogr.*, 1991, **558**, 405–414.
25. R. M. Black and R. W. Read, Improved methodology for the detection and quantitation of urinary metabolites of sulphur mustard using gas chromatography-tandem mass spectrometry, *J. Chromatogr. B: Biomed. Sci. Appl.*, 1995, **665**, 97–105.
26. R. M. Black and R. W. Read, Biological fate of sulphur mustard, 1,1-thiobis(2- chloroethane): identification of β-lyase metabolites and hydrolysis products in human urine, *Xenobiotica*, 1995, **25**, 167–173.
27. R. W. Read and R. M. Black, Analysis of β-lyase metabolites of sulfur mustard in urine by electrospray liquid chromatography-tandem mass spectrometry, *J. Anal. Toxicol.*, 2004, **28**, 346–351.

28. R. W. Read and R. M. Black, Analysis of the sulfur mustard metabolite 1,1′-sulfonylbis[2-S-(N-acetylcysteinyl)ethane] in urine by negative ion electrospray liquid chromatography-tandem mass spectrometry, *J. Anal. Toxicol.*, 2004, **28**, 352–356.
29. E. M. Jakubowski, F. R. Sidell, R. A. Evans, M. A. Carter, J. R. Keeler, J. D. McMonagle, A. Swift, J. R. Smith and T. W. Dolzine, Quantification of thiodiglycol in human urine after an accidental sulfur mustard exposure, *Toxicol. Methods*, 2000, **10**, 143–150.
30. J. R. Barr, C. L. Pierce, J. R. Smith, B. R. Capacio, A. R. Woolfit, M. I. Solano, J. V. Wooten, S. W. Lemire, J. D. Thomas, D. H. Ash and D. L. Ashley, Analysis of urinary metabolites of sulfur mustard in two individuals after accidental exposure, *J. Anal. Toxicol.*, 2008, **32**, 10–16.
31. M. Halme, M. Karjalainen, H. Kiljunen and P. Vanninen, Development and validation of efficient stable isotope dilution LC-HESI-MS/MS method for the verification of β-lyase metabolites in human urine after sulfur mustard exposure, *J. Chromatog. B*, 2011, **879**, 908–914.
32. J. D. Daly, C. M. O'Hehir and G. M. Frame, A sensitive method for quantitation of β-lyase metabolites of sulfur mustard as 1,1′-sulfonylbis[2-(methylthio)ethane] (SBMTE) in human urine by isotope dilution liquid chromatography-positive ion-electrospray-tandem mass spectrometry, *J. Chromatogr. B*, 2007, **850**, 120–127.
33. M. K. Reddy, C. Nixon, S. A. Wyatt and T. R. Croley, A robust high-throughput sample preparation and liquid chromatography/tandem mass spectrometry method for the quantitation of β-lyase metabolites of sulfur mustard as 1,1′-sulfonylbis-[2-(methylthio)ethane] in human urine, *Rapid Commun. Mass Spectrom.*, 2013, **27**, 1128–1134.
34. I. A. Rodin, A. V. Braun, E. I. Savelieva, I. V. Rybalchenko, I. A. Ananieva and O. E. Shpigun, Rapid method for the detection of metabolite of sulfur mustard 1,1′-sulfonylbis[2-S-(N-acetylcysteinyl)ethane] in plasma and urine by liquid chromatography-negative electrospray-tandem mass spectrometry, *J. Liq. Chromatogr. Relat. Technol.*, 2011, **34**, 1676–1685.
35. C. Li, J. Chen, Q. Liu, J. Xie and H. Li, Simultaneous quantification of seven plasma metabolites of sulfur mustard by ultra high performance liquid chromatography-tandem mass spectrometry, *J. Chromatogr. B*, 2013, **917–918**, 100–107.
36. A. Fidder, D. Noort, A. L. de Jong, H. C. Trap, L. P. A. de Jong and H. P. Benschop, Monitoring of in vitro and in vivo exposure to sulfur mustard by GC/MS determination of the N-terminal valine adduct in hemoglobin after a modified Edman degradation, *Chem. Res. Toxicol.*, 1996, **9**, 788–792.
37. H. P. Benschop, G. P. van der Schans, D. Noort, A. Fidder, R. H. Mars-Groenendijk and L. P. A. de Jong, Verification of exposure to sulfur mustard in two casualties of the Iran-Iraq conflict, *J. Anal. Toxicol.*, 1997, **21**, 249–251.

38. R. M. Black, R. J. Clarke, J. M. Harrison and R. W. Read, Biological fate of sulphur mustard: identification of valine and histidine adducts in haemoglobin from casualties of sulphur mustard poisoning, *Xenobiotica*, 1997, **27**, 499–512.
39. D. Noort, A. Fidder, H. P. Benschop, L. P. A. de Jong and J. R. Smith, Procedure for monitoring exposure to sulfur mustard based on a modified Edman degradation of globin, *J. Anal. Toxicol.*, 2004, **28**, 311–315.
40. Z. Nie, Q. Liu and J. Xie, Improvements in monitoring the N-terminal valine adduct in human globin after exposure to sulfur mustard and synthesis of reference chemicals, *Talanta*, 2011, **85**, 1154–1159.
41. H. von Stedingk, P. Rydberg and M. Törnqvist, A new modified Edman procedure for analysis of N-terminal valine adducts in hemoglobin by LC-MS/MS, *J. Chromatogr. B*, 2010, **878**, 2483–2490.
42. D. Noort, A. Fidder, A. G. Hulst, A. R. Woolfitt, D. Ash and J. R. Barr, Retrospective detection of exposure to sulfur mustard: Improvements on an assay for liquid chromatography-tandem mass spectrometry analysis of albumin/sulfur mustard adducts, *J. Anal. Toxicol.*, 2004, **28**, 333–338.
43. T. M. Andacht, B. G. Pantazides, B. S. Crow, A. Fidder, D. Noort, J. D. Thomas, T. A. Blake and R. C. Johnson, An enhanced throughput method for quantification of sulfur mustard aducts to human serum albumin via isotope dilution tandem mass spectrometry, *J. Anal. Toxicol.*, 2014, **38**, 8–15.
44. J. R. Smith, B. R. Capacio, W. D. Korte, A. R. Woolfitt and J. R. Barr, Analysis for plasma protein biomarkers following an accidental human exposure to sulfur mustard, *J. Anal. Toxicol.*, 2008, **32**, 17–24.
45. B. R. Capacio, J. R. Smith, M. T. DeLion, D. R. Anderson, J. S. Graham, G. E. Platoff and W. D. Korte, Monitoring sulfur mustard exposure by gas chromatography-mass spectrometry analysis of thiodiglycol cleaved from blood proteins, *J. Anal. Toxicol.*, 2004, **28**, 306–310.
46. R. J. Lawrence, J. R. Smith, B. L. Boyd and B. R. Capacio, Improvements in the methodology of monitoring sulfur mustard exposure by gas chromatography-mass spectrometry analysis of cleaved and derivatized blood protein adducts, *J. Anal. Toxicol.*, 2008, **32**, 31–36.
47. H. Xu, Z. Nie, Y. Zhang, C. Li, L. Yue, W. Yang, J. Chen, Y. Dong, Q. Liu, Y. Lin, B. Wu, J. Feng, H. Li, L. Guo and J. Xie, Four sulfur mustard exposure cases: Overall analysis of four types of biomarkers in clinical samples provides positive implication for early diagnosis and treatment monitoring, *Toxicol. Rep.*, 2014, **1**, 533–543.
48. R. M. Black and J. M. Harrison, The chemistry of organophosphorus nerve agents, in *Patai's Chemistry of Functional Groups, Online*, ed. I. Marek, John Wiley & Sons Ltd., Chichester, UK, 2009.
49. R. M. Black and R. W. Read, Biological markers of exposure to organophosphorus nerve agents, *Arch. Toxicol.*, 2013, **87**, 421–437.
50. J. P. Langenberg, M. J. van der Schans and D. Noort, Assessment of nerve agent exposure: existing and emerging methods, *Bioanalysis*, 2009, **1**, 729–739.

51. L. M. Schopfer and O. Lockridge, Analytical approaches for monitoring exposure to organophosphorus and carbamate agents through analysis of protein adducts, *Drug Test. Anal.*, 2012, **4**, 246–261.
52. G. L. Ellman, K. D. Courtney, V. Andres Jr. and R. M. Featherstone, A new and rapid colorimetric determination of acetylcholinesterase activity, *Biochem. Pharmacol.*, 1961, **7**, 88–95.
53. F. Worek, U. Mast, D. Kiderlen, C. Diepold and P. Eyer, Improved determination of acetylcholinesterase activity in human whole blood, *Clin. Chim. Acta*, 1999, **288**, 73–90.
54. M. L. Shih, J. R. Smith, J. D. McMonagle, T. W. Dolzine and V. C. Gresham, Detection of metabolites of toxic alkylmethylphosphonates in biological samples, *Biol. Mass Spectrom.*, 1991, **20**, 717–723.
55. S.-Å. Fredriksson, L.-G. Hammarström, L. Henriksson and H.-Å. Lakso, Trace determination of alkyl methylphosphonic acids in environmental and biological samples using gas chromatography/negative-ion chemical ionization mass spectrometry and tandem mass spectrometry, *J. Mass Spectrom.*, 1995, **30**, 1133–1143.
56. W. J. Driskell, M. Shih, L. L. Needham and D. B. Barr, Quantitation of organophosphorus nerve agent metabolites in human urine using isotope dilution gas chromatography-tandem mass spectrometry, *J. Anal. Toxicol.*, 2002, **26**, 6–10.
57. J. R. Barr, W. J. Driskell, L. S. Aston and R. A. Martinez, Quantitation of metabolites of the nerve agents sarin, soman, cyclohexylsarin, VX, and Russian VX in human urine using isotope-dilution gas chromatography-tandem mass spectrometry, *J. Anal. Toxicol.*, 2004, **28**, 372–378.
58. J. Riches, I. Morton, R. W. Read and R. M. Black, The trace analysis of alkyl alkylphosphonic acids in urine using gas chromatography-ion trap negative ion tandem mass spectrometry, *J. Chromatogr. B*, 2005, **816**, 251–258.
59. R. Subramaniam, A. Östin, C. Nilsson and C. Åstot, Direct derivatization and gas chromatography-tandem mass spectrometry identification of nerve agent biomarkers in urine samples, *J. Chromatogr. B*, 2013, **928**, 98–105.
60. Y. Lin, J. Chen, L. Yan, L. Guo, B. Wu, C. Li, J. Feng, Q. Liu and J. Xie, Determination of nerve agent metabolites in human urine by isotope-dilution gas chromatography-tandem mass spectrometry after solid phase supported derivatization, *Anal. Bioanal. Chem.*, 2014, **406**, 5213–5220.
61. I. A. Rodin, A. V. Braun, I. A. Anan'eva, O. A. Schpigun, E. I. Savel'eva, I. V. Rybal'chenko, S. L. Bolotov and G. M. Rodchenkov, Detection of nerve agent markers by liquid chromatography-mass spectrometry, *J. Anal. Chem.*, 2011, **66**, 1417–1422.
62. H. John, F. Worek and H. Thiermann, LC-MS-based procedures for monitoring of toxic organophosphorus compounds and verification of pesticide and nerve agent poisoning, *Anal. Bioanal. Chem.*, 2008, **391**, 97–116.

63. F. L. Ciner, C. E. McCord, R. W. Plunkett Jr, M. F. Martin and T. R. Croley, Isotope dilution LC/MS/MS for the detection of nerve agent exposure in urine, *J. Chromatogr. B*, 2007, **846**, 42–50.
64. D. B. Mawhinney, E. I. Hamelin, R. Fraser, S. S. Silva, A. J. Pavlopoulos and R. J. Kobelski, The determination of organophosphonate nerve agent metabolites in human urine by hydrophilic interaction liquid chromatography tandem mass spectrometry, *J. Chromatogr. B*, 2007, **852**, 235–243.
65. L. L. Swaim, R. C. Johnson, Y. Zhou, C. Sandlin and J. R. Barr, Quantification of organophosphorus nerve agent metabolites using a reduced-volume, high-throughput sample processing format and liquid chromatography-tandem mass spectrometry, *J. Anal. Toxicol.*, 2008, **32**, 774–777.
66. J. Y. Lee and Y. H. Lee, Rapid screening and determination of nerve agent metabolites in human urine by LC-MS/MS, *J. Anal. Chem.*, 2014, **69**, 909–916.
67. Q. Wang, J. Xie, M. Gu, J. Feng and J. Ruan, Gas chromatographic-mass spectrometric method for quantitation of trimethylsilyl derivatives of nerve agent degradation products in human plasma, using strong anion-exchange solid-phase extraction, *Chromatographia*, 2005, **62**, 167–173.
68. E. I. Hamelin, N. D. Schulze, R. L. Shaner, R. M. Coleman, R. J. Lawrence, B. S. Crow, E. M. Jakubowski and R. C. Johnson, Quantitation of five organophosphorus nerve agent metabolites in serum using hydrophilic interaction liquid chromatography and tandem mass spectrometry, *Anal. Bioanal. Chem.*, 2014, **406**, 5195–5202.
69. M. Polhuijs, J. P. Langenberg and H. P. Benschop, New method for retrospective detection of exposure to organophosphorus anticholinesterases: application to alleged sarin victims of Japanese terrorists, *Toxicol. Appl. Pharmacol.*, 1997, **146**, 156–161.
70. M. J. van der Schans, M. Polhuijs, C. van Dijk, C. E. A. M. Degenhardt, K. Pleijsier, J. P. Langenberg and H. P. Benschop, Retrospective detection of exposure to nerve agents: analysis of phosphofluoridates originating from fluoride-induced reactivation of phosphylated BuChE, *Arch. Toxicol.*, 2004, **78**, 508–524.
71. C. E. A. M. Degenhardt, K. Pleijsier, M. J. van der Schans, J. P. Langenberg, K. E. Preston, M. I. Solano, V. L. Maggio and J. R. Barr, Improvements of the fluoride reactivation method for the verification of nerve agent exposure, *J. Anal. Toxicol.*, 2004, **28**, 364–371.
72. K. E. Holland, M. I. Solano, R. C. Johnson, V. L. Maggio and J. R. Barr, Modifications to the organophosphorus nerve agent-protein adduct refluoridation method for retrospective analysis of nerve agent exposures, *J. Anal. Toxicol.*, 2008, **32**, 116–124.
73. J. A. van der Meer, H. C. Trap, D. Noort and M. J. van der Schans, Comprehensive gas chromatography with time of flight MS and large volume introduction for the detection of fluoride-induced regenerated nerve agent in biological samples, *J. Chromatogr. B*, 2010, **878**, 1320–1325.

74. E. M. Jakubowski, J. M. McGuire, R. A. Evans, J. L. Edwards, S. W. Hulet, B. J. Benton, J. S. Forster, D. C. Burnett, W. T. Muse, K. Matson, C. L. Crouse, R. J. Mioduszewski and S. A. Thomson, Quantitation of fluoride ion released sarin in red blood cell samples by gas chromatography-chemical ionization mass spectrometry using isotope dilution and large-volume injection, *J. Anal. Toxicol.*, 2004, **28**, 357–363.
75. J. M. McGuire, J. T. Taylor, C. E. Byers, E. M. Jakubowski and S. A. Thomson, Determination of VX-G analogue in red blood cells via gas chromatography-tandem mass spectrometry following an accidental exposure to VX, *J. Anal. Toxicol.*, 2008, **32**, 73–77.
76. T. K. Adams, B. R. Capacio, J. R. Smith, C. E. Whalley and W. D. Korte, The application of the fluoride reactivation process to the detection of sarin and soman nerve agent exposures in biological samples, *Drug Chem. Toxicol.*, 2004, **27**, 77–91.
77. A. Fidder, A. G. Hulst, D. Noort, R. de Ruiter, M. J. van der Schans, H. P. Benschop and J. P. Langenberg, Retrospective detection of exposure to organophosphorus anti-cholinesterases: Mass spectrometric analysis of phosphylated human butyrylcholinesterase, *Chem. Res. Toxicol.*, 2002, **15**, 582–590.
78. K. Tsuge and Y. Seto, Detection of human butyrylcholinesterase-nerve gas adducts by liquid chromatography-mass spectrometric analysis after in gel chymotryptic digestion, *J. Chromatogr. B*, 2006, **838**, 21–30.
79. M. J. van der Schans, A. Fidder, D. van Oeveren, A. G. Hulst and D. Noort, Verification of exposure to cholinesterase inhibitors: generic detection of OPCW Schedule 1 nerve agent adducts to human butyrylcholinesterase, *J. Anal. Toxicol.*, 2008, **32**, 125–130.
80. D. Noort, A. Fidder, M. J. van der Schans and A. G. Hulst, Verification of exposure to organophosphates: Generic mass spectrometric method for detection of human butyrylcholinesterase adducts, *Anal. Chem.*, 2006, **78**, 6640–6644.
81. J. L. S. Sporty, S. W. Lemire, E. M. Jakubowski, J. A. Renner, R. A. Evans, R. F. Williams, J. G. Schmidt, M. J. van der Schans, D. Noort and R. C. Johnson, Immunomagnetic separation and quantification of butyrylcholinesterase nerve agent adducts in human serum, *Anal. Chem.*, 2010, **82**, 6593–6600.
82. J. S. Knaack, Y. Zhou, C. W. Abney, J. T. Jacob, S. M. Prezioso, K. Hardy, S. W. Lemire, J. Thomas and R. C. Johnson, A high-throughput diagnostic method for measuring human exposure to organophosphorus nerve agents, *Anal. Chem.*, 2012, **84**, 9470–9477.
83. B. G. Pantazides, C. M. Watson, M. D. Carter, B. S. Crow, J. W. Perez, T. A. Blake, J. D. Thomas and R. C. Johnson, An enhanced butyrylcholinesterase method to measure organophosphorus nerve agent exposure in humans, *Anal. Bioanal. Chem.*, 2014, **406**, 5187–5194.
84. C. W. Abney, J. L. S. Knaack, A. A. I. Ali and R. C. Johnson, Novel dual-mode immunomagnetic method for studying reactivation of nerve-agent inhibited butyrylcholinesterase, *Chem. Res. Toxicol.*, 2013, **26**, 775–782.

85. M. D. Carter, B. S. Crow, B. G. Pantazides, C. M. Watson, J. D. Thomas, T. A. Blake and R. C. Johnson, Direct quantitation of methyl phosphonate adducts to human serum butyrylcholinesterase by immunomagnetic-UHPLC-MS/MS, *Anal. Chem.*, 2013, **85**, 11106–11111.
86. W. Jiang, E. A. Murashko, Y. A. Dubrovskii, E. P. Podolskaya, V. N. Babakov, J. Mikler, F. Nachon, P. Masson, L. M. Schopfer and O. Lockridge, Matrix assisted laser desorption/ionization time-of-flight mass spectrometry of titanium oxide-enriched peptides for detection of aged organophosphorus adducts on human butyrylcholinesterase, *Anal. Biochem.*, 2013, **439**, 132–141.
87. R. M. Black, J. M. Harrison and R. W. Read, The interaction of sarin and soman with plasma proteins: the identification of a novel phosphonylation site, *Arch. Toxicol.*, 1999, **73**, 123–126.
88. E. S. Peeples, L. M. Schopfer, E. G. Duysen, R. Spaulding, T. Voelker, C. M. Thompson and O. Lockridge, Albumin, a new biomarker of organophosphorus toxicant exposure, identified by mass spectrometry, *Toxicol. Sci.*, 2005, **83**, 303–312.
89. N. H. Williams, J. M. Harrison, R. W. Read and R. M. Black, Phosphylated tyrosine in albumin as a biomarker of exposure to organophosphorus nerve agents, *Arch. Toxicol.*, 2007, **81**, 627–639.
90. R. W. Read, J. R. Riches, J. A. Stevens, S. J. Stubbs and R. M. Black, Biomarkers of organophosphorus nerve agent exposure: comparison of phosphylated butyrylcholinesterase and phosphylated albumin after oxime therapy, *Arch. Toxicol.*, 2010, **84**, 25–36.
91. Y. Bao, Q. Liu, J. Chen, Y. Lin, B. Wu and J. Xie, Quantification of nerve agent adducts with albumin in rat plasma using liquid chromatography-isotope dilution tandem mass spectrometry, *J. Chromatogr. A*, 2012, **1229**, 164–171.
92. W. Jiang, Y. A. Dubrovskii, E. P. Podolskaya, E. A. Murashko, V. Babakov, F. Nachon, P. Masson, L. M. Schopfer and O. Lockridge, PHOS-select iron affinity beads enrich peptides for the detection of organophosphorus adducts on albumin, *Chem. Res. Toxicol.*, 2013, **26**, 1917–1925.
93. D. R. W. Verstappen, A. G. Hulst, A. Fidder, N. P. E. Vermeulen and D. Noort, Interactions of organophosphates with keratins in the cornified epithelium of human skin, *Chem.–Biol. Interact.*, 2012, **197**, 93–102.
94. L. M. Schopfer, H. Grigoryan, B. Li, F. Nachon, P. Masson and O. Lockridge, Mass spectral characterization of organophosphate-labeled, tyrosine-containing peptides: characteristic mass fragments and a new binding motif for organophosphates, *J. Chromatogr. B*, 2010, **878**, 1297–1311.
95. M. Minami, D.-M. Hui, M. Katsumata, H. Inagaki and C. A. Boulet, Method for the analysis of the methylphosphonic acid metabolites of sarin and its ethanol-substituted analogue in urine as applied to the victims of the Tokyo sarin disaster, *J. Chromatogr. B: Biomed. Sci. Appl.*, 1997, **695**, 237–244.

96. T. Nakajima, K. Sasaki, H. Ozawa, Y. Sekijima, H. Morita, Y. Fukushima and N. Yanagisawa, Urinary metabolites of sarin in a patient of the Matsumoto sarin incident, *Arch. Toxicol.*, 1998, **72**, 601–603.
97. M. Nagao, T. Takatori, Y. Matsuda, M. Nakajima, H. Iwase and K. Iwadate, Definitive evidence for the acute sarin poisoning diagnosis in the Tokyo subway, *Toxicol. Appl. Pharmacol.*, 1997, **144**, 198–203.
98. Y. Matsuda, M. Nagao, T. Takatori, H. Niijima, M. Nakajima, H. Iwase, M. Kobayashi and K. Iwadate, Detection of the sarin hydrolysis product in formalin-fixed brain tissues of victims of the Tokyo subway terrorist attack, *Toxicol. Appl. Pharmacol.*, 1998, **150**, 310–320.
99. H. Tsuchihashi, M. Katagi, M. Nishikawa and M. Tatsuno, Identification of metabolites of nerve agent VX in serum collected from a victim, *J. Anal. Toxicol.*, 1998, **22**, 383–388.
100. M. I. Solano, J. D. Thomas, J. T. Taylor, J. M. McGuire, E. M. Jakubowski, S. A. Thomson, V. L. Maggio, K. E. Holland, J. R. Smith, B. Capacio, A. R. Woolfitt, D. L. Ashley and J. R. Barr, Quantification of nerve agent VX-butyrylcholinesterase adduct biomarker from an accidental exposure, *J. Anal. Toxicol.*, 2008, **32**, 68–72.
101. D. H. Ash, S. W. Lemire, S. C. McGrath, L. G. McWilliams and J. R. Barr, Multianalyte quantification of five sesqui- and ethyl ether oxy-mustard metabolites in human urine by liquid chromatography-atmospheric pressure chemical ionization-tandem mass spectrometry, *J. Anal. Toxicol.*, 2008, **32**, 44–50.
102. S. W. Lemire, J. R. Barr, D. L. Ashley, C. T. Olson and T. L. Hayes, Quantitation of biomarkers of exposure to nitrogen mustards in urine from rats dosed with nitrogen mustards and from an unexposed human population, *J. Anal. Toxicol.*, 2004, **28**, 320–326.
103. M. K. Reddy, G. Mills, C. Nixon, S. A. Wyatt and T. R. Croley, High-throughput sample preparation and simultaneous column regeneration liquid chromatography-tandem mass spectrometry method for determination of nitrogen mustard metabolites in human urine, *J. Chromatogr. B*, 2011, **879**, 2383–2388.
104. D. Noort, A. Fidder and R. Jansen, Covalent binding of nitrogen mustards to the cysteine-34 residue in human serum albumin, *Arch. Toxicol.*, 2002, **76**, 83–88.
105. T.-H. Yeo, M.-L. Ho and W.-K. Loke, Development of a liquid chromatography – multiple reaction monitoring procedure for concurrent verification of exposure to different forms of mustard agents, *J. Anal. Toxicol.*, 2008, **32**, 51–56.
106. J. V. Wooten, D. L. Ashley and A. M. Calafat, Quantitation of 2-chlorovinylarsonous acid in human urine by automated solid-phase microextraction-gas chromatography-mass spectrometry, *J. Chromatogr. B*, 2002, **772**, 147–153.
107. N. L. Koryagina, E. S. Ukolova, E. I. Savel'eva, N. G. Voitenko, O. I. Orlova, R. O. Jenkins and N. V. Goncharov, High-sensitivity determination of

2-chlorovinylarsonous acid in biomedical samples for retrospective detection of exposure to lewisite upon antidotal therapy, *Spectroscopy*, 2011, **26**, 1–10.
108. M. T. Naseri, M. Shamsipur, M. Babri, H. Saeidian, M. Sarabadani, D. Ashrafi and N. Taghizadeh, Determination of lewisite metabolite 2-chlorovinylarsonous acid in urine by use of dispersive derivatization liquid-liquid microextraction followed by gas chromatography-mass spectrometry, *Anal. Bioanal. Chem.*, 2014, **406**, 5221–5230.
109. R. D. Stanelle, W. J. McShane, E. N. Dodova, R. S. Pappas and R. Kobelski, Rapid analysis of Lewisite metabolites in urine by high-performance liquid chromatography-inductively coupled plasma-mass spectrometry, *J. Anal. Toxicol.*, 2010, **34**, 122–128.
110. I. Rodin, A. Braun, A. Stavrianidi, O. Shpigun and I. Rybalchenko, Lewisite metabolites detection in urine by liquid chromatography-tandem mass spectrometry, *J. Chromatogr. B*, 2011, **879**, 3788–3796.
111. A. Fidder, D. Noort, A. G. Hulst, L. P. A. de Jong and H. P. Benschop, Biomonitoring of exposure to lewisite based on adducts to haemoglobin, *Arch. Toxicol.*, 2000, **74**, 207–214.
112. G. D. Byrdt, R. C. Paule, L. C. Sander, L. T. Sniegoski, E. White V and H. T. Bausum, Determination of 3-quinuclidinyl benzilate (QNB) and its major metabolites in urine by isotope dilution gas chromatography mass/spectrometry, *J. Anal. Toxicol.*, 1992, **16**, 182–187.
113. D. Noort, A. G. Hulst, A. Fidder, R. A. van Gurp, L. P. A. de Jong and H. P. Benschop, In vitro adduct formation of phosgene with albumin and hemoglobin in human blood, *Chem. Res. Toxicol.*, 2000, **13**, 719–726.
114. S. L. Youso, G. A. Rockwood, J. P. Lee and B. A. Logue, Determination of cyanide exposure by gas chromatography-mass spectrometry analysis of cyanide-exposed plasma proteins, *Anal. Chim.Acta.*, 2010, **677**, 24–28.
115. E. I. Hamelin, W. Bragg, R. L. Shaner, L. S. Swaim and R. C. Johnson, Comparison of high-resolution and tandem mass spectrometry for the analysis of nerve agent metabolites in urine, *Rapid Commun. Mass Spectrom.*, 2013, **27**, 1697–1704.
116. F. Zydel, J. R. Smith, V. S. Pagnotti, R. J. Lawrence, C. N. McEwen and B. R. Capacio, Rapid screening of chemical warfare nerve agent metabolites in urine by atmospheric solids analysis probe – mass spectroscopy (ASAP-MS), *Drug Test. Anal.*, 2012, **4**, 308–311.

CHAPTER 7

The Impact of New Technologies on the Elucidation of Chemical Warfare Agent Toxicology

JONATHAN DAVID*[a] AND HARALD JOHN[b]

[a]CBR Division, Dstl, Porton Down, Salisbury, Wiltshire, SP4 0JQ, UK;
[b]Bundeswehr Institute of Pharmacology and Toxicology, Neuherbergstrasse 11, 80937 Munich, Germany
*E-mail: jdavid@dstl.gov.uk

7.1 Introduction

Over the years, scientific methods continue to develop and advance in their complexity. In the last two decades, partly due to increases in computing power, many novel, multiplexed or data rich technologies have arrived on the market. These technologies are applicable to all aspects of the biological sciences and in general terms have given scientists the ability to study numerous biological or chemical variables simultaneously. In the field of toxicology this includes the discovery of (i) how compounds interact with organisms, (ii) how compounds interact with each other, (iii) increased sensitivity of methodologies, and (iv) the interplay of the previous three points. As the number of experimental variables increases so does the necessary computing power and mathematical algorithms needed for data interpretation. For some technologies their development can often outstrip the data analysis

Issues in Toxicology No. 27
Chemical Warfare Toxicology, Volume 2: Management of Poisoning
Edited by Franz Worek, John Jenner, and Horst Thiermann

Published by the Royal Society of Chemistry, www.rsc.org

Table 7.1 Publications relating to the use of transcriptomic and proteomic approaches to elucidate CWA toxicology.

CWA	Acronym	Transcriptomics publications	Proteomics publications
Tabun	GA		
Sarin	GB	Damodaran *et al.* (2006)	Hoffman *et al.* (2014)
		Damodaran *et al.* (2006)	
		Pachiappan *et al.* (2009)	
		Spradling *et al,* (2011)	
		Spradling *et al.* (2011)	
Soman	GD	Dillman *et al.* (2009)	
Cyclosarin	GF		
	VX	Blanton *et al.* (2004)	
		Gao *et al.* (2013)	
Sulphur mustard	HD	Zhang *et al.* (2002)	Dillman *et al.* (2003)
		Rogers *et al.* (2004)	An *et al.* (2006)
		Sabourin *et al.* (2004)	Mol *et al.* (2008)
		Dillman *et al.* (2005)	Mehrani *et al.* (2009)
		Platteborze (2005)	Everley *et al.* (2010)
		Dillman *et al.* (2006)	Mehrani *et al.* (2011)
		Rogers *et al.* (2008)	Yue *et al.* (2014)
		Gerecke *et al.* (2009)	
		Price *et al.* (2009)	
		Najafi *et al.* (2014)	
Nitrogen mustard	HN2	Kisby *et al.* (2006)	
Lewisite	L	Platteborze (2005)	
Phosgene		Sciuto *et al.* (2005)	
		Leikauf *et al.* (2013)	
Chlorine		Leikauf *et al.* (2012)	
		Price *et al.* (2012)	
Ricin		DaSilva *et al.* (2003)	
		Wong *et al.* (2007)	
		David *et al.* (2009)	
Abrin		Bhaskar *et al.* (2012)	

tools needed to determine biological or chemical meaning from the data. This chapter considers the current impact of these technologies in the field of chemical warfare agent (CWA) toxicology, highlighting successes and suggesting avenues for future research. The majority of information available is currently in the area of transcriptomics and proteomics (see Table 7.1). As such, this chapter will focus on these technologies, whilst also suggesting areas where researchers could improve the knowledge gained from these data rich technologies.

7.2 Transcriptomics

The genetic information of a system is encoded in its DNA and this is transcribed into to a single stranded RNA before translation into functional proteins. Transcriptomics is the study of any or all of the RNA molecules in a test system (cell, tissue or organism). Many types of RNA molecules exist and can be broadly categorised into three classes: (i) protein synthesis RNAs [*e.g.* messenger RNA (mRNA), transfer RNA *etc.*]; (ii) post-transcriptional modification RNAs (*e.g.* small nuclear RNA, guide RNA *etc.*); and (iii) regulatory RNAs (*e.g.* micro RNA, PIWI-interacting RNA, small interfering RNA *etc.*). It is possible to study all of these RNA molecules using multiplexed technologies, but the focus over recent years has been on those involved in protein synthesis, specifically mRNA. In the past few years, study of the regulatory RNAs has become more prevalent as more is discovered about their biological importance.[1] These regulatory RNAs have yet to be studied in depth for CWA toxicology but are discussed further in Section 7.2.2.2. In the context of this diverse set of RNA molecules, the majority of research in the field of CWA toxicology has studied mRNA molecules involved in protein synthesis.[2]

The levels of mRNA in a biological system can be enumerated using several experimental techniques, which have been reviewed elsewhere.[3] To date, the most commonly used tool to study the global mRNA response to CWAs is the microarray (see Figure 7.1). The first use of microarray technology for the investigation of gene expression was described in 1995 to probe 45 genes from the model plant *Arabidopsis*.[4] Following this proof of principle study, the technology was used to examine human responses, with early microarrays covering over 1000 features.[5] Current technologies can represent the entire human genome and feature generation can be carried out using methods from crude oligonucleotide spotting through to photolithography, electrochemistry and inkjet technologies. The aim of all of these technologies is to deposit a known oligonucleotide (feature) in a known position on a solid surface (usually silicon chips or glass slides). The length of the oligonucleotide sequence tends to range from 25 to 60 bases (termed 25–60-mers) based on a trade-off between sensitivity *versus* specificity. Fluorescently labelled sample nucleic acids are hybridised to these immobilised oligonucleotides and the fluorescence of each feature measured using a high resolution scanner. By comparing differently labelled samples (a two colour experimental design), it is possible to carry out a ratio based analysis between samples (*e.g.* CWA exposed *versus* un-exposed). One colour experimentation allows quantification of RNA in the samples compared with a standard curve or ratio based analysis against other one colour measurements. Microarray experimental design is complex and the data analysis even more so. In order to standardise the reporting of microarray data the Minimal Information About a Microarray Experiment (MIAME) standard was introduced by the Microarray Gene Expression Database (MGED) Society.[6] Despite the introduction of more recent multiplexed technologies, such as next generation sequencing (see Section 7.2.2.1), microarrays remain a useful research tool to investigate CWA toxicology.

7.2.1 The Use of Microarrays to Study CWA Toxicology

The use of microarrays to investigate CWA toxicology is well established with numerous publications describing the use of this technique to probe transcriptional changes following CWA exposure. For some agents, such as

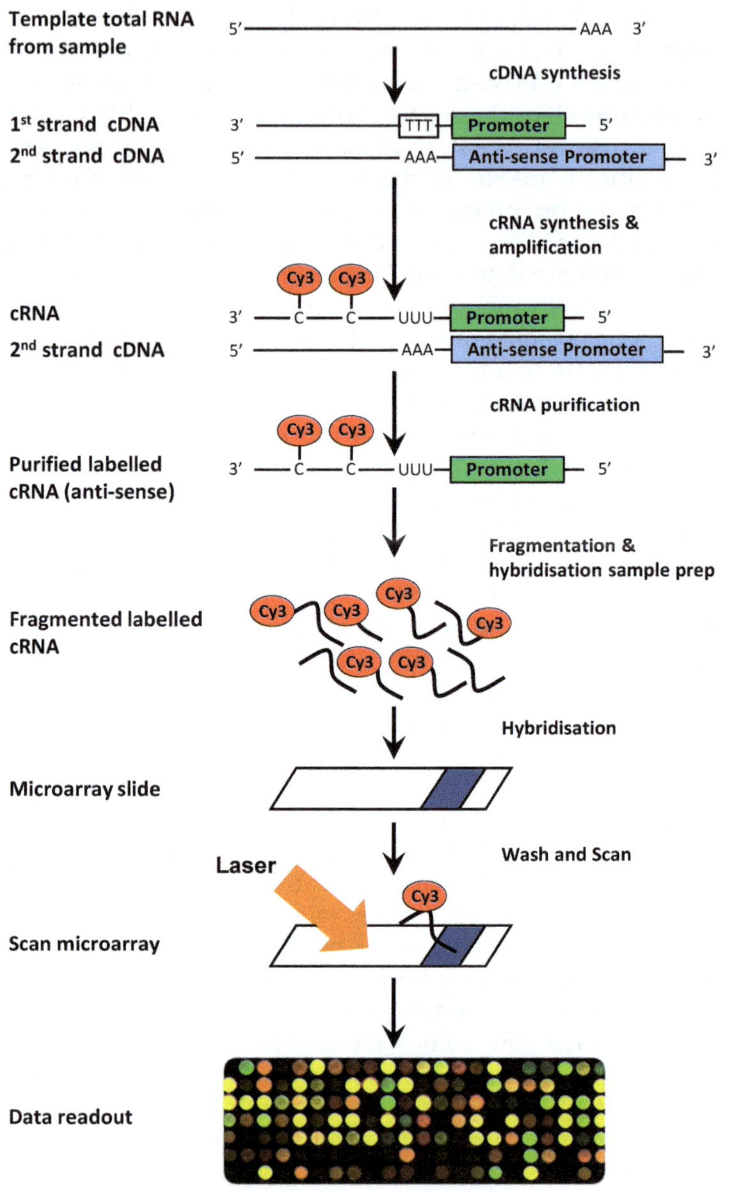

Figure 7.1 Schematic of standard microarray process; cRNA synthesis and hybridisation to oligonucleotide microarrays. Total RNA is reverse transcribed to cDNA. cRNA is synthesised and amplified from the template, incorporating a fluorescent dye (*i.e.* Cy3). cRNA is purified, fragmented and hybridised to an oligonucleotide microarray. Following hybridisation, slides are washed and scanned to determine a fluorescent reading for each microarray feature.

nerve agents, critical molecular mechanisms have been well characterised using classical techniques.[7,8] For other agents, such as the blister agents, the molecular mechanism is diverse and still poorly understood.[9,10] A significant driver behind toxicology, certainly for CWAs, is the development of medical countermeasures to overcome toxic effects. Without a clear understanding of the totality of the toxicological effects of CWAs, researchers are limited in the design of medical countermeasures due to lack of understanding. Transcriptomics offers the researcher the ability to probe the total transcribed host response to CWAs and subsequently to down-select new targets for therapeutic intervention. Even for the well characterised agents where toxicology has been established using classical methods, transcriptomics can still offer further insight into the response following exposure. Intriguingly, the normal toxicological considerations within experimental design (animal model, dose, and long and short term effects) are still present in transcriptomics and make data interpretation an essential and complex step. The advancements in computational power and analyses in the field of toxicology (to date led and driven by transcriptomics) may yet be able to solve these issues (see Section 7.4) that still remain. The power of transcriptomics to analyse the total experimental response to CWA exposure is in no doubt, and is now considered for the different classes of CWAs.

7.2.1.1 Nerve Agents

The effects of nerve agents on synaptic junctions is well characterised but numerous studies have used transcriptomics to research the global toxicological effects of this class of CWA. However, not all agents have been investigated using transcriptomics. Tabun (GA) and cyclosarin (GF) remain unexplored using this technique, and the opportunity to do so endures. The most well studied agent by transcriptomics is sarin (GB; see Table 7.1). Early studies using small scale northern blot methods to probe mRNA levels made little headway into the toxicology of GB, but did show the applicability of measuring mRNA levels to probe the toxicological response.[11–13] The first full scale transcriptomic analysis of GB occurred in 2006 with the profiling of the rat brain at early and late time points post-exposure.[14,15] Seeking to differentiate short term and longer term responses, the initial study mapped the transcriptome at 15 min and 3 months after exposure in a Sprague–Dawley rat intra-muscular model of GB exposure.[15] The experimental design in this study used two different doses for the time points [0.5 × lethal dose, 50% (LD_{50}) for the 15 min time point and 1 × LD_{50} for the 3 month time point] with no clear explanation for the differences in doses. Furthermore, short term clinical signs were significantly different between the two groups, making comparisons difficult. The comprehensive analysis of the differentially expressed genes (66 genes at 15 min and 38 genes at 3 months) grouped genes into biologically functional categories for functional analysis. Chemokines, cytoskeletal and cell adhesion molecules, and calcium and ion channels were identified at the early time point and various neurological functional transcripts were identified after 3 months (GABAnergic signalling, neurotransmitter early genes and synaptic vesicle proteins). Care must be taken in the interpretation of these data due to the low numbers of genes returned (~3–5%) from a non-whole genome microarray (~1200 genes). However, this study demonstrated the power of transcriptomics to validate known toxicology (synaptic effects; Synj1 and Snygr1) and identify potential new avenues (chemokine involvement; Cmkbr3, Cxcr4, CX-3C and Ltn). The work was continued in the rat brain using the same platform to identify the early activation of degenerative and regenerative pathways.[14] A feature of both of these publications was an admission of the limitations of placing sole emphasis on mRNA expression and the importance of biologically validating the results using classical techniques. A further limitation highlighted was the extraction of mRNA from a whole organ and the inadvertent pooling of signals from a variety of cell types. Addressing this issue, further studies of GB toxicology in the brain have looked at single neuronal cell types.[16] By analysing more transcripts on a larger microarray platform, a larger number of significantly altered genes were identified (224 genes $p \leq 0.01$). By studying a single cell type the authors postulated an ETS2 driven mechanism for GB neuropathology and moved towards hypothesis validation using western blots and double immunofluorescence assays. Single dose experiments gave variable outputs but a repeated dosing model consistently down-regulated neurodegenerative gene profiles following exposure. The most recent transcriptomic work involving sarin was carried out in 2011, again focussing on the response in brain tissue in a rat model.[17,18] In these studies, the response to sarin was compared with controls, with both groups treated with atropine sulphate, 2-pryridine aldoxime methylchloride and diazepam after onset of seizures (and corresponding time matched controls for the saline exposed group). This therapeutic combination is proven to increase survival but long term neurological damage may still occur.[19,20] By examining the piriform cortex, known to be particularly sensitive to pathology following sarin exposure, the biological pathways were mapped over a time course (15 min, and 1, 3, 6 and 24 h post-exposure).[18] In brief, an early response (15 min) was characterised by dysregulation of metabolic pathways (glutamate, inositol and phospholipid metabolism). These transcriptional findings corroborate the temporal model of nerve agent exposure induced neuropathology.[20] A full discussion of this can be found in Spradling *et al.* 2011.[18] Novel findings were also presented, indicating the importance of the inflammatory response in this brain region following sarin exposure. The complete transcriptional map lends support to other limited polymerase chain reaction (PCR) based studies that had eluded to inflammatory mRNA increases following exposure.[21] The inflammatory response (cell mediated immune response, immune cell trafficking, TREM1 signalling, and IL-6 and IL-10 signalling) was observed across all time points. Specifically, TNF-α, IL-1β and IL-6 were expressed as early as 15 min post-exposure and continued to be expressed for the duration of the study. Subsequently, the inflammatory response was postulated as a novel target for therapeutic intervention but has yet to be explored. This comprehensive mapping of the response to sarin highlights the ability of transcriptomics to confirm known mechanisms, identify novel mechanisms and distinguish temporal profiles, providing essential toxicological data to maximise understanding.

Having characterised the importance of the inflammatory response in the piriform cortex the work was continued in other brain regions.[17] The hippocampus and amygdala shared a similar severity of transcriptional regulation to the piriform cortex, while the septum and thalamus returned fewer genes with altered expression levels following sarin exposure and treatment (atropine sulphate, 2-pryridine aldoxime methylchloride and diazepam). The same TNF-α, IL-1β and IL-6 inflammatory response was seen across all brain regions. A full description of gene changes over time in each brain region is well documented in the original manuscript.[17] With the transcriptional mapping of five brain regions in response to $1 \times LD_{50}$ of sarin complete, the identification of the neuro-inflammatory response is presented as a promising candidate for combination therapy to prevent or limit sarin induced neurodegeneration. Despite the promising identification of targets, these have yet to be explored for potential therapeutics. This is perhaps one of the biggest problems presented following transcriptional mapping (and holds true for most CWAs discussed in this text). Research groups carrying out transcriptomics generate vast quantities of data and present future hypotheses for testing. These may not be subsequently executed by the wider research community. It is unclear whether this is due to the complexity of the data or the lack of current data exploitation pathways from these technologies. The use of transcriptional data to drive subsequent experimental testing using classical methods is a key step to display the power of these technologies. Suggestions to maximise the potential of these data are discussed in Section 7.4.

Other nerve agents have been the focus of less transcriptomic research compared with sarin. Classical acetylcholinesterase (AChE) effects are similar for all nerve agents but it has been suggested that soman may present alternative downstream effects due to the dealkylation of soman adducts.[2] In order to investigate this, Dillman *et al.* investigated the neurodegenerative effects of soman in rat hippocampi in a similar fashion to that previously discussed for sarin.[22] In this study a longer time course was utilised (7 days). Principal component analysis (PCA) suggested a return to normal levels of gene expression in the brain at later time points (72 h onwards), but some differences were still observed. The neuro-inflammatory response was typical of this profile, with large increases soon after exposure resolving to basal levels by 168 h (TNF-α, IL-6 and IL-10). At later time points, pathways involved in RNA repair mechanisms (RNA damage and repair, RNA post transcriptional modification and genetic disorders) were observed alongside cellular regeneration (cellular development, connective tissue development, cell to cell signalling and interaction). This perhaps suggests that at later time points the host attempts to repair those mechanisms altered by soman in the brain. A therapeutic intervention to move these time points forward and drive early resolution may be a future avenue for therapy development.

Additionally, VX has also been investigated using transcriptomics. An early study in 2004 also followed a longer time course (2 weeks), observing similar returns of gene expression to basal levels at later time points.[23] Rather than inflammation, the work identified neuronal genes outside of the classical cholinesterase pathway as changed following VX exposure (0.1–0.6 × LD_{50}). This clearly demonstrates that non-cholinergic pathways are significant in nerve agent exposure and should be explored further. These alterations were confirmed in a study using human neuronal cell lines across a 72 h time course.[24] Inflammatory markers were not observed due to the use of a specific neuronal cell model rather than *in vivo* derived whole tissue. Gene specific observations were compared with known neurological disorders (CDH2 for Huntington's disease, RTN4 for schizophrenia and Parkinson's, and NTRK2 for Alzheimer's and Parkinson's, amongst others). Perhaps more notably, pathway analysis identified the neuregulin signalling pathway. Involvement of this pathway was heavily supported by numerous transcripts mapping to the pathway, and the pathway has been identified as particularly important in schizophrenia.[25] This specific research demonstrates another major advantage of transcriptomics as an approach to develop therapeutics. By identifying the most essential pathways/genes in CWA exposure and comparing these to known pathways/genes from public health diseases (where the market is larger) it may be that therapeutic developments in public health disorders can be used directly for CWA applications, offering a fast track to licensing. It is clear that transcriptomics has been a useful tool in the study of nerve agent toxicology and has suggested several avenues for future research for therapeutic interventions (neuroinflammation, neuregulin *etc.*). With the aforementioned bottleneck for the exploitation of transcriptomic data by the wider research community it will be interesting to see if these hypotheses are developed further in future years.

7.2.1.2 Vesicants

The CWA vesicants, sulphur mustard (HD), nitrogen mustard (HN2) and lewisite (L) have a less well characterised mechanism compared with nerve agents, with numerous host responses observed.[26–28] These are described in more detail in Chapter 2 in Volume 1 and Chapter 4 in this book. These observed host responses make them ideal agents to study using multiplexed technologies, such as transcriptomics. The bulk of CWA vesicant research using transcriptomics has focused on HD. Initial studies used relatively limited microarray platforms (representing 2304 genes), but were able to use this technology to propose a model of HD induced apoptosis in human Jurkat cells.[29] Transcriptomics identified caspases and the Bcl family as dysregulated following HD exposure, ultimately leading to the discovery that HD apoptosis is driven by Akt modulation. Despite this early success using microarray technology, other studies at the time used more classical techniques to try and observe the whole transcriptome in response to HD. Platteborze initially used differential display PCR technology (the precursor to microarrays) to investigate the molecular mechanism of HD induced intracellular events in human T lymphocytes.[30] Subsequently, Platteborze adopted microarray technology to continue to investigate the vesicating properties of HD in keratinocyte cell lines.[31] Both technologies identified genes from the NADH pathway, supplying NAD^+ for DNA damage repair mechanisms,[32] and ubiquitin transcripts for degradation of abnormal proteins. As with the nerve agents, studies then focussed on animal models of exposure, but for vesicants they investigated both skin and lung injury.[33–35] In the mouse ear skin model, a variety of doses—low (0.005–0.01 mg) and high (0.08–0.16 mg)—have been characterised for the response to HD.[33,36] These studies identified inflammation, apoptosis and cell cycle regulation as key biological pathways with a strong bias towards up-regulation over down-regulation. Following the elucidation of the response to HD in the mouse ear model, transcriptomics was used to investigate potential topical therapeutic treatments.[34] The treatments provided a physiological benefit, decreased ear weight, which correlated with gene expression profiles derived by microarray. The biological pathways associated with this correlation were cell cycle regulation, inflammation, signal transduction, and cytoskeletal and cell adhesion processes. The elucidation of the response specifically following treatment was not reported as many of the genes involved in the correlation were not above the two fold expression change normally used as a cut-off for biological significance.[34] This cut off is an arbitrary fold change and it may be that by probing the genes altered by treatment but below the two fold cut-off, the molecular effects could be elucidated. This approach was adopted by Gerecke *et al.*, who also investigated the effects of HD on the mouse ear model but this time with MMP-2 and MMP-9 inhibitors as treatments.[37] Histopathology showed no difference between treated and untreated HD exposed groups, but transcriptomics was able to identify activation of several repair processes in the treatment groups. The mouse ear model research again shows the utility of transcriptomics to map the host response to injury and to probe for the efficacy of treatment at the molecular level. Using mRNA levels as an indicator of efficacy should be practiced with care as mRNA is not necessarily the appropriate marker compared with translated proteins and physiological effects. However, as a molecular biomarker (either for specific genes or pathways) to map the response (*i.e.* differences in regulation of inflammation following treatment), transcriptomics has shown its utility in this field.

Comparative transcriptomics has investigated the commonalities between HD skin injuries and thermal burns in a swine model.[38,39] These studies identified inflammatory and immune cascades, along with cellular movement, as pathways significantly altered following HD exposure. As both studies compared HD injury to thermal burns it was possible to identify therapeutic targets in advanced clinical trials for burns treatments that may be used for HD injury. These include the CXCR4 antagonist AMD3100, the FGFR2 agonist palifermin and the IL-1 receptor antagonist Kineret.[38] Alternatively, the differences between thermal and HD induced burns may present additional targets for therapy, as suggested by Everley and Dillman.[2] The role of inflammation has also been seen in murine liver tissue along with cell-cycle dysregulation.[40] Anand *et al.* were able to suppress this inflammatory response by orally administering a pre-treatment of DRDE-07 [*S*-2(2-amino-ethylamino) ethyl phenyl sulphide].[40] Another major concern for HD induced injury is the lung. Initial studies were performed in a rat model exposed by intravenous administration to 1–5 × LD_{50}.[35] The data revealed a p53 driven DNA damage pathway as the initial transcriptional response to injury progressing to apoptosis at later time points. The conclusion drawn by Dillman *et al.* suggested that future research efforts should focus on long term carcinogenesis studies to elucidate the impact of mutations caused by this DNA damage.[35] These studies have now been continued by Najafi *et al.*, who studied the transcriptome of veterans of the Iran–Iraq war of 1984–88.[41] Despite only investigating three human subjects, this is the first and only transcriptional profiling of human subjects exposed to HD. After 25 years post-exposure there were 122 genes returned from a pan-genome test panel. Of these 122 genes, airway remodelling was a key observation from the data. However, only approximately 2% of the returned transcripts were directly involved in this pathway and gene ontology analysis did not indicate any predominant biological responses.[41]

Other vesicants have also been transcriptionally profiled, including L and HN2.[31,42] Similar to the other vesicant research (excluding the long term human study of Najafi *et al.*[41]), these studies returned a bias of up-regulated transcripts over those that were down-regulated. The more rapid skin penetration of L, compared with HD, was observed at the transcriptional level with apoptotic signals observed earlier than those seen for HD exposure.[31] As well as several similarities with HD, a key difference was observed for the re-structuring of the extracellular matrix, which was not seen in HD exposure. The ability to dissect key mechanistic differences between vesicants may prove critical in understanding the options for therapeutic intervention. Commonalities on the other hand may provide a target for a single therapy for all vesicating agents. DNA damage and apoptosis have been observed for all vesicants, including HN2.[42] Whether an intervention at this stage is possible remains to be seen. It is likely that this response is indicative of the catastrophic damage caused by vesicant CWAs. Thus, it may be that focusing efforts on earlier molecular events may provide more utility in the hunt for therapeutics.

Transcriptomics has again shown its utility for mapping the toxicological effects of a class of CWAs. For vesicant research there appears to have been a stronger focus on extrapolation of the transcriptomic data towards therapeutic target identification and subsequent testing. This is perhaps driven by both the complex and varied nature of vesicant injury and the lack of medical options beyond supportive care. Either way, the research into vesicant toxicology using transcriptomics appears more directed and is showing promise for increased understanding and development of therapies.

7.2.1.3 Toxic Industrial Chemicals

Transcriptomics for the toxicology of toxic industrial chemicals (TIC) has so far been sparse. Of particular relevance to CWAs has been research studying the effects of phosgene and chlorine. The effects of inhaled phosgene on mice were first studied in 2005 by Sciuto *et al.*[43] This Affymetrix microarray paper has since been used by other groups adopting *in silico* approaches to generate protein–protein interaction networks for phosgene injury and gene networks for oxidative stress.[44,45] The use of transcriptomics datasets in this way is discussed in more detail in Section 7.4, which demonstrates the power of these data rich experiments. The original work by Sciuto *et al.* looked to identify phosgene induced transcriptional changes in CD-1 male mice after an exposure of 8 ppm phosgene for 20 min.[43] By mapping the response across a 3 day time course the authors identified the important early response of genes involved in the antioxidant response, specifically those of the glutathione synthesis and redox pathways. These data were cross validated against a previous study measuring glutathione related proteins in bronchoalveolar lavage fluid (BALF).[46] The biochemical data correlated with the transcriptomics and serve to validate the importance of these pathways in response to phosgene. Whilst the transcriptomics study focussed on glutathione pathways, it also identified other transcripts that changed in response to phosgene.[43] These included those involved in angiogenesis, cell adhesion and cell cycle regulation amongst others, but these were not explored or validated further. In 2013, transcriptomics was again used to study the effects of phosgene on the mouse lungs.[47] The aim of this work was not to characterise the functional response to phosgene but rather to determine underlying host genetic determinants of susceptibility to phosgene by exposing some 43 mouse strains to 1 ppm phosgene for 24 h. The different transcriptional responses between a sensitive murine strain (SM/J) and a resistant strain (129X1/SvJ) are reported but not interrogated in depth. These data offer the opportunity for future exploration as outlined in the methods reviewed in Section 7.4.

This same approach of identifying genetic determinants of susceptibility has also been used for chlorine exposure.[48] A sensitive strain (C57/BLKS/J) was compared to a resistant strain (C57/BL/10J) following a dose of 45 ppm chlorine over 24 h. Following exposure, the sensitive strain had increased transcriptional activity of transcription factors and cell death with decreased activity of protein transport and development of the vasculature. Conversely, the resistant strain had increased expression of cell adhesion and cytoskeletal organisation genes. The transcriptomics data from this study were used to validate the expression levels of candidate susceptibility genes and as such have not been explored rigorously. Exploitation of these data provides an opportunity for further insight into chlorine toxicology. Moving away from murine models of TIC exposure, transcriptomics has been performed on skin biopsies from swine (*Sus scofa*) following exposure to 2.9 g l^{-1} of chlorine for 30 min.[49] By mapping the response over 24 h, common biological functions across all time points were reported following exposure: cancer, cellular growth, cell death, cellular movement, cardiovascular disease, genetic disorders, and skeletal and muscular disorders. By analysing canonical pathways three common pathways were identified and, more specifically, candidate therapeutic targets that were expressed at all time points following exposure. These genes were IL-1A, IL-1B and IL-6, with IL-1 identified as a priority candidate for therapeutic exploitation.[49] It is clear that there is a growing body of transcriptomics data available to study the toxicology of TICs. Transcriptomics has also been shown to be a valid approach to help progress research towards therapeutic interventions.[43,49] However, not all of the data have been fully exploited, offering the potential to yield further toxicologically relevant information from these studies.

7.2.1.4 Toxins

Plant derived toxins may also be considered CWAs, with ricin and abrin being the most commonly associated with potential uses in warfare.[50–52] The ribosome inactivating toxin of the *Ricinus communis* plant is the most well characterised of these, with a well known mechanism of action.[51] Transcriptomics has been carried out by several research groups to identify the host response to ricin. Initial efforts were limited by the available technology at the time and used custom microarray platforms covering portions of the whole genome (1178 probes).[53] Within the bounds of these limitations it was possible to elucidate the host response mechanism to a $1 \times LD_{50}$ (14 μg kg^{-1}) aerosolised ricin challenge in the Balb/c mouse. Several gene targets were identified including those of the inflammatory response (*i.e.* IL-6, MCP3 and ICAM1), which may offer potential therapeutic targets, and those that were indicative of the damage caused by the toxin (*i.e.* apoptosis and DNA repair mechanisms).[53] Furthermore, the study identified genes with altered expression early on following exposure—egr-1, cish-3 and c-myc—that may act as biomarkers for ricin induced injury. Following on from the early identification of the role of inflammation in response to ricin, other groups specifically studied this response.[54,55] A whole genome approach was able to identify the same strong inflammatory bias observed in primary human tracheal cells.[54] Specific correlations were seen for IL-6 and egr-1. In these human cells the inflammatory response seen at the transcriptional level was postulated to be driven by NF-κB and p38 MAPK, and these were identified as potential therapeutic targets. In order to investigate the specific inflammatory response in a murine model, studies were carried out in 2009 using a specific custom inflammatory microarray platform, again in the Balb/c mouse.[55] This study characterised the inflammatory response more fully to a low dose aerosol exposure of 11 μg kg^{-1} ($\sim 0.8 \times LD_{50}$). The specific response involved TNF-α, IL-1β, the IL-1 pathway, CCL4, CCL6 and CCL10, and macrophage and lymphocyte activators. This work was also able to elucidate the role of extracellular matrix remodelling and cell–cell adhesion pathways. Ricin caused a dysregulation of MMPs, TIMPS and focal adhesion networks, offering a new avenue for therapeutic intervention.[55] Initial characterisation of the whole genome response in mice has also been carried out for another ribosome inactivating protein, derived from *Abrus precatorius*, abrin.[56] Divergently from the ricin studies, which focussed on the lung response, the microarray for abrin exposed mice investigated the response in the brain tissue following intraperitoneal injection of 1–2 × LD_{50} (2.83 and 5.66 μg kg^{-1}). The investigation of brain tissues aimed to determine the role of the CNS in the observed neurological effects of abrin in human cases.[56–58] A rapid inflammatory and immune response was seen in the brain with specific modulation of immune cell migration: chemotaxis, antigen processing and presentation, and cell adhesion molecules.[56] Thus it appears that the toxins abrin and ricin may share a similar toxicology at the mRNA level, with inflammation the major response to the toxins in several tissue types. By targeting any similarities it may be possible to yield a therapeutic intervention against both toxins that is effective in numerous tissues, independent of route of exposure.

7.2.2 Alternative RNA Based Approaches

Microarray technology has proved its worth in studying CWA toxicology but as time progresses other newer technologies become available to researchers. These technologies have yet to be fully applied to CWA toxicology but have the potential to surpass microarrays. These alternative RNA approaches will now be considered.

7.2.2.1 RNA Sequencing Transcriptomics

Transcriptomics methods by microarray are limited by the fact that the target sequence (probe) must be based on prior knowledge of transcripts for its design. This inevitably biases the microarray towards known sequences rather than previously unidentified transcripts. An alternative methodology that does not suffer from these limitations and is currently overtaking microarray for the study of transcriptomics is termed RNA sequencing (RNA-Seq). RNA-Seq uses next generation sequencing platforms to sequence cDNA libraries synthesised from the isolated sample RNA. The comparison of microarray technology *versus* RNA-Seq has been reviewed extensively elsewhere and RNA-Seq is generally considered to have surpassed microarray for use in transcriptomics.[3,59,60] With regard to non-CWA dose–response toxicology, the differences between the two technologies have been directly addressed in the literature.[61] The comparative study by Black *et al.* identified that the differences are complex and the results diverse. Overall comparison of the technologies identified similar biological processes. The correlation between the technologies was highest when analysis was based upon fold change values, compared to a lower correlation when performed on *p*-values. The impact of this observation was that RNA-Seq returned fewer statistically significant genes at low doses compared with microarray.

Importantly, the authors identified that microarray normalisation and analysis strategies have matured over many years whilst RNA-Seq is not yet fully developed.[61] Taking this further, it is suggested here that researchers should move to RNA-Seq with care and expert guidance for data handling and analysis for this new transcriptomics technique. For CWA toxicology, RNA-Seq has yet to be carried out, and if researchers begin to use this tool, a full understanding of the complex and computationally intense data analysis pipelines should be understood prior to study design. RNA-Seq has successfully been used in the wider field of toxicology, showing its utility, and this is reviewed elsewhere.[62] As predicted by RNA-Seq advocates, in certain studies the technology has been able to identify novel transcripts, including unannotated novel exons, providing novel insights into toxicology.[63] Thus RNA-Seq has the potential to yield novel insights into CWA toxicology in the future.

7.2.2.2 RNA Interference

As discussed in Section 7.2 there are many types of RNA molecule other than mRNA that may be investigated under the banner of transcriptomics (*i.e.* microRNAs). These can be measured using specific microarray and RNA-Seq methodologies. Similarly to RNA-Seq, these methods have yet to be employed on CWA toxicology to determine the role of these molecules in the host response to CWAs. A further use of this class of RNA molecule is as a research tool to target specific genes and reduce the translation of these mRNA molecules. This approach is termed RNA interference (RNAi). Discovered by Fire *et al.* in 1998 the technique has been used extensively for post transcriptional gene silencing.[64] This technique has been used in the study of CWAs, albeit in a limited number of studies. For HD toxicology, microarray technology identified the importance of the inflammatory response following exposure.[33,36,37] Inflammation is known to be driven by NF-κB, p38 and p53, and as such these were targeted by RNAi transfection in human keratinocytes.[65] Target protein knockdown using RNAi was successful (78–92%) and specific downstream effects were observed. Analysis of cytokine levels indicated that only p38 inhibition lowered cytokine production. Inhibition of NF-κB had no effect on cytokine production but did partially inhibit cell death in response to HD. On the other hand, p53 inhibition potentiated cell death, indicating a more complex role for this molecule in HD induced skin injury. This work was advanced by studying downstream effectors of p38, namely MAPK activated kinase 2 (MK2).[66] The inhibition of p38 by RNAi again reduced production of all cytokines tested (TNF-α, IL-1β, IL-6 and IL-8). Direct inhibition of MK2 by RNAi only reduced TNF-α and IL-6. These papers studying HD toxicology show the power of transcriptomics (to identify inflammatory pathways) and RNAi (to explore the specifics of the pathway) to elucidate the toxicology of CWAs in a rational and logical pipeline from global expression to specific therapeutic targets. This pipeline has also been used in the study of abrin induced apoptosis.[67] A microarray identified prohibin (PHB) as an up-regulated gene target in response to abrin exposure in the Jurkat cell line. PHB was subsequently knocked down by RNAi leading to a decrease in apoptosis by approximately 10–17% dependent on dose (1 nM and 0.1 nM, respectively). The authors suggested that PHB is therefore involved in abrin induced apoptosis and is a potential therapeutic target. From these limited but successful studies, it is clear that by coupling transcriptomics to specific RNA knockdown techniques it is possible to identify and modulate the host response to alter the toxicity of CWAs. This approach may yet yield significant inroads into CWA toxicology if suitable targets can be identified from the large datasets generated.

7.2.3 Transcriptomics Conclusion

It is clear that transcriptomics has been able to identify key players in the host response to CWAs. Broadly, the field (with some obvious exceptions) appears to operate based on one of two approaches: (i) the characterisation of the transcriptome for an agent with apparent minimal exploitation of the data; or (ii) characterisation of the transcriptome with a bias towards already known or favoured arms of the response derived from other methods. Neither of these approaches is inappropriate but rather allows individual research groups to further specific research goals. Perhaps an unexplored avenue of research is the ability to use these legacy datasets for other aims (see Section 7.4). However, transcriptomics has confirmed known mechanisms and characterised previously unknown areas of CWA toxicology across all classes of CWA. As these techniques become more commonplace, the exploitation pipeline of these data rich experiments is becoming better established.

Transcriptomics has been carried out on the majority of CWAs (with the exception of GA and GF) in a variety of *in vivo* and *in vitro* models. To date these studies have been carried out predominantly in classical models of CWA toxicology (*i.e.* rat, mouse, human neuronal cell lines *etc.*). The choice of model is driven to some extent by the widespread use of the model for CWA toxicology studies.[68–70] A further driver is the limitation of the transcriptomics technology itself. Microarray platforms can be developed for any model organism, but unsurprisingly, this has predominantly been biased towards human, rat and mouse models, where larger sections of the research community could engage. As the technology has developed, more species are now catered for by microarray platforms, including the chicken, guinea pig and large white pig.[39,71,72] With the advent of next generation sequencing, the range of species available to study using transcriptomics will continue to improve. However, characterising the toxicology of every agent in every model may yield vast amounts of data for a potentially incremental reward. It may be more prudent to focus efforts on the establishment of a pipeline to successfully exploit transcriptomics data towards a biologically meaningful end-point. This end-point may be a fuller mechanistic understanding of toxicity or a therapeutic intervention. Either way, transcriptomics has demonstrated huge potential to help elucidate CWA toxicology.

7.3 Proteomics

Proteomics denominates the (semi)quantitative description of all proteins of a biological system (*e.g.* cells, organs, fluids) under defined conditions. A proteome obtained under condition I can be compared with the proteome of an identical system obtained under a different condition II. Relevant variations might include age, sex, effect of drugs and toxicants, nutrient supply, or the presence and status of any disease. Following this differential approach changes in protein content are analysed with respect to parameters such as total amount, occurrence of novel compounds or variations in diverse post-translational modifications (PTMs). Resulting differences may point out essential effects caused by the modified conditions. The same idea is followed within the context of peptidomics, which is focussed on differential detection of peptides analysed in the blood and urine.[73–79] Any differences may provide valuable insight to understand biological, pathophysiological, pharmacological or toxicological processes at the molecular level. As seen for transcriptomics, such information is essential for defining new drug targets or candidates for the treatment of poisoning, or finding biomarkers as diagnostic targets.[80,81] In contrast to techniques characterising influences at the DNA and RNA level, analysis of the proteome covers proteins after maturation and secretion, and protein–protein interactions. Specifically, direct covalent reactions between proteins and toxicants can be unravelled. Therefore, proteome analysis considers differences in translation and degradation not detectable from mRNA levels and thus helps to generate a more complete picture of any functional changes in a biological system.

Success of interpretation strictly depends on the use of electronic databases containing concise, detailed and extensive information on all aspects of the natural proteins and their function, thus linking their role in regulatory processes to other compounds. Several decades of detailed pathophysiological research have helped to characterise most CWAs, but knowledge of their effects on regulatory pathways and mechanisms of long term action is limited. This applies especially for vesicants like HD. Therefore, proteome analysis can be specifically applied to decipher the effects of HD in mouse *in vivo* studies,[82] in cultured HEK (human embryonic kidney) and HaCaT cells ("human adult calcium and temperature", immortal cultured human keratinocytes)[83–85] and patients' BALF or plasma.[86,87]

7.3.1 The Principle Strategy of Proteomics

The principle technical strategy for proteome analysis comprises (i) selection of a relevant biological system, (ii) (selective) isolation or separation of the protein fraction, (iii) (semi)quantitative determination of differences, (iv) identification of proteins of interest, (v) interpretation of biological context, and (vi) sometimes targeted quantification of selected marker proteins and peptides. The described approach is specified as *bottom-up* proteomics (identification and characterisation of proteins after enzymatic cleavage) and distinguished from *top-down* proteomics [direct mass spectrometry (MS) analysis of separated proteins without prior proteolysis].[88,89] The latter strategy preserves all of the information on the intact protein (*e.g.* PTM, total length, mutations *etc.*) whereas the first variant only covers part of the sequence. Nevertheless, both principles are valuable and applicability depends on the instruments available.[88–91] Whereas *shotgun* proteomics intends to unravel all differences in the proteome without any protein pre-selection, approaches following *targeted* proteomics analyse only a limited number of selected proteins that are of special interest. These targets might include a group of phosphorylated (phosphoproteomics[90,92,93]), glycosylated (glycoproteomics[90]) or chemically modified proteins. Selective detection of phosphorylated butyrylcholinesterase (BChE) from body fluids of different donors represents an example of targeted proteomics to characterise the effects of organophosphorus poisons such as pesticides and nerve agents.[94]

For two decades, proteomics approaches have advanced life science research based on extraordinary progress in analytical instrumentation and bioinformatics.[95,96] Analysis of a proteome requires tools best designed for enhanced throughput, high resolution, reproducibility and robustness. Meanwhile, numerous special variations were introduced providing ingenious tools for improved throughput, selectivity and quantitation.[84,97–102] Common, highly sophisticated and well engineered techniques include electrophoresis, typically performed as high resolving two-dimensional gel electrophoresis (2D-GE) for intact proteins and capillary electrophoresis (CE) for peptides,[78,79,103] as well as liquid chromatography (LC) for proteins and peptides.[76,77] Techniques suitable for CWA proteomics are summarised below.

7.3.2 Two-Dimensional Gel Electrophoresis

2D-GE is the most widespread technique for separation of complex protein mixtures. In 2D-GE, a protein sample is separated in two steps in one gel. The first step (first dimension) represents isoelectrical focusing (IEF), allowing analyte separation in an electric field based on individual isoelectric points (pI). Zwitterionic proteins migrate in a strip containing an immobilised pH gradient. When entering the pH zone corresponding to the protein's pI the analyte loses its net charge, becomes electric neutral and thus does not migrate further. Proteins distributed in the IEF strip are then denatured and treated with sodium dodecylsulphate (SDS) thereby coating the unfolded protein with negatively charged SDS molecules to an extent approximately proportional to its molecular weight (MW). In the second step (second dimension) proteins are separated by means of an electric current based on differing MWs. Following this step, proteins appear as defined spots that can be visualised by diverse methods such as Coomassie Blue or the more sensitive silver staining. With respect to the method's resolution, no other approach is more powerful. Images of separated proteins related to condition I are obtained and can be compared with images of samples originated from condition II. Elaborated software tools enable quantitative assessment and allow differential expression analysis.[104] However, 2D-GE alone does not allow protein identification or analysis of small proteins and peptides with MWs below 10 kDa, thereby losing important information on processed proteins and resulting regulatory peptides. Analysing the peptide content (peptidomics) thus requires CE or LC for efficient separation.[73] No studies investigating the peptidome after CWA treatment have been described in the literature so far, even though suggestions of the effects on peptide secretion can be found.[18] Accordingly, this fascinating field of research will not be discussed further.

7.3.3 Mass Spectrometry

Following 2D-GE and spot identification, the major challenge lies in characterisation of the corresponding proteins. For that purpose, proteolysis is required to cut the entire protein into smaller peptides. The choice of the proteolytic enzyme determines the predictable cleavage sites. Trypsin is the most commonly applied protease, cutting at the C-terminus of lysine and arginine residues. Resulting small cleavage products are extracted from the gel by diverse washing steps and subjected to MS based analysis. Modern MS techniques like matrix assisted laser desorption/ionisation time of flight (MALDI-TOF) MS and electrospray ionisation (ESI) MS, typically coupled to high performance liquid chromatography (HPLC), provide the best suited technical properties for protein identification.[90] The basic technical principles of MALDI and ESI MS are described in a variety of easily available proteomic textbooks. Due to the fundamental and far reaching importance of these two soft ionisation methods, the inventors were honoured with the Nobel Prize in Chemistry in 2002 [Koichi Tanaka for soft laser desorption (SLD), which is related to MALDI, and John Fenn for ESI], but it was Franz Hillenkamp and Michael Karas who elaborated and made MALDI-TOF MS an optimum method for protein and peptide analysis.[105,106] Development and establishment of these techniques for routine analysis marked the start of the rapidly growing research efforts in proteomics. Accordingly, protein identification in CWA toxicology research has also made use of MALDI[82,83,85–87,107] and ESI MS.[84,94,97,108]

7.3.3.1 Matrix Assisted Laser Desorption/Ionisation Mass Spectrometry

The most conventional way to identify a protein is by analysing the peptide mass fingerprint (PMF). Following the MALDI MS approach, the entire number of extracted peptides after in-gel proteolysis is detected creating a characteristic pattern of signals similar to a barcode that can be interpreted by an automatic database search. This process compares the mass of the detected peptides with theoretical expectations that are deduced from database listed amino acid sequences subjected to virtual *in silico* cleavage with the protease of choice. The grade of matching (score) determines the feasibility of accuracy for protein identification. Plausibility increases with the number of assigned peptides. The PMF approach was successfully used in CWA research after 2D-GE to elaborate the effects of HD on diverse keratins,[83] tubulins,[84] haptoglobin[86,87] and apolipoprotein.[86] Furthermore, an increase of prolactin in the gonads of air breathing catfish was documented by PMF as an effect of exposure to malathion, an organophosphorus pesticide with endocrine disruptor activity.[107] In addition to simple PMF analysis, more modern MALDI MS instruments also provide the technical prerequisites for mass spectrometric fragmentations (MS/MS) by collision induced dissociation (CID) or laser induced dissociation (LID), as well as by post-source decay (PSD). For MS/MS a peptide signal detected in the PMF spectrum is selected (precursor ion) and subjected to fragmentation, resulting in a series of product ions. As peptide fragmentation follows some common, well described rules, product ions provide relevant information to elucidate (parts of) the entire amino acid sequence of the selected peptide (sequence tags). These tags are assigned by sophisticated platform specific software tools in combination with protein databases such as Mascot from Matrix Science, which is the most often applied in proteomics research. Combination of PMF with MS/MS of one or more peptides tremendously enhances the plausibility of correct protein identification.

Protein identification can be restricted by impurities (presence of additional proteins) that have not been separated in 2D-GE. Such impurities cause mixed PMF spectra that are more difficult to interpret. Therefore, consideration of additional MS/MS spectra is of essential relevance to overcome the drawback of non-optimum purity. Furthermore, low sequence coverage, denominating the ratio of the detected (recovered) protein sequence to its entire length, might make correct identification difficult. Coverages of only 20–40% are not unusual in bottom-up proteomics and may be caused by: (i) peptide cleavage products that are too small to be detected by MALDI MS; (ii) ion suppression (reduction of signal intensity) caused by too many cleavage products or any matrix compounds; (iii) unknown modifications of the protein that are not considered in the electronic database search; (iv) amino acid sequences of peptides not favouring ionisation due to too many negatively charged side chains or PTM; (v) incomplete in-gel proteolysis of the protein; (vi) incomplete recovery of peptide cleavage products from the gel; or (vii) unknown mutations at the protein level. Therefore, consideration of additional MS/MS spectra is of essential relevance for identification. Significant improvements in data interpretation can be achieved by MALDI MS instruments that provide higher resolution (≥12 000), typically realised by reflector mode technologies (see common textbooks). The more accurately the mass of a peptide is measured the more exact the correlation to theoretical prognosis will be. A highly impressive overview of the relevance of mass accuracy and matching scores has been given by McHugh and Arthur,[96] and Dodds *et al.*[109] Accordingly, reflector mode instruments are more appropriate than older linear mode analysers, but the most valuable mass spectrometers are MALDI-TOF/TOF MS, which provide additional opportunities for reliable MS/MS experiments. Despite all of the general limitations, MALDI MS represents a rapid, cheap, sensitive and indispensable tool for protein identification.

7.3.3.2 Electrospray Ionisation Mass Spectrometry

ESI, typically performed in the positive mode for peptides and proteins, represents the ideal interface for measurements of analytes in solution. Therefore, it is feasible for direct on-line coupling to any liquid separation technique such as LC or CE. Conventional triple quadrupole and ion trap ESI mass spectrometers have demonstrated suitability for such proteome analyses. Whereas MALDI MS analysis allows simultaneous detection of a large number of peptides within seconds, sensitive LC-ESI MS/MS requires about 1 h. The longer time consuming chromatographic step is a major advantage and allows efficient separation of the peptide mixture thus enabling mass spectrometric detection of more peptides due to fewer ion suppression effects. Less abundant peptides could therefore be detected that otherwise might be lost in MALDI MS analyses, typically relinquishing prior separation. Therefore, proteome analysis is also often performed by LC-ESI MS/MS using capillary columns for nano-LC dimension (inner diameter ≈75 µm, flow 200 nl min^{-1}) that provide optimum chromatographic resolution and sensitivity.[101] Coupling to high resolution MS/MS yields fragment spectra best suited for database searches, allowing (partial) peptide sequencing and identification of the original proteins.[110] Most modern mass analysers provide superior characteristics for more exact peptide detection and protein identification. Time of flight (TOF), Fourier transform ion cyclotron resonance (FT-ICR) and especially the Orbitrap analyser allow detection with maximum resolution of up to 150 000 and are predestined for top-down proteomics.[88,90,101,111–113] In addition to having the highest resolution, FT-ICR and Orbitrap technologies also provide prerequisites for improved fragmentation techniques [electron capture dissociation (ECD) and electron transfer dissociation (ETD)] suited very well for top-down proteomics of intact proteins and their PTM.[91,113] Accordingly, proteome analysis of guinea pig brainstem after *in vivo* challenge with sarin,[97] proteins from HaCaT cell cultures after HD treatment,[84] DNA adducts from rat derma exposed to HD,[108] and protein adducts formed in human plasma with organophosphorus poisons were analysed using the Orbitrap technology.[94]

7.3.4 Special Analytical Feature for Relative or Absolute Protein/Peptide Quantification

The more conservative approaches for elaboration of differentially expressed proteins are based on stained 2D-GE gels that are analysed with respect to different colour intensities. Alternative methods for relative and absolute protein quantification have been introduced in the last decade based on diverse reagents for labelling of selected amino acids (*e.g.* ICAT,[99] MeCAT,[114] iTRAQ[92]) or *in vitro* inclusion of stable isotope labelled amino acids into proteins (SILAC).[92,93,98] Simultaneous identification, quantification and comparison of two proteomes can be performed by MS appropriate for differentiation between *e.g.* ^{12}C and ^{13}C, ^{1}H and ^{2}H, ^{14}N and ^{15}N, and ^{16}O and ^{18}O, as well as for quantitative detection of metal ions by inductively coupled plasma MS (ICP-MS). These two techniques will be introduced briefly as they have also been applied to CWA proteomics.[84,97]

7.3.4.1 Stable Isotope Labelling by Amino Acids in Cell Culture

SILAC was developed by the working group of Matthias Mann and is applicable to cell cultures for relative protein quantification.[98] As necessary for growth and proliferation, cultured cells are fed essential amino acids required for protein biosynthesis. Of two test cultures, one culture is fed normal naturally occurring amino acids (condition I) and for the other at least one stable isotope labelled amino acid is supplied (condition II). Labelled amino acids represent common chemical structures of natural amino acids, but contain *e.g.* deuterium (^{2}H), ^{13}C or ^{15}N without changing the chemical and physiological properties with respect to protein biosynthesis.[92,93,98,115] After a certain number of cell doublings, respective natural amino acids will be replaced by their isotope labelled analogues causing altered molecular weights of proteins and their peptide breakdown products after proteolysis. Harvested purified proteins of one culture used as a control (condition I) and the other one manipulated by any factor (condition II *e.g.* CWA exposed) are mixed in equal parts, prepared and analysed by MS. Peptides containing labelled and non-labelled amino acids differ by characteristic mass shifts in MS and MS/MS detection but show nearly identical chromatographic properties and fragmentation patterns. Therefore, relative peak areas in LC-MS/MS or relative MS signal intensities in simple MS analysis allow relative protein/peptide quantification and characterisation of the effect of any factor applied. This technique was applied to identify the effects of HD on HaCaT cells by targeting phosphorylated proteins.[84] In this study, Everley and Dillman used arginine and lysine labelled with ^{13}C and ^{15}N and allowed at least five population doublings before treatment with HD.[84] Relative protein quantification by LC-ESI MS/MS was performed after SDS-PAGE, in-gel cleavage with trypsin and isolation of phosphopeptides.

7.3.4.2 Isobaric Tagging for Relative and Absolute Quantification

The fascinating technology of isobaric tagging for relative and absolute quantification (iTRAQ) was developed by the working group of Pappin and is suitable for relative and absolute quantification of proteins in complex mixtures.[92,100,115] Peptides produced by proteolysis of purified proteins obtained from diverse conditions are subjected to separate chemical derivatisation using special amine reactive tagging reagents that modify primary amino groups at the N-termini and lysine residue side chains. Coupling to NH_2 moieties is based on the well known amine specific reaction with the *N*-hydroxy succinimide (NHS) coupling group. NHS is connected to the isobaric tag comprised of a carbonyl *balance group* [–C(O)–] prolonged by a *reporter group* (*N*-methyl-piperazinidyl derivative; see Figure 7.2). These parts of the tag contain ^{13}C, ^{15}N and ^{18}O heavy isotopes to differing extents and composition, yielding four different masses for the four *reporter groups* (MW 114, 115, 116 and 117) and four different masses for the *balance group* (MW 31, 30, 29, and 28), but in total exhibiting the same molecular weight (MW 145). Therefore, resulting peptide derivatives possess identical masses (isobaric precursor) in combination with identical chromatographic behaviour in LC-ESI MS/MS analysis. Nevertheless, differentiation of the individual tags is possible by MS/MS, producing tag specific characteristic fragments of the labelled *reporter group* after CID (*m*/*z* 114.1, 115.1, 116.1 and 117.1).[100] The variety of tagging reagents not only allows simultaneous analysis of a binary sample mixture (condition I and II) but also enables multiplexed simultaneous comparative analysis of up to four samples (conditions I–IV).[100] Recently, special iTRAQ reagents commercially offered by a common MS provider (AB Sciex Ltd.) promised analysis of eight samples simultaneously. Hoffmann *et al.* applied this multiplexed procedure to elucidate the effects on the guinea pig brainstem proteome after *in vivo* treatment with lethal doses of sarin.[97]

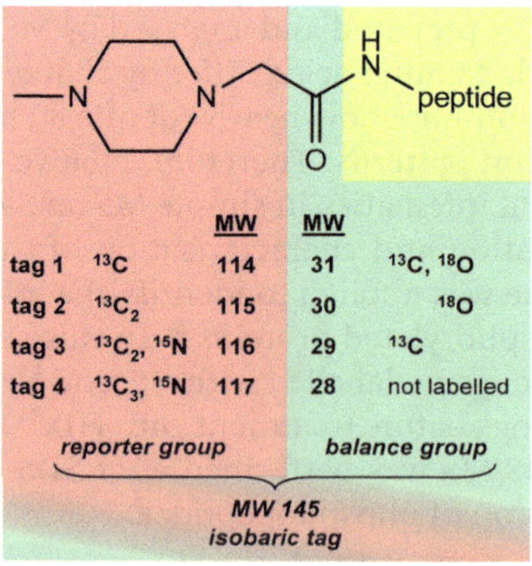

Figure 7.2 iTRAQ reagents suitable for relative and absolute quantification of proteins. iTRAQ technology enables labelling of N-termini and lysine residue side chains by attachment of an isobaric tag. Four different reagents corresponding to tags 1–4 are added to four samples each for quantitative comparison. Differentiation of the individual isobaric tags is possible by MS/MS, producing tag specific characteristic fragments of the labelled *reporter group* after CID (*m*/*z* 114.1, 115.1, 116.1 and 117.1).

7.3.5 Proteomic Research of CWAs

Based on the techniques described above some more general proteomics studies investigating the effects of CWAs were performed. In most cases HD was tested,[82–87,108] whereas a minority dealt with organophosphorus agents, and it is these that will be introduced first.[94,97,107]

7.3.5.1 *Organophosphorus Agents*

Organophosphorus agents include nerve agents and pesticides that might cause fatal harm by inhibition of AChE in the acute phase, block neuropathy target esterase (NTE), which is relevant for chronic effects of pesticides, and react with BChE, thus producing valuable markers for verification analysis.[116] As the main mechanisms of toxicity are well characterised and sufficient antidotal treatment is established, the need for more detailed proteome analysis seems to be less imperative. Nevertheless, some studies have been performed. Hoffmann *et al.* identified a number of proteins isolated from guinea pig brainstem that were influenced by an acute high dose exposure to sarin *in vivo* ($2 \times LD_{50}$).[97] By considering a 20% change in relative protein abundance as significant, they found 40 proteins that were increased and 33 decreased. The majority of proteins were derived from the cytosol and cytoskeleton, and were of primary relevance in metabolism and neuronal degeneration and regeneration. Based on these data, sarin was found to induce glutamate excitotoxicity, destabilisation of cytoskeletal proteins and hamper ongoing axonal regeneration. Marsillach *et al.* reported on a highly focussed targeted proteomic approach detecting organophosphorus agent adducts with BChE isolated from the plasma of persons who potentially had been exposed to organophosphorus agents.[94] The use of selective immunomagnetic separation (IMS) for BChE extraction followed by proteolytic cleavage with chymotrypsin and LC-ESI MS/MS analysis of the resulting derivatised dodecapeptide enabled rapid and sensitive monitoring of exposure. Incorporation of diverse organophosphorus agents was tested, including tricresylphosphate (which has been suggested to play a role in the quite unspecific symptoms of aerotoxic syndrome in pilots and flight attendants after *in vivo* biotransformation to cyclic saligenin cresyl phosphate, although actual exposure has not been verified) and organophosphorus pesticides in agricultural workers.[94] Such organophosphorus pesticides do not only affect humans but also the ecosystem. Diverse organophosphorus pesticides used for agricultural purposes reach the aquatic environment and thus chronically affect aquatic organism, *e.g.* as endocrine disruptors.[107] Such chemicals, including malathion, interfere with physiological systems especially during the critical developmental and reproductive stages. To elaborate these effects Laldinsangi *et al.* investigated the gonads (testis and ovary) of air breathing catfish after *in vivo* exposure to malathion for 21 days.[107] Up-regulation of prolactin in the ovaries and down-regulation of progonadoliberin-2 and cytochrome P450 1A1 was found by 2D-GE and MALDI MS. Even though this study is quite different from common CWA studies, it represents an interesting example for the use of proteomics techniques to characterise the effects of poisons in non-mammalian organisms.

7.3.5.2 HD and Alkylating Agents

Numerous questions concerning effective and more targeted therapy for HD poisoning remain open and thus provoke more comprehensive proteomics research than that found for organophosphorus poisoning, especially with respect to skin and skin cells. Accordingly, An *et al.* investigated alterations of protein expression in mouse ear skin after dermal challenge with HD *in vivo*.[82] Fifteen proteins were identified by MALDI MS after 2D-GE, including up-regulation of apolipoprotein A-I and prealbumin, and down-regulation of peroxiredoxin 6, actin, glutathione *S*-transferase and proteins involved in the oxidative stress response, apoptosis and energy metabolism. Using 1D- and 2D-GE in combination with MALDI MS, Dillman *et al.* showed that HD and N-Lost induce diverse intermolecular crosslinks to homodimers and heterodimers of keratin 14 and keratin 5 in cultured HEK cells that involve about 1–10% of total keratins.[83] Such aggregations correlate with intermediate filament network collapses and are postulated to perturb the hemidesmosomes that attach basal keratinocytes to the basement membrane at the epidermal–dermal junction.[83] In another study using HEK cells under HD exposure, proteins of the cellular and secreted fraction were analysed by the same techniques, yielding a variety of up- and down-regulated molecules (*e.g.* α- and β-tubulin) that was observable even 16 h after exposure.[84] Mol *et al.* also reported on proteomics studies with HEK cells exposed to HD.[85] Diverse cytokeratins, actins, galectin-7 and stratifin were found to be alkylated, as demonstrated by radiolabelled HD bound to proteins, separated by 2D-GE, monitored by autoradiography and identified by MALDI MS. Furthermore, analysis of differential expression revealed changes in heat shock protein 27, ribosomal protein P0 and diverse cytokeratins again. However, achieving practical benefit from these discoveries for therapy still remains a future challenge. The working group of Dillman also monitored changes in phosphoprotein expression caused by HD treatment of HaCaT cells.[84] This targeted proteome analysis for PTM was based on the SILAC concept (use of labelled arginine and lysine) and applied phosphorylation selective extraction of peptides after protein proteolysis by immobilised metal ion affinity chromatography (IMAC).[117] More than 2300 non-redundant phosphorylation sites were identified by LC-ESI MS/MS on an Orbitrap system correlating to HD induced elevated phosphorylation in diverse signalling pathways such as NF-κB, LIG1 and DNA damage.[84] Altered structures might be of importance for therapy. Mehrani *et al.* reported on two studies investigating the effects on the proteome in plasma and BALF of human victims of HD poisoning suffering from chronic lung diseases.[86,87] Trying to find any diagnostic marker reflecting the long term effects of HD and characterising the state of disease, proteins from the plasma as well as from BALF were analysed by 2D-GE and MALDI MS allowing comparison of sick (n = 20) and healthy people ($n = 20$).[86,87] Interestingly, it was found that isoforms of α1 haptoglobin and amyloid A1 were detected in the plasma of patients whereas healthy people did not show these proteins.[87] In BALF, significantly elevated concentrations of isoforms of vitamin D binding protein, haptoglobin and fibrinogen were detected, whereas reduced amounts were found for calcyphosine, surfactant protein A and transthyretin. Furthermore, apolipoprotein A1 and S100 calcium binding protein A8 were identified in patient's BALF exclusively.[86] Therefore, the authors concluded that ongoing tissue remodelling occurs in HD patients, which is potentially of relevance for patient care, therapy and diagnostic monitoring.

7.3.5.3 Protein Adducts as Biomarkers

Apart from general proteomics studies, numerous reports are focussed on the selective detection of proteins modified by covalent reactions with diverse CWAs (protein adducts), including nerve agents and HD. These procedures might be considered as somehow *targeted* proteomics approaches for selective evidence of a CWA *in vitro* and *in vivo*. Organophosphorus nerve agents and structurally related pesticides are known to react with (phosphylate) the serine residue of the active centre of BChE and AChE, forming adducts and causing enzyme inhibition.[116] Furthermore, binding to tyrosine and serine residues in albumin as well as to lysine residues in ubiquitin and some additional proteins has been documented.[118,119] In each case, the analytical strategy requires purified protein, typically isolated from plasma by affinity chromatography, which is proteolytically cleaved to generate an internal peptide product that still carries the bound agent. These modified peptides are separated by LC, ionised by ESI and fragmented by CID. The most sensitive detection of diagnostic fragments is performed in the multiple reaction monitoring (MRM) mode of triple quadrupole mass analysers. Detection of these analytes may provide evidence for an alleged use of nerve agents and is therefore a valuable tool for verification analysis. These procedures were applied to prove nerve agent exposures in the case of the terrorist attack on the Tokyo subway in 1995 and for the current Syrian Arab Republic conflict at the time of writing (2014).[120] Similar approaches were introduced for HD adducts with albumin[121–124] and haemoglobin[125–127] that are suitable to prove HD poisoning. Even though all of these reliable methods are of high forensic relevance they will not be presented in more detail as they target well known protein derivatisations in a highly selective way, thus not providing general proteome information. In contrast, more global approaches identifying novel protein adducts will be essential to elaborate additional targets of poison relevant for understanding pathophysiology or for establishment of novel biomarkers of exposure. Following such a non-targeted approach, Lockridge and Schopfer looked for additional mammalian plasma proteins and special amino acid motif targets for organophosphate binding.[128] Similarly, Mol *et al.* identified a number of protein targets, including several cytokeratins (5, 6, 14, 16 and 17), alkylated by radiolabelled HD in exposed HEK cells.[85]

7.3.6 Proteomics Conclusion

Differential proteome analysis represents a state of the art analytical approach to unravel changes in protein expression caused by any toxicant. Nevertheless, protein identification by MS and MS/MS strictly depends on the quality of the spectra and algorithms used for the database search. Despite the reliability and robustness of modern MS instruments, protein assignment should be scrutinised and interpreted with care, in order to not follow false results. *Shotgun proteomics* approaches are beneficial if there is no idea of the specific effects. Less complex and presumably more reliable samples might be obtained when focussing on diverse protein subgroups for *targeted proteomics*. Selective sample preparation for this targeted approach allows analysis of special sub-domains of proteomics such as phosphoproteomics,[90,92] glycoproteomics,[90,129] immunoproteomics,[130] metaproteomics for microbial function[131] or metallomics for metalloproteins.[132] The latter field, accessible by ICP-MS, might be highly relevant when looking for protein targets of CWA that contain metals, such as arsenic in L. Even though stable isotope labelling techniques like iTRAQ and SILAC are highly sophisticated and valuable for protein quantification, the trial of alternative derivatisation technologies might provide additional and reliable information. A well known possibility for selective derivatisation of cysteine residues in proteins has been established as isotope coded affinity tags (ICAT), which were developed by the working group of Aebersold.[99] Proteins of two samples (conditions I and II) are modified by two reagents of related chemical structure that contain either a deuterated heavy chain or a non-deuterated light chain. As these tags are also biotin labelled, they are accessible for extraction on avidin columns after combination of derivatised protein mixtures and subsequent proteolysis. Extracted peptides containing the tagged cysteine residues are analysed by LC-ESI MS/MS for identification and relative quantification based on the signal intensities of the isotopic labels. Even though this technique was introduced about 15 years ago,[99] it has not been applied to CWA proteome research so far. Despite the cysteine selective mechanism for labelling, it surely represents a versatile tool for relative quantification. A quite novel and important approach, metal-coded affinity tags (MeCAT), has been introduced, allowing quantitative proteomics.[114] Thiol groups of cysteine residues of the intact protein (top-down approach) or primary amino groups of peptides (bottom-up approach) are chemically labelled with lanthanide bearing chelators (rare earth metals such as holmium and thulium) predestined for highly selective and sensitive analysis by ICP-MS in an absolute manner (element MS). Measurement of proteins separated by gel electrophoresis is possible by simple flow injection of dissolved gel spots. Protein identification is realised by common MS/MS experiments. From the technical point of view, CWA related proteomics research might further profit from the use of orthogonal liquid separation techniques for multi-dimensional chromatography.[90] This modification promises to provide much improved chromatographic resolution, allowing detection of less abundant peptides. Enhanced throughput and more detailed MS/MS data might be obtained when applying ultra-performance liquid chromatography (using a stationary phase of sub-2 μm particles) coupled to MS of elevated energy (UPLC MS^E).[81] Thus, despite limited forays into proteomics it is clear that there are numerous techniques still available to probe CWA toxicology at the protein level.

7.4 *In silico* Approaches

The application of new technologies to elucidate CWA toxicology has the ability to generate vast amounts of data. Understandably, research groups aim to publish against specific hypotheses (*i.e.* the involvement of the glutathione pathway in phosgene induced injury[43]) or generate new hypotheses (the involvement of neuro-inflammation following nerve agent exposure[17,18,22]). However, these approaches leave large amounts of data un-investigated. Thanks to various open access initiatives, complete datasets are available on public databases such as the Gene Expression Omnibus (GEO), MIAM-Express, ExPASy and Proteomics Identifications Database (PRIDE). These databases offer the opportunity for others to exploit the data to further understand CWA toxicology. The field of proteomics is not as well advanced as that for transcriptomics and as such the discussion here will focus on transcriptomic approaches. These methods tend to focus on bioinformatics to identify commonalities across agents or diseases. Soon after the inception of microarray technology, clustering algorithms were used to study 15 hepatotoxins and to compare their profiles to the clinical chemistry and histopathology.[133] By clustering gene expression profiles it was possible to group compounds based on their shared expression profiles, potentially opening the door for generic treatments. It was also possible to identify clusters of genes that correlated with clinical chemistry and histopathology data, allowing the identification of biomarkers. Following this proof of principal, the authors suggested the use of a database of expression profiles in order to study toxicology, which has ultimately been provided by initiatives such as GEO.

Now that datasets are deposited in these databases they have been successfully re-analysed to study CWA toxicology. For example, new algorithms have been designed for generating biologically meaningful toxicological data from multi-parameter experiments (both time and dose dependent).[134] The software GO-Quant was developed specifically for toxicogenomics and used the HD exposed murine lung data generated by Dillman *et al.*[35] This *in silico* approach to re-analyse the data from the GEO was able to validate the original findings and also identify more detailed biological functions in response to HD. The GO-Quant programme was able to quantify biological processes across time and doses and present a clear picture of the changes occurring across these variables. The dose response analysis approach identified the M-phase of the mitotic cycle as a key response to HD 24 h after exposure, coupled with a decrease in immune cell activation.[134] The time dependent analysis revealed cell cycle arrest, tissue development and protein ubiquitination as all increasing over time after exposure. The *in silico* method has added further valuable insight into this dataset but, as freely admitted by the authors, it was not the intent to describe why these functional alterations occurred but rather to publish a novel method for biological interpretation.[134]

Other *in silico* approaches using CWA GEO data have also furthered the understanding of CWA toxicology. The phosgene dataset generated by Sciuto *et al.* has been used as an oxidative stress comparator dataset for the investigation of cigarette smoke.[43,45] The driver of the research was to identify a biomarker panel to characterise asthma and cigarette smoke induced gene expression. The output was a candidate list of 26 genes indicative of oxidative stress in these two conditions. This list was then compared against the phosgene dataset after it had been identified from GEO as a dataset showing signals of oxidative stress. Eighteen of the 26 markers held true for phosgene and were able to identify activating transcription factor 3 as an early marker of phosgene induced injury because it was up-regulated at 30 min post-exposure. The study also identified MMP3 and TIMP1 as up-regulated in response to phosgene. These were not identified by the original publication.[43] The *in silico* strategy employed showed that gene expression levels can be successfully compared and commonalities observed across platforms, species and challenges (here defined as cigarette smoke, asthma and phosgene).[45] This approach should be applied directly to more CWA datasets in order to gain further understanding of the toxicology and, ultimately, identify generic targets for therapeutic intervention.

A common limitation placed on the transcriptomics datasets found in the GEO is that a map of mRNA it is not directly related to the translated proteins of the host. *In silico* analysis allows extrapolation of transcript data to infer protein–protein interactions. The phosgene dataset generated by Sciuto *et al.* was used to investigate this approach.[43,44] Re-analysis from the GEO identified 582 differentially expressed genes. These genes were then mapped to a protein–protein interaction (PPI) network. Combined with gene set enrichment analysis, the re-analysis from GEO was able to identify the spliceosome, glutathione metabolism and cell cycle dysregulation following phosgene exposure. The PPI network was able to identify four phosgene specific biomarkers: F3, Meis1, Pvf and Cdc6. These biomarkers have yet to be validated experimentally. This is a common observation with *in silico* approaches where publication of novel algorithms or software is often the aim of the mathematically or computationally driven research groups. The data generated under this research that feed into CWA toxicology will ultimately need to be tested and validated by life scientists. It is this interaction between the life sciences and bioinformatics that is currently lacking. If this can be overcome, then the potential to take large steps forward in our understanding may be realised by these types of study.

7.5 Overall Conclusion

The use of new multiplexed technologies such as transcriptomics and proteomics has covered a variety of chemical agents. There are still some substantial areas for improvement to fill existing gaps, especially in the area of proteomics (see Table 7.1). However, the continued profiling of responses to CWAs in a variety of models may not yield large steps forward in the understanding of the toxicology of these agents. Work to date has shown that, whilst these experiments continue to generate vast amounts of data, these data are not necessarily fully exploited. This is both in terms of a successful downstream analysis pipeline, allowing classical techniques to build upon the hypotheses generated, and in terms of fully understanding the data. It is suggested here that the field could consider two options for advancement.

The first of these is an increase in CWA proteomics research and the comparison of these data with existing transcriptional data. Any comparison will be subject to the usual toxicological experimental design challenges regarding choices about animal model, dosing regimen, long *versus* short term exposure effects, *etc.* It would perhaps be prudent to design future proteomics experiments closely based on the existing transcriptomics data. This would allow both the discovery of the protein response and subsequently a comparison between the transcribed and translated response. This would provide several critical analyses from one experiment. If this approach is not used, then any comparison will continue to be dogged by comments that platforms and technologies do not support each other. The link between the transcribed and translated response is one of contention and appropriate proteomics experiments could provide the solution in this area. Whilst it is not necessarily expected that a direct overlay of results would be achieved, it would provide a step forward in understanding the role of each technology in investigating CWAs. The second option is the increased exploitation of legacy data. Small steps have been made in this area (as outlined in Section 7.4), but there is significant room for advancement. The datasets generated by these technologies can be re-analysed to provide novel understanding or hypotheses. This is especially important in the field of CWA toxicology where facilities and access mean that the body of researchers able to carry out CWA animal research is small. Scientist from other areas (non-CWA toxicology, bioinformatics, protein modelling, *etc.*) should be encouraged to utilise the existing legacy data to derive new avenues of scientific research. The onus of instigating this interaction may lie with CWA toxicologists to engage these fields to ensure maximum use of their data.

Despite these suggestions for advancement in the field, it is clear that transcriptomics and proteomics have, and continue to, offer an understanding of CWA toxicology at the molecular level. The power of these technologies to observe multiple parameters cannot be denied. Rather than be seen as complex novel technologies it is imperative that they are seen as just another tool in the toxicologist's experimental tool-kit. It is in this way and by coupling them to classical techniques that they add most value to the research of CWA toxicology.

References

1. K. V. Morris and J. S. Mattick, The rise of regulatory RNA, *Nat. Rev. Genet.*, 2014, **15**, 423–437.
2. P. A. Everley and J. F. Dillman, III, Genomics and proteomics in chemical warfare agent research: Recent studies and future applications, *Toxicol. Lett.*, 2010, **198**, 297–303.
3. Z. Dong and Y. Chen, Transcriptomics: advances and approaches, *Sci. China: Life Sci.*, 2013, **56**, 960–967.
4. M. Schena, D. Shalon, R. W. Davis and P. O. Brown, Quantitative monitoring of gene expression patterns with a complementary-DNA microarray, *Science*, 1995, **270**, 467–470.
5. M. Schena, D. Shalon, R. Heller, A. Chai, P. O. Brown and R. W. Davis, Parallel human genome analysis: aicroarray-based expression monitoring of 1000 genes, *Proc. Natl. Acad. Sci. U. S. A.*, 1996, **93**, 10614–10619.
6. A. Brazma, P. Hingamp, J. Quackenbush, G. Sherlock, P. Spellman, C. Stoeckert, J. Aach, W. Ansorge, C. A. Ball, H. C. Causton, T. Gaasterland, P. Glenisson, F. C. P. Holstege, I. F. Kim, V. Markowitz, J. C. Matese, H. Parkinson, A. Robinson, U. Sarkans, S. Schulze-Kremer, J. Stewart, R. Taylor, J. Vilo and M. Vingron, Minimum information about a microarray experiment (MIAME) – toward standards for microarray data, *Nat. Genet.*, 2001, **29**, 365–371.
7. O. Soukup, G. Tobin, U. K. Kumar, J. Binder, J. Proska, D. Jun, J. Fusek and K. Kuca, Interaction of Nerve Agent Antidotes with Cholinergic Systems, *Curr. Med. Chem.*, 2010, **17**, 1708–1718.
8. M. Moshiri, E. Darchini-Maragheh and M. Balali-Mood, Advances in toxicology and medical treatment of chemical warfare nerve agents, *Daru, J. Pharm. Sci.*, 2012, **20**, 81.
9. K. Ghabili, P. S. Agutter, M. Ghanei, K. Ansarin, Y. Panahi and M. M. Shoja, Sulfur mustard toxicity: history, chemistry, pharmacokinetics, and pharmacodynamics, *Crit. Rev. Toxicol.*, 2011, **41**, 384–403.
10. M. P. Shakarjian, D. E. Heck, J. P. Gray, P. J. Sinko, M. K. Gordon, R. P. Casillas, N. D. Heindel, D. R. Gerecke, D. L. Laskin and J. D. Laskin, Mechanisms Mediating the Vesicant Actions of Sulfur Mustard after Cutaneous Exposure, *Toxicol. Sci.*, 2010, **114**, 5–19.
11. T. V. Damodaran, M. A. Bilska, A. A. Rahman and M. B. Abou-Donia, Sarin causes early differential alteration and persistent overexpression in mRNAs coding for glial fibrillary acidic protein (GFAP) and vimentin genes in the central nervous system of rats, *Neurochem. Res.*, 2002, **27**, 407–415.
12. T. V. Damodaran, K. H. Jones, A. G. Patel and M. B. Abou-Donia, Sarin (nerve agent GB)-induced differential expression of mRNA coding for the acetylcholinesterase gene in the rat central nervous system, *Biochem. Pharmacol.*, 2003, **65**, 2041–2047.
13. T. V. Damodaran, A. A. Mecklai and M. B. Abou-Donia, Sarin causes altered time course of mRNA expression of alpha tubulin in the central nervous system of rats, *Neurochem. Res.*, 2002, **27**, 177–181.

14. T. V. Damodaran, S. T. Greenfield, A. G. Patel, H. K. Dressman, S. K. Lin and M. B. Abou-Donia, Toxicogenomic studies of the rat brain at an early time point following acute sarin exposure, *Neurochem. Res.*, 2006, **31**, 367–381.
15. T. V. Damodaran, A. G. Patel, S. T. Greenfield, H. K. Dressman, S. M. Lin and M. B. Abou-Donia, Gene expression profiles of the rat brain both immediately and 3 months following acute satin exposure, *Biochem. Pharmacol.*, 2006, **71**, 497–520.
16. A. Pachiappan, M. M. Thwin, L. W. Keong, F. K. Lee, J. Manikandan, V. Sivakumar and P. Gopalakrishnakone, ETS2 Regulating Neurodegenerative Signaling Pathway of Human Neuronal (SH-SY5Y) Cells Exposed to Single and Repeated Low-Dose Sarin (GB), *Chem. Res. Toxicol.*, 2009, **22**, 990–996.
17. K. D. Spradling, L. A. Lumley, C. L. Robison, J. L. Meyerhoff and J. F. Dillman, III, Transcriptional responses of the nerve agent-sensitive brain regions amygdala, hippocampus, piriform cortex, septum, and thalamus following exposure to the organophosphonate anticholinesterase sarin, *J. Neuroinflammation*, 2011, **8**, 84.
18. K. D. Spradling, L. A. Lumley, C. L. Robison, J. L. Meyerhoff and J. F. Dillman, III, Transcriptional analysis of rat piriform cortex following exposure to the organophosphonate anticholinesterase sarin and induction of seizures, *J. Neuroinflammation*, 2011, **8**, 83.
19. M. A. Brown and K. A. Brix, Review of health consequences from high-, intermediate- and low-level exposure to organophosphorus nerve agents, *J. Appl. Toxicol.*, 1998, **18**, 393–408.
20. J. H. McDonough and T. M. Shih, Neuropharmacological mechanisms of nerve agent-induced seizure and neuropathology, *Neurosci. Biobehav. Rev.*, 1997, **21**, 559–579.
21. S. Chapman, T. Kadar and E. Gilat, Seizure duration following sarin exposure affects neuro-inflammatory markers in the rat brain, *Neurotoxicology*, 2006, **27**, 277–283.
22. J. F. Dillman, III, C. S. Phillips, D. M. Kniffin, C. P. Tompkins, T. A. Hamilton and R. K. Kan, Gene Expression Profiling of Rat Hippocampus Following Exposure to the Acetylcholinesterase Inhibitor Soman, *Chem. Res. Toxicol.*, 2009, **22**, 633–638.
23. J. L. Blanton, J. A. D'Ambrozio, J. E. Sistrunk and E. G. Midboe, Global changes in the expression patterns of RNA isolated from the hippocampus and cortex of VX exposed mice, *J. Biochem. Mol. Toxicol.*, 2004, **18**, 115–123.
24. X. Gao, H. Lin, R. Ray and P. Ray, Toxicogenomic Studies of Human Neural Cells Following Exposure to Organophosphorus Chemical Warfare Nerve Agent VX, *Neurochem. Res.*, 2013, **38**, 916–934.
25. A. Buonanno, The neuregulin signaling pathway and schizophrenia: from genes to synapses and neural circuits, *Brain Res. Bull.*, 2010, **83**, 122–131.
26. F. R. Tang and W. K. Loke, Sulfur mustard and respiratory diseases, *Crit. Rev. Toxicol.*, 2012, **42**, 688–702.

27. M. Ghanei and A. A. Harandi, Molecular and cellular mechanism of lung injuries due to exposure to sulfur mustard: a review, *Inhalation Toxicol.*, 2011, **23**, 363–371.
28. M. Ghanei, Z. Poursaleh, A. A. Harandi, S. E. Emadi and S. N. Emadi, Acute and chronic effects of sulfur mustard on the skin: a comprehensive review, *Cutaneous Ocul. Toxicol.*, 2010, **29**, 269–277.
29. P. Zhang, P. Ng, D. Caridha, R. A. Leach, L. V. Asher, M. J. Novak, W. J. Smith, S. L. Zeichner and P. K. Chiang, Gene expressions in Jurkat cells poisoned by a sulphur mustard vesicant and the induction of apoptosis, *Br. J. Pharmacol.*, 2002, **137**, 245–252.
30. P. L. Platteborze, Effects of sulfur mustard on transcription in human epidermal keratinocytes: analysis by mRNA differential display, *J. Appl. Toxicol.*, 2003, **23**, 249–254.
31. P. L. Platteborze, The transcriptional effects of the vesicants lewisite and sulfur mustard on human epidermal keratinocytes, *Toxicol. Mech. Methods*, 2005, **15**, 185–192.
32. H. L. Meier, C. L. Gross and B. Papirmeister, 2,2′-Dichlorodiethyl sulphide (sulfur mustard) decreases NAD+ levels in human leukocytes, *Toxicol. Lett.*, 1987, **39**, 109–122.
33. J. V. Rogers, Y. W. Choi, R. C. Kiser, M. C. Babin, R. P. Casillas, J. J. Schlager and C. L. K. Sabourin, Microarray analysis of gene expression in murine skin exposed to sulfur mustard, *J. Biochem. Mol. Toxicol.*, 2004, **18**, 289–299.
34. J. F. Dillman, A. I. Hege, C. S. Phillips, L. D. Orzolek, A. J. Sylvester, C. Bossone, C. Henemyre-Harris, R. C. Kiser, Y. W. Choi, J. J. Schlager and C. L. Sabourin, Microarray analysis of mouse ear tissue exposed to bis-(2-chloroethyl) sulfide: gene expression profiles correlate with treatment efficacy and an established clinical endpoint, *J. Pharmacol. Exp. Ther.*, 2006, **317**, 76–87.
35. J. F. Dillman, C. S. Phillips, L. M. Dorsch, M. D. Croxton, A. I. Hege, A. J. Sylvester, T. S. Moran and A. M. Sciuto, Genomic analysis of rodent pulmonary tissue following bis-(2-chloroethyl) sulfide exposure, *Chem. Res. Toxicol.*, 2005, **18**, 28–34.
36. C. L. K. Sabourin, J. V. Rogers, Y. W. Choi, R. C. Kiser, R. P. Casillas, M. C. Babin and J. J. Schlager, Time- and dose-dependent analysis of gene expression using microarrays in sulfur mustard-exposed mice, *J. Biochem. Mol. Toxicol.*, 2004, **18**, 300–312.
37. D. R. Gerecke, M. Chen, S. S. Isukapalli, M. K. Gordon, Y.-C. Chang, W. Tong, I. P. Androulakis and P. G. Georgopoulos, Differential gene expression profiling of mouse skin after sulfur mustard exposure: extended time response and inhibitor effect, *Toxicol. Appl. Pharmacol.*, 2009, **234**, 156–165.
38. J. V. Rogers, J. N. McDougal, J. A. Price, F. M. Reid and J. S. Graham, Transcriptional responses associated with sulfur mustard and thermal burns in porcine skin, *Cutaneous Ocul. Toxicol.*, 2008, **27**, 135–160.

39. J. A. Price, J. V. Rogers, J. N. McDougal, M. Q. Shaw, F. M. Reid and J. S. Graham, Transcriptional changes in porcine skin at 7 days following sulfur mustard and thermal burn injury, *Cutaneous Ocul. Toxicol.*, 2009, **28**, 129–140.
40. T. Anand, R. Vijayaraghavan, P. V. L. Rao, I. Bansal and B. K. Bhattacharya, Attenuation of sulfur mustard toxicity by S-2 (2-aminoethylamino) ethyl phenyl sulfide (DRDE-07) in mouse liver, *Toxicol. Mech. Methods*, 2011, **21**, 596–605.
41. A. Najafi, A. Masoudi-Nejad, A. A. I. Fooladi, M. Ghanei and M. R. Nourani, Microarray gene expression analysis of the human airway in patients exposed to sulfur mustard, *J. Recept. Signal Transduction*, 2014, **34**, 283–289.
42. G. E. Kisby, A. Olivas, M. Standley, X. Lu, P. Pattee, J. O'Malley, X. Li, J. Muniz and S. R. Nagalla, Genotoxicants target distinct molecular networks in neonatal neurons, *Environ. Health Perspect.*, 2006, **114**, 1703–1712.
43. A. M. Sciuto, C. S. Phillips, L. D. Orzolek, A. I. Hege, T. S. Moran and J. F. Dillman, Genomic analysis of murine pulmonary tissue following carbonyl chloride inhalation, *Chem. Res. Toxicol.*, 2005, **18**, 1654–1660.
44. Z. Liu, F. Gao, L. Hou, Y. Qian and R. Tian, Network Clusters Analysis Based on Protein-Protein Interaction Network Constructed in Phosgene-Induced Acute Lung Injury, *Lung*, 2013, **191**, 545–551.
45. R. J. Freishtat, A. S. Benton, A. M. Watson, Z. Wang, M. C. Rose and E. P. Hoffman, Delineation of a Gene Network Underlying the Pulmonary Response to Oxidative Stress in Asthma, *J. Invest. Med.*, 2009, **57**, 756–764.
46. A. M. Sciuto, M. B. Cascio, T. S. Moran and J. S. Forster, The fate of antioxidant enzymes in bronchoalveolar lavage fluid over 7 days in mice with acute lung injury, *Inhalation Toxicol.*, 2003, **15**, 675–685.
47. G. D. Leikauf, V. J. Concel, K. Bein, P. Liu, A. Berndt, T. M. Martin, K. Ganguly, A. S. Jang, K. A. Brant, R. A. Dopico, Jr., S. Upadhyay, C. Cario, Y. P. P. Di, L. J. Vuga, E. Kostem, E. Eskin, M. You, N. Kaminski, D. R. Prows, D. L. Knoell and J. P. Fabisiak, Functional Genomic Assessment of Phosgene-Induced Acute Lung Injury in Mice, *Am. J. Respir. Cell Mol. Biol.*, 2013, **49**, 368–383.
48. G. D. Leikauf, H. Pope-Varsalona, V. J. Concel, P. Liu, K. Bein, A. Berndt, T. M. Martin, K. Ganguly, A. S. Jang, K. A. Brant, R. A. Dopico, Jr., S. Upadhyay, Y. P. P. Di, Q. Li, Z. Hu, L. J. Vuga, M. Medvedovic, N. Kaminski, M. You, D. C. Alexander, J. E. McDunn, D. R. Prows, D. L. Knoell and J. P. Fabisiak, Integrative Assessment of Chlorine-Induced Acute Lung Injury in Mice, *Am. J. Respir. Cell Mol. Biol.*, 2012, **47**, 234–244.
49. J. A. Price, J. V. Rogers, J. L. Plahovinsak, M. Q. S. Wendling, M. R. Perry, F. M. Reid and J. S. Graham, Toxicogenomic analysis of chlorine vapor-induced porcine skin injury, *Cutaneous Ocul. Toxicol.*, 2012, **31**, 323–331.

50. K. J. Dickers, S. M. Bradberry, P. Rice, G. D. Griffiths and J. A. Vale, Abrin poisoning, *Toxicol. Rev.*, 2003, **22**, 137–142.
51. G. D. Griffiths, Understanding Ricin from a Defensive Viewpoint, *Toxins*, 2011, **3**, 1373–1392.
52. S. Olsnes, The history of ricin, abrin and related toxins, *Toxicon*, 2004, **44**, 361–370.
53. L. DaSilva, D. Cote, C. Roy, M. Martinez, S. Duniho, M. L. M. Pitt, T. Downey and M. Dertzbaugh, Pulmonary gene expression profiling of inhaled ricin, *Toxicon*, 2003, **41**, 813–822.
54. J. Wong, V. Korcheva, D. B. Jacoby and B. E. Magun, Proinflammatory responses of human airway cells to ricin involve stress-activated protein kinases and NF-kappa B, *Am. J. Physiol.*, 2007, **293**, L1385–L1394.
55. J. David, L. J. Wilkinson and G. D. Griffiths, Inflammatory gene expression in response to sub-lethal ricin exposure in Balb/c mice, *Toxicology*, 2009, **264**, 119–130.
56. A. S. B. Bhaskar, N. Gupta and P. V. L. Rao, Transcriptomic profile of host response in mouse brain after exposure to plant toxin abrin, *Toxicology*, 2012, **299**, 33–43.
57. V. Sahni, S. K. Agarwal, N. P. Singh and S. Sikdar, Acute demyelinating encephalitis after jequirity pea ingestion (Abrus precatorius), *Clin. Toxicol.*, 2007, **45**, 77–79.
58. R. Sahoo, A. Hamide, S. D. Amalnath and B. S. Narayana, Acute demyelinating encephalitis due to Abrus precatorius poisoning - complete recovery after steroid therapy, *Clin. Toxicol.*, 2008, **46**, 1071–1073.
59. J. H. Malone and B. Oliver, Microarrays, deep sequencing and the true measure of the transcriptome, *BMC Biol.*, 2011, **9**, 34.
60. Z. Wang, M. Gerstein and M. Snyder, RNA-Seq: a revolutionary tool for transcriptomics, *Nat. Rev. Genet.*, 2009, **10**, 57–63.
61. M. B. Black, B. B. Parks, L. Pluta, T.-M. Chu, B. C. Allen, R. D. Wolfinger and R. S. Thomas, Comparison of Microarrays and RNA-Seq for Gene Expression Analyses of Dose-Response Experiments, *Toxicol. Sci.*, 2014, **137**, 385–403.
62. M. Chen, M. Zhang, J. Borlak and W. Tong, A Decade of Toxicogenomic Research and Its Contribution to Toxicological Science, *Toxicol. Sci.*, 2012, **130**, 217–228.
63. B. A. Merrick, D. P. Phadke, S. S. Auerbach, D. Mav, S. M. Stiegelmeyer, R. R. Shah and R. R. Tice, RNA-Seq Profiling Reveals Novel Hepatic Gene Expression Pattern in Aflatoxin B1 Treated Rats, *PLoS One*, 2013, **8**, e61768.
64. A. Fire, S. Q. Xu, M. K. Montgomery, S. A. Kostas, S. E. Driver and C. C. Mello, Potent and specific genetic interference by double-stranded RNA in Caenorhabditis elegans, *Nature*, 1998, **391**, 806–811.
65. A. L. Ruff and J. F. Dillman, III, Sulfur Mustard Induced Cytokine Production and Cell Death: investigating the Potential Roles of the p38, p53, and NF-kappa B Signaling Pathways with RNA Interference, *J. Biochem. Mol. Toxicol.*, 2010, **24**, 155–164.

66. E. C. K. Yego and J. F. Dillman, III, Cytokine regulation by MAPK activated kinase 2 in keratinocytes exposed to sulfur mustard, *Toxicol. In Vitro*, 2013, **27**, 2067–2075.
67. Y.-H. Liu, K. Peck and J.-Y. Lin, Involvement of Prohibitin Upregulation in Abrin-Triggered Apoptosis, *J. Evidence-Based Complementary Altern. Med.*, 2012, 605154.
68. P. M. Lundy, M. G. Hamilton, T. W. Sawyer and J. Mikler, Comparative protective effects of HI-6 and MMB-4 against organophosphorous nerve agent poisoning, *Toxicology*, 2011, **285**, 90–96.
69. D. Rocksen, D. Elfsmark, V. Heldestad, K. Wallgren, G. Cassel and A. G. Nyberg, An animal model to study health effects during continuous low-dose exposure to the nerve agent VX, *Toxicology*, 2008, **250**, 32–38.
70. T. M. Shih and J. H. McDonough, Organophosphorus nerve agents-induced seizures and efficacy of atropine sulfate as anticonvulsant treatment, *Pharmacol., Biochem. Behav.*, 1999, **64**, 147–153.
71. A. A. Gheyas and D. W. Burt, Microarray resources for genetic and genomic studies in chicken: a review, *Genesis*, 2013, **51**, 337–356.
72. R. Jain, B. Dey and A. K. Tyagi, Development of the first oligonucleotide microarray for global gene expression profiling in guinea pigs: defining the transcription signature of infectious diseases, *BMC Genomics*, 2012, **13**, 520.
73. M. Soloviev and P. Finch, Peptidomics: bridging the gap between proteome and metabolome, *Proteomics*, 2006, **6**, 744–747.
74. P. Schulz-Knappe, M. Raida, M. Meyer, E. A. Quellhorst and W. G. Forssmann, Systematic isolation of circulating human peptides: the concept of peptide trapping, *Eur. J. Med.Res.*, 1996, **1**, 223–236.
75. P. SchulzKnappe, M. Schrader, L. Standker, R. Richter, R. Hess, M. Jurgens and W. G. Forssmann, Peptide bank generated by large-scale preparation of circulating human peptides, *J. Chromatogr. A*, 1997, **776**, 125–132.
76. E. Machtejevas, H. John, K. Wagner, L. Standker, G. Marko-Varga, W. G. Forssmann, R. Bischoff and K. K. Unger, Automated multi-dimensional liquid chromatography: sample preparation and identification of peptides from human blood filtrate, *J. Chromatogr. B: Anal. Technol. Biomed. Life Sci.*, 2004, **803**, 121–130.
77. M. Schrader and P. Schulz-Knappe, Peptidomics technologies for human body fluids, *Trends Biotechnol.*, 2001, **19**, S55–S60.
78. S. Wittke, T. Kaiser and H. Mischak, Differential polypeptide display: the search for the elusive target, *J. Chromatogr. B: Anal. Technol. Biomed. Life Sci.*, 2004, **803**, 17–26.
79. T. Kaiser, H. Kamal, A. Rank, H. J. Kolb, E. Holler, A. Ganser, B. Hertenstein, H. Mischak and E. M. Weissinger, Proteomics applied to the clinical follow-up of patients after allogeneic hematopoietic stem cell transplantation, *Blood*, 2004, **104**, 340–349.

80. M. A. M. Rodrigo, O. Zitka, S. Krizkova, A. Moulick, V. Adam and R. Kizek, MALDI-TOF MS as evolving cancer diagnostic tool: a review, *J. Pharm. Biomed. Anal.*, 2014, **95**, 245–255.
81. Y.-Y. Zhao and R.-C. Lin, UPLC-MSE application in disease biomarker discovery: the discoveries in proteomics to metabolomics, *Chem.-Biol. Interact.*, 2014, **215**, 7–16.
82. W.-H. An, Y.-X. Zhong, X.-Y. Ying, H.-N. Shi and Y. Ying, Identification of differential proteins of pinnal skin of mice poisoned by sulfur mustard, *Zhongguo Yaolixue Yu Dulixue Zazhi*, 2006, **20**, 152–156.
83. J. F. Dillman, K. L. McGary and J. J. Schlager, Sulfur mustard induces the formation of keratin aggregates in human epidermal keratinocytes, *Toxicol. Appl. Pharmacol.*, 2003, **193**, 228–236.
84. P. A. Everley and J. F. Dillman, III, A Large-Scale Quantitative Proteomic Approach To Identifying Sulfur Mustard-Induced Protein Phosphorylation Cascades, *Chem. Res. Toxicol.*, 2010, **23**, 20–25.
85. M. A. E. Mol, R. M. van den Berg and H. P. Benschop, Proteomic assessment of sulfur mustard-induced protein adducts and other protein modifications in human epidermal keratinocytes, *Toxicol. Appl. Pharmacol.*, 2008, **230**, 97–108.
86. H. Mehrani, M. Ghanei, J. Aslani and L. Golmanesh, Bronchoalveolar lavage fluid proteomic patterns of sulfur mustard-exposed patients, *Proteomics: Clin. Appl.*, 2009, **3**, 1191–1200.
87. H. Mehrani, M. Ghanei, J. Aslani and Z. Tabatabaei, Plasma proteomic profile of sulfur mustard exposed lung diseases patients using 2-dimensional gel electrophoresis, *Clin. Proteomics*, 2011, **8**, 2–2.
88. Z. R. Gregorich, Y.-H. Chang and Y. Ge, Proteomics in heart failure: top-down or bottom-up?, *Pflugers Arch.*, 2014, **466**, 1199–1209.
89. A. D. Catherman, O. S. Skinner and N. L. Kelleher, Top Down proteomics: facts and perspectives, *Biochem. Biophys. Res. Commun.*, 2014, **445**, 683–693.
90. J. R. Yates, C. I. Ruse and A. Nakorchevsky, Proteomics by Mass Spectrometry: approaches, Advances, and Applications, *Annu. Rev. Biomed. Eng.*, 2009, **11**, 49–79.
91. M. Sarbu, R. M. Ghiulai and A. D. Zamfir, Recent developments and applications of electron transfer dissociation mass spectrometry in proteomics, *Amino Acids*, 2014, **46**, 1625–1634.
92. T. B. Schreiber, N. Maeusbacher, S. B. Breitkopf, K. Grundner-Culemann and H. Daub, Quantitative phosphoproteomics – an emerging key technology in signal-transduction research, *Proteomics*, 2008, **8**, 4416–4432.
93. C. Pan, F. Gnad, J. V. Olsen and M. Mann, Quantitative phosphoproteome analysis of a mouse liver cell line reveals specificity of phosphatase inhibitors, *Proteomics*, 2008, **8**, 4534–4546.
94. J. Marsillach, E. J. Hsieh, R. J. Richter, M. J. MacCoss and C. E. Furlong, Proteomic analysis of adducted butyrylcholinesterase for biomonitoring organophosphorus exposures, *Chem.-Biol. Interact.*, 2013, **203**, 85–90.

95. S. Cristoni and L. R. Bernardi, Bioinformatics in mass spectrometry data analysis for proteomics studies, *Expert Rev. Proteomics*, 2004, **1**, 469–483.
96. L. McHugh and J. W. Arthur, Computational Methods for Protein Identification from Mass Spectrometry Data, *PLoS Comput. Biol.*, 2008, **4**, e12.
97. M. M. A. Hoffmann, M. Makley, J. J. Schlager, T. Snider and J. Gearhart, Quantitative proteomic analysis of the Guinea Pig Brainstem following exposure to Sarin, *J. Proteomics Bioinf.*, 2014, **7**, 8.
98. S. E. Ong, B. Blagoev, I. Kratchmarova, D. B. Kristensen, H. Steen, A. Pandey and M. Mann, Stable isotope labeling by amino acids in cell culture, SILAC, as a simple and accurate approach to expression proteomics, *Mol. Cell. Proteomics*, 2002, **1**, 376–386.
99. S. P. Gygi, B. Rist, S. A. Gerber, F. Turecek, M. H. Gelb and R. Aebersold, Quantitative analysis of complex protein mixtures using isotope-coded affinity tags, *Nat. Biotechnol.*, 1999, **17**, 994–999.
100. P. L. Ross, Y. L. N. Huang, J. N. Marchese, B. Williamson, K. Parker, S. Hattan, N. Khainovski, S. Pillai, S. Dey, S. Daniels, S. Purkayastha, P. Juhasz, S. Martin, M. Bartlet-Jones, F. He, A. Jacobson and D. J. Pappin, Multiplexed protein quantitation in Saccharomyces cerevisiae using amine-reactive isobaric tagging reagents, *Mol. Cell. Proteomics*, 2004, **3**, 1154–1169.
101. M. Ramstrom and J. Bergquist, Miniatuized proteomics and pepitdomics using capillary liquid separation and high mass spectrometry, *FEBS Lett.*, 2004, **567**, 92–95.
102. K. Wagner, T. Miliotis, G. Marko-Varga, R. Bischoff and K. K. Unger, An automated on-line multidimensional HPLC system for protein and peptide mapping with integrated sample preparation, *Anal. Chem.*, 2002, **74**, 809–820.
103. H. Mischak, T. Kaiser, M. Walden, M. Hillmann, S. Wittke, A. Herrmann, S. Knueppel, H. Haller and D. Fliser, Proteomic analysis for the assessment of diabetic renal damage in humans, *Clin. Sci.*, 2004, **107**, 485–495.
104. K. S. Lilley and D. B. Friedman, All about DIGE: quantification technology for differential-display 2D-gel proteomics, *Expert Rev. Proteomics*, 2004, **1**, 401–409.
105. M. Karas, D. Bachmann, U. Bahr and F. Hillenkamp, Matrix-assisted ultraviolet-laser desorption of nonvolatile compounds, *Int. J. Mass Spectrom. Ion Processes*, 1987, **78**, 53–68.
106. M. Karas and F. Hillenkamp, Laser desorption ionisation of proteins with molecular masses exceeding 10000 daltons, *Anal. Chem.*, 1988, **60**, 2299–2301.
107. C. Laldinsangi, K. Vijayaprasadarao, A. Rajakumar, R. Murugananthkumar, Y. Prathibha, C. C. Sudhakumari, S. K. Mamta, A. Dutta-Gupta and B. Senthilkumaran, Two-dimensional proteomic analysis of gonads of air-breathing catfish, Clarias batrachus after the exposure of endosulfan and malathion, *Environ. Toxicol. Pharmacol.*, 2014, **37**, 1006–1014.

108. L. Yue, Y. Wei, J. Chen, H. Shi, Q. Liu, Y. Zhang, J. He, L. Guo, T. Zhang, J. Xie and S. Peng, Abundance of Four Sulfur Mustard-DNA Adducts ex Vivo and in Vivo Revealed by Simultaneous Quantification in Stable Isotope Dilution-Ultrahigh Performance Liquid Chromatography-Tandem Mass Spectrometry, *Chem. Res. Toxicol.*, 2014, **27**, 490–500.
109. E. D. Dodds, B. H. Clowers, P. J. Hagerman and C. B. Lebrilla, Systematic characterization of high mass accuracy influence on false discovery and probability scoring in peptide mass fingerprinting, *Anal. Biochem.*, 2008, **372**, 156–166.
110. G. Alves, A. Y. Ogurtsov, S. Kwok, W. W. Wu, G. Wang, R.-F. Shen and Y.-K. Yu, Detection of co-eluted peptides using database search methods, *Biol. Direct*, 2008, **3**, 1–16.
111. K. Adermann, H. John, L. Standker and W. G. Forssmann, Exploiting natural peptide diversity: novel research tools and drug leads, *Curr. Opin. Biotechnol.*, 2004, **15**, 599–606.
112. M. Thevis and D. A. Volmer, Recent instrumental progress in mass spectrometry: advancing resolution, accuracy, and speed of drug detection, *Drug Test. Anal.*, 2012, **4**, 242–245.
113. E. B. Erba, Investigating macromolecular complexes using top-down mass spectrometry, *Proteomics*, 2014, **14**, 1259–1270.
114. U. Bergmann, R. Ahrends, B. Neumann, C. Scheler and M. W. Linscheid, Application of Metal-Coded Affinity Tags (MeCAT): absolute Protein Quantification with Top-Down and Bottom-Up Workflows by Metal-Coded Tagging, *Anal. Chem.*, 2012, **84**, 5268–5275.
115. L. R. Zieske, A perspective on the use of iTRAQ (TM) reagent technology for protein complex and profiling studies, *J. Exp. Bot.*, 2006, **57**, 1501–1508.
116. H. John, F. Balszuweit, K. Kehe, F. Worek and H. Thiermann, *Toxicokinetics of Chemical Warfare Agents: Nerve Agents and Vesicants*, 2009.
117. M. Belew and J. Porath, Immobilized metal-ion affinity-chromatography – effect of solute structure, ligand density and salt concentration on the retention of peptides, *J. Chromatogr.*, 1990, **516**, 333–354.
118. H. John, F. Breyer, J. O. Thumfart, H. Hoechstetter and H. Thiermann, Matrix-assisted laser desorption/ionization time-of-flight mass spectrometry (MALDI-TOF MS) for detection and identification of albumin phosphylation by organophosphorus pesticides and G- and V-type nerve agents, *Anal. Bioanal. Chem.*, 2010, **398**, 2677–2691.
119. C. Schmidt, F. Breyer, M.-M. Blum, H. Thiermann, F. Worek and H. John, V-type nerve agents phosphonylate ubiquitin at biologically relevant lysine residues and induce intramolecular cyclization by an isopeptide bond, *Anal. Bioanal. Chem.*, 2014, **406**, 5171–5185.
120. A. Fidder, A. G. Hulst, D. Noort, R. de Ruiter, M. J. van der Schans, H. P. Benschop and J. P. Langenberg, Retrospective detection of exposure to organophosphorus anti-cholinesterases: mass spectrometric analysis of phosphylated human butyrylcholinesterase, *Chem. Res. Toxicol.*, 2002, **15**, 582–590.

121. D. Noort, A. G. Hulst, L. P. A. de Jong and H. P. Benschop, Alkylation of human serum albumin by sulfur mustard in vitro and in vivo: mass spectrometric analysis of a cysteine adduct as a sensitive biomarker of exposure, *Chem. Res. Toxicol.*, 1999, **12**, 715–721.
122. D. Noort, A. Fidder, A. G. Hulst, L. P. A. de Jong and H. P. Benschop, Diagnosis and dosimetry of exposure to sulfur mustard: development of a standard operating procedure for mass spectrometric analysis of haemoglobin adducts: exploratory research on albumin and keratin adducts, *J. Appl. Toxicol.*, 2000, **20**, S187–S192.
123. T.-H. Yeo, M.-L. Ho and W.-K. Loke, Development of a liquid chromatography-multiple reaction monitoring procedure for concurrent verification of exposure to different forms of mustard agents, *J. Anal. Toxicol.*, 2008, **32**, 51–56.
124. T. M. Andacht, B. G. Pantazides, B. S. Crow, A. Fidder, D. Noort, J. D. Thomas, T. A. Blake and R. C. Johnson, Enhanced Throughput Method for Quantification of Sulfur Mustard Adducts to Human Serum Albumin *Via* Isotope Dilution Tandem Mass Spectrometry, *J. Anal. Toxicol.*, 2014, **38**, 8–15.
125. D. Noort, A. G. Hulst, H. C. Trap, L. P. A. deJong and H. P. Benschop, Synthesis and mass spectrometric identification of the major amino acid adducts formed between sulphur mustard and haemoglobin in human blood, *Arch. Toxicol.*, 1997, **71**, 171–178.
126. D. Noort, E. R. Verheij, A. G. Hulst, L. P. A. deJong and H. P. Benschop, Characterization of sulfur mustard induced structural modifications in human hemoglobin by liquid chromatography tandem mass spectrometry, *Chem. Res. Toxicol.*, 1996, **9**, 781–787.
127. E. O. Price, J. R. Smith, C. R. Clark, J. J. Schlager and M. L. Shih, MALDI-ToF/MS as a diagnostic tool for the confirmation of sulfur mustard exposure, *J. Appl. Toxicol.*, 2000, **20(suppl. 1)**, S193–S197.
128. O. Lockridge and L. M. Schopfer, Review of tyrosine and lysine as new motifs for organophosphate binding to proteins that have no active site serine, *Chem.-Biol. Interact.*, 2010, **187**, 344–348.
129. H. Liu, N. Zhang, D. Wan, M. Cui, Z. Liu and S. Liu, Mass spectrometry-based analysis of glycoproteins and its clinical applications in cancer biomarker discovery, *Clin. Proteomics*, 2014, **11**, 14–14.
130. J. Wang, F. Zhao, C.-X. Yu, D. Xiao, L.-J. Song, X.-R. Yin, S. Shen, W.-Q. Hua, J.-Z. Zhang, H.-F. Zhang, L.-H. He, C.-Y. Qian, W. Zhang, Y.-L. Xu and J. Yang, Identification of proteins inducing short-lived antibody responses from excreted/secretory products of Schistosoma japonicum adult worms by immunoproteomic analysis, *J. Proteomics*, 2013, **87**, 53–67.
131. D.-Z. Wang, Z.-X. Xie and S.-F. Zhang, Marine metaproteomics: current status and future directions, *J. Proteomics*, 2014, **97**, 27–35.
132. C. G. Vogiatzis and G. A. Zachariadis, Tandem mass spectrometry in metallomics and the involving role of ICP-MS detection: a review, *Anal. Chim. Acta*, 2014, **819**, 1–14.

133. J. F. Waring, R. A. Jolly, R. Ciurlionis, P. Y. Lum, J. T. Praestgaard, D. C. Morfitt, B. Buratto, C. Roberts, E. Schadt and R. G. Ulrich, Clustering of hepatotoxins based on mechanism of toxicity using gene expression profiles, *Toxicol. Appl. Pharmacol.*, 2001, **175**, 28–42.
134. X. Yu, W. C. Griffith, K. Hanspers, J. F. Dillman, III, H. Ong, M. A. Vredevoogd and E. M. Faustman, A system-based approach to interpret dose- and time-dependent microarray data: quantitative integration of gene ontology analysis for risk assessment, *Toxicol. Sci.*, 2006, **92**, 560–577.

CHAPTER 8

Chemical Defence Against Fentanyls

CHRISTOPHER D. LINDSAY[a], JAMES R. RICHES[a], NEIL ROUGHLEY[a], AND CHRISTOPHER M. TIMPERLEY*[a]

[a]Defence Science and Technology Laboratory (Dstl), Porton Down, Salisbury, Wiltshire, SP4 0JQ, UK
*E-mail: cmtimperley@dstl.gov.uk

8.1 Introduction

Fentanyls differ from most classical chemical warfare (CW) agents, which are typically gases or liquids at ambient temperature (see Chapter 1 in Volume 1).[1,2] Fentanyls are solids used in human and veterinary medicine to cause general anaesthesia (loss of sensation accompanied by unconsciousness) and analgesia (a reduction in pain sensitivity). Some have lethality comparable to organophosphorus nerve agents if misused outside the clinic in the absence of medical support. Only a few fentanyls are produced worldwide; they are produced batch-wise in multi-kilogram amounts, and marketed as medicines. However, fentanyls are potentially dual-use—medicinal and military—and could be directed to cause harm. This chapter frames fentanyls in the context of defence and security, and describes their biological effects and chemistry to help facilitate protective and international arms control efforts against these toxic chemicals.

Issues in Toxicology No. 27
Chemical Warfare Toxicology, Volume 2: Management of Poisoning
Edited by Franz Worek, John Jenner, and Horst Thiermann

Published by the Royal Society of Chemistry, www.rsc.org

8.2 Brief History

The evolution of fentanyl returns to Dr Paul Janssen (1926–2003),[3] founder of the Belgium company Janssen Pharmaceutica and developer of over 80 pharmaceuticals (many important to anaesthesiology). The scientific career of Janssen attests to a brilliant man who was driven to develop new medicines.[4] In 1953, he recognised morphine, the main alkaloid in latex obtained from the seed pods of the opium poppy *Papaver somniferum*,[5] as the standard analgesic for pain relief. Yet morphine had two disadvantages: it depressed respiration by inhibiting the responsiveness of the brain to high blood concentrations of carbon dioxide (the stimulus for breathing) and also induced addiction.[6] At a dose exceeding that necessary to induce analgesia, morphine caused narcosis (a state of stupor, drowsiness, or unconsciousness).[7,8] It also caused constipation, hence its use to treat severe diarrhoea.[9]

Janssen discovered many compounds were potent analgesics if they included features common to morphine: an aromatic group linked to a carbon atom or non-basic tertiary nitrogen atom, and further linked through several carbon atoms to a tertiary, or in some instances, a secondary, basic nitrogen atom. He recalled meperidine (pethidine), an atropine like anti-spasmodic/anti-diarrhoeal drug introduced into human medicine previously, in 1939. Clinical experience had suggested that meperidine was similar in action to morphine but less potent. Surveying the structure of meperidine, Janssen concluded that the piperidine ring was one of the features of both morphine and meperidine vital for analgesic efficacy. He focussed on meperidine as a template for the synthesis of newer compounds, rather than morphine, because of its greater structural simplicity.[4] His goal was to discover molecules more potent than morphine but with a more specific analgesic and anti-diarrhoeal action and fewer side-effects. He sought compounds of high potency because he believed they might display high specificity and low toxicity.

The Janssen team realised that meperidine had about a tenth of the analgesic potency of morphine and assumed this was because it was unable to penetrate the central nervous system (CNS) easily.[4] Suspecting that meperidine was too hydrophilic, they sought more lipophilic derivatives, hypothesising that they might enter the CNS more readily. They replaced the methyl group on the piperidine nitrogen atom with a 3-hydroxy-3-phenylpropyl group to generate, in 1957, a substance they named phenoperidine. This had a greater lipophilicity and a stronger analgesic action than meperidine, presumably due to greater penetration of the blood–brain barrier.[4] Further elaboration of phenoperidine resulted, in 1960, in the discovery of fentanyl, which was found to be 80–100 times more potent an analgesic than morphine to humans, and was introduced into clinical practice 3 years later.[4] The chemical design process starting with morphine and arriving at fentanyl is summarised in Figure 8.1.

After discovering fentanyl, the Janssen team, by making structural changes to its skeleton,[3,4] crafted carfentanil in 1974 (introduced into veterinary

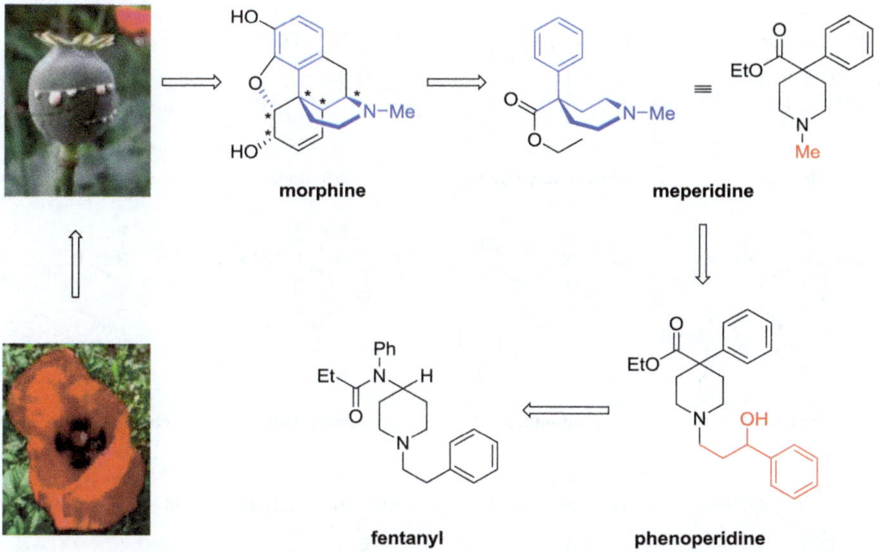

Figure 8.1 The poppy species from which opium is extracted, *Papaver somniferum* (bottom left), is not known to grow in the wild; it has been domesticated for its seeds, which are used for food, and for its dried sap, which yields opium (from the Greek *opion* meaning 'poppy juice').[10] For centuries humans have bred the species to enhance the size of the capsule that contains the seeds and the opium rich sap. Once the petals have fallen, opium is harvested from the green capsule. Horizontal scores are made in it and a creamy sap appears on its outer surface (top left). This sap dries brown or black and is collected using a curved scraper. It is kneaded into balls that are dried in the sun to reduce the water content from 30% to 10% by weight. The opium obtained contains over 30 alkaloids, including codeine, noscapine and papaverine. A major component (10% by weight) is (−)-morphine (named in honour of Morpheus, the Greek god of dreams; top middle) from which Janssen designed meperidine (top right), further elaborated to give phenoperidine (bottom right), and later remodelled to provide fentanyl (bottom middle).[4] (In the Janssen patent for fentanyl[11] it was first named 'phentanyl'.) Morphine has five asymmetric centres (marked with asterisks) and this geometry is central to its pharmacological action; (+)-morphine with the opposite geometry at all five centres is inactive as an analgesic.[8,12]

practice in 1986),[13,14] sufentanil in 1974 (introduced into clinical medicine in Europe in 1979 and the USA in 1985),[13,14] and alfentanil in 1976 (introduced in Europe in 1983 and the USA in 1987).[3,15] Two regions of the fentanyl molecule were altered to produce these compounds: the apex of the piperidine ring (H → CO_2Me or CH_2OMe) or the piperidinyl *N*-substituent (phenethyl → 2-thienylethyl or tetrazolidinone system) (Figure 8.2).[15] A piperidinyl 3-methyl substituent gave two diastereomers of 3-methylfentanyl whose activities contrasted: the *cis*-isomer was six times more potent than fentanyl, while the *trans*-isomer was equipotent to fentanyl [ascertained from effective dose, 50% (ED_{50}) values after intravenous injection to mice].[16] *Cis*-3-methyl

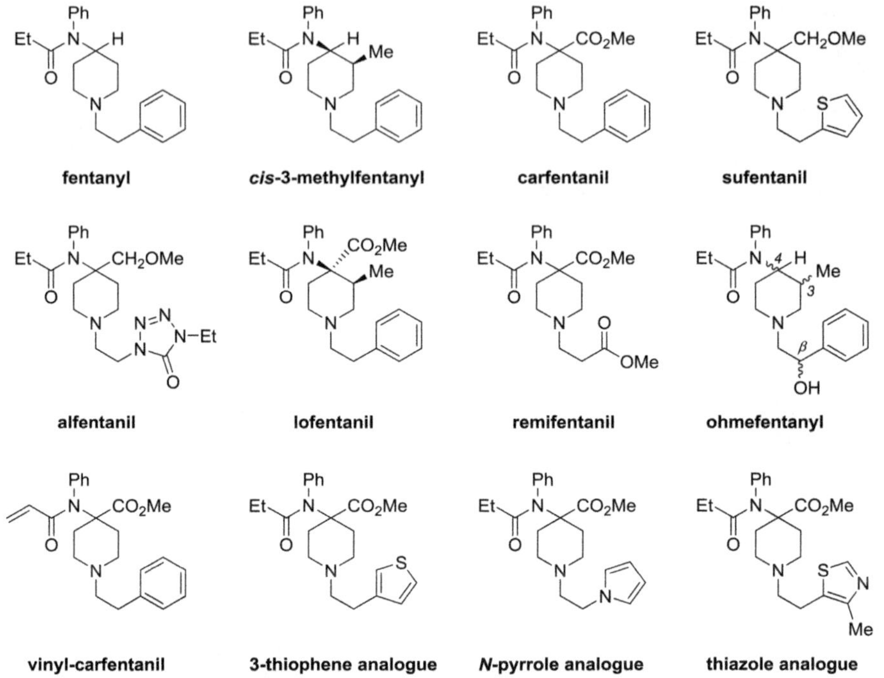

Figure 8.2 Fentanyl compounds relevant to defence and security. Fentanyl, sufentanil and remifentanil are analgesic–anaesthetics used in humans, whilst carfentanil is used in veterinary medicine to tranquillise large mammals.[3] These structures were arrived at from structure–activity relationships published by Janssen.[3,11–16,18] Relative analgesic potencies of analogues of fentanyl with different RCON groups are: meperidine 1; MeCON 50; EtCON 700; *n*-PrCON 90. An *N*-phenethyl tail is optimal: NCH_2Ph 0.7; NCH_2CH_2Ph 700; $NCH_2CH_2CH_2Ph$ 14; an NMe substituent produces a virtually inactive analogue. The bottom row shows fentanyls of similar analgesic potency to carfentanil, most likely based on their structural similarity to carfentanil, possessing high toxicity to humans and low therapeutic ratios. Vinyl-carfentanil and related analogues have been studied by Chinese researchers.[19,20] An optimised synthesis of a key precursor of the 'thiazole analogue' has been reported by Russian chemists[21] linked to military fentanyl research.[22]

substitution of carfentanil gave the extremely potent and long lasting analgesic lofentanil.[3] Modification of carfentanil by replacing the *N*-piperidinyl tail NCH_2CH_2Ph with $NCH_2CH_2CO_2Me$ was performed by GlaxoSmithKline much later to produce the fast acting and metabolically labile analogue, remifentanil, introduced into clinical medicine in the 1990s.[17]

Ohmefentanyl[23–26] is an analogue of *cis*-3-methylfentanyl that binds selectively to the μ-opioid receptor (see Section 8.8.4) and Chinese researchers, who first synthesised it in the 1970s, have recorded that it has an analgesic potency 6300 times that of morphine in mice (determined after intraperitoneal injection using the hotplate test).[27–31] It has three chiral centres and exists as a mixture of eight stereoisomers (F9201–F9208) that have different pharmacological properties.[26] The most active (F9204) has the (+)-*cis*-3*R*,4*S*,β*S* configuration and is a 28 fold more powerful painkiller in mice than fentanyl[28] (in the ohmefentanyl series, isomers with the β*S*-hydroxy group are more potent than those with the β*R*-hydroxy group[32]). Analogues of ohmefentanyl[33–35] with 18 000 times the analgesic potency of morphine, measured using the hotplate test in mice after subcutaneous administration, are also known.[34]

Another potent analgesic is vinyl-carfentanil.[19,20] This compound is one of several related analogues that must be considered in the context of chemical defence. In a similar category are several analogues, equipotent as analgesics to carfentanil (ED_{50} by the mouse hotplate test), reported by the US company Anaquest.[15] These include a 3-thiophene analogue, an *N*-pyrrole analogue, and a thiazole analogue. The latter requires the precursor 5-(2-chloroethyl)-4-methylthiazole (Heminvirin® or Clomethiazole®, a drug used as a hypnotic, tranquiliser, and anticonvulsant). Optimised synthesis (400 g batch) of this precursor compound was reported in 1999 by Russian chemists[21] known to have been involved in Russian military research on fentanyls.[22] The "thiazole analogue" shown in Figure 8.2 might thus be important from a defence standpoint (although it might not). The current status and future prospects for pharmaceutical applications of fentanyl related compounds and derivatives have been reviewed.[36] The next section focuses on the medicinal uses of fentanyl compounds.

8.3 Medicinal Uses

Fentanyl is a high affinity μ-opioid receptor agonist.[36,37] A dose of 100 μg to humans is approximately equivalent in analgesic activity to 10 mg of morphine or 75 mg of meperidine.[38] The main actions of therapeutic value are analgesia and sedation. Alterations in respiratory rate and alveolar ventilation may exceed in duration the analgesic effect. As the dose is increased, the decrease in pulmonary exchange becomes greater, and large doses may produce apnoea (suspension of breathing). The onset of action is almost immediate when the drug is delivered intravenously; however, the maximal analgesic and respiratory depression effect may not be noted for several minutes.[38] The analgesic effect usually lasts 30–60 min after a single intravenous dose of up to 100 μg. Following intramuscular application, the onset of action is around 8 min and the duration of action from 1 to 2 h.[38] Fentanyl administration to humans at doses of up to 50 μg kg^{-1} does not cause clinically significant histamine release.[38,39] Fentanyl in analgesic (2–10 μg kg^{-1}) or anaesthetic (30–100 μg kg^{-1}) doses rarely causes decreases in blood pressure.[40] Fentanyl has minimal effects on cardiovascular function.[40,41] The pharmacokinetics of fentanyl can be described by a three compartment model, with a distribution time of 1.7 min, redistribution time of 13 min, and terminal elimination time of 219 min.[38] The volume distribution for fentanyl is 4 l kg^{-1}.[38]

The clinical use of fentanyl is increasing, although supporting facts and figures are hard to obtain; fentanyl prescriptions jumped from 2.6 to 7.6 million from 2000 to 2008.[37] Fentanyl citrate is marketed as oral transmucosal lozenges (Actiq®) and buccal tablets (Fentora®).[37] The free base is formulated in transdermal patches (Duragesic®) and injectable formulations. Lozenges, tablets, and patches are used as an adjunctive treatment[38] to manage breakthrough pain in cancer patients receiving opioid medication, most frequently oral morphine for treatment of persistent pain. Injectable formulations usually contain fentanyl citrate for intravenous, intramuscular, or epidural administration.

Fentanyl citrate[38] was introduced in the 1980s as the favoured analgesic–anaesthetic for major operations, such as cardiac surgery,[40] at intravenous doses of 50–150 μg kg^{-1} or more,[41] despite breathing having to be supported by mechanical ventilation. The total amount of fentanyl injected is often limited to 100 μg kg^{-1}, because more than 140 μg kg^{-1} is likely to result in prolonged post-operative respiratory depression.[39] Toxicological parameters for fentanyl compounds are given in Table 8.1.

Sufentanil citrate (Sufenta®) is used in human medicine as an analgesic–anaesthetic for certain major surgical procedures,[42] including open heart surgery, as it maintains good cardiovascular stability[39,43] compared with other analgesic–anaesthetic combinations. Like fentanyl, it is a μ-opioid receptor agonist (see Section 8.8.4). An intravenous dose to humans of ≥8 μg kg^{-1} is needed for anaesthesia.[44]

Lofentanil is about 20 times more potent than fentanyl (from a comparison of lowest ED_{50} values obtained from tail withdrawal tests in rats).[3] Lofentanil's duration of action in this test at a dosage equal to twice the lowest ED_{50} is not less than 600 min, in comparison with 30 min for fentanyl, 34 min for sufentanil, and 60 min for carfentanil.[3] Despite its high activity, its use in human medical procedures could be justified only if respiration could be assisted mechanically long after its use. For this reason, the use of lofentanil in human medicine has not found favour,[3] with preference being given to less potent and shorter acting analogues, such as alfentanil and remifentanil (remifentanil hydrochloride is marketed as Ultiva®). Alfentanil has a shorter duration of

Table 8.1 Toxicological data for fentanyl compounds compared with pethidine[3]

Compound	Lowest ED_{50}[a] (mg kg^{-1})	LD_{50}[b] (mg kg^{-1})	Safety ratio[b]	Potency ratio (in relation to pethidine)[b]	Peak effect (min)
Pethidine	6.2	29	5	1	4
Morphine	3.2	223	71	2	30
Alfentanil	0.04	48	1080	140	1
Fentanyl	0.01	3.1	277	560	4
Sufentanil	0.0007	18	26 716	9200	8
Lofentanil	0.0006	0.07	112	10 400	8
Carfentanil	0.0004	3.1	8460	16 600	10

[a]Lowest ED_{50} values in the tail withdrawal test in rats.
[b]LD_{50} values, safety margins, and potency ratio for intravenous administration.

action than fentanyl and sufentanil, and remifentanil is also short acting due to facile metabolism in the human body[17] (see Section 8.10.2).

Carfentanil citrate is marketed under the trade name Wildnil® for specialist veterinary use.[45] Intramuscular delivery *via* a tranquilliser dart causes rapid immobilisation and anaesthesia in large animals;[45] doses of ~20 μg kg^{-1} can immobilise polar bears (*Ursus maritimus*).[46] Carfentanil is extremely potent and can cause respiratory paralysis and apnoea in the absence of forced ventilation.[47] Naltrexone hydrochloride antidote (see Section 8.8.3) must be immediately available to restore the function of the animal, and this substance or another 'opioid antagonist' must be injected promptly (*e.g.* 100 mg of naltrexone hydrochloride for each 1 mg of carfentanil citrate[45]). The animals revive, usually without complication, and are reintroduced into the wild. Carfentanil has been used only at extremely low doses in humans in positron emission tomography mapping of μ-opioid receptors throughout the body.[48] Its high toxicity to humans is discussed more fully later in this chapter (see Section 8.8.1). Military interest in fentanyls as human incapacitating agents is discussed next.

8.4 Military Interest

The concept of rapid knock-down and resuscitation for hostage rescue prompted military research into fentanyls during the Cold War (the state of political tension and military rivalry between the Soviet bloc countries and Western powers from 1945 to 1990). Narcosis was a physical effect viewed by some countries as desirable for military exploitation and even popularised in fiction. In the 1959 Ian Fleming novel *Goldfinger*, Auric Goldfinger obsessed with gold, advocates "a highly concentrated opiate… the symptoms are a deep and instant sleep" to enable a raid on Fort Knox, the United States Bullion Depository.[49] (The word *opiate* indicates a plant substance and *opioid* a synthetic, although the terms are often interchanged. The term opioid is also used to describe all compounds with morphine like action. In this chapter the words are used appropriately.)

Opiates and opioids are active when inhaled (*e.g.* morphine, fentanyl, sufentanil, alfentanil)[50–53] and to an extent thermally stable (like certain other pharmaceuticals[54]). Consideration of opium smoking in ancient civilisations indicates that opiates may be administered by inhalation, by inhaling smoke from burning opium. Pedanius Dioskurides, a physician, pharmacologist and botanist, and author of *De Materia Medica*, a five volume encyclopaedia on herbal medicines, commented on the latex (*opos*) and total plant extract (*mekonium*), and the use of oral and pipe smoked opium to induce euphoria and sedation, in about A.D. 77.[8] Opium and opioids have influenced human creativity and artistry,[55–58] as a result of low doses engendering a trance like state. The mysterious poem *Kubla Khan* was composed by the British writer Samuel Taylor Coleridge (1772–1834) "in a sort of reverie brought on by two grains of opium taken to check a dysentery" from an oral dose of laudanum (from the Latin verb *laudere* 'to praise'). A tincture of opium containing

~10% w/w powdered opium (equivalent to 1% morphine) had been discovered to have painkilling properties by the 16th century Swiss–German alchemist Paracelsus. Laudanum intake, common in the 18–19th centuries, often fostered lifelong addiction. Indeed, human reliance on opium as a drug has been a precipitant of conflict and violence throughout history, *e.g.* spanning the Opium Wars that occurred in the mid-19th century between Britain and China, to the modern American War on Drugs, aiming to discourage the production, distribution, and consumption of psychoactive drugs deemed illegal by participating Governments and the United Nations.

Fentanyl is absorbed by human lung[50] and nasal[59] tissue. Its inhalation toxicology in humans has been discussed.[60] The rapid onset of narcosis of fentanyl upon inhalation differs insubstantially from that after intravenous injection.[51–53] A study of the effect of fentanyl aerosol on mice breathing patterns and respiratory variables has shown that in this species the lowest ED_{50} and lethal dose, 50% (LD_{50}) were very close.[61] The authors concluded mainly for this reason that: "this type of sedative should not be used as an incapacitating agent". A follow-on study by some of the same authors on the effects of the smoke of fentanyl and some analogues on mice, showed that the smoke caused respiratory depression and had high acute toxicity.[62]

The expected narrow safety margin in humans for fentanyl and its analogues in inhalable droplet/particulate form contrasts with the situation for riot control agents (RCAs),[63] which do not act on the CNS but on the peripheral nervous system (PNS). Not listed in the Schedules of Chemicals controlled under the Chemical Weapons Convention (CWC), like fentanyl compounds and their chemical precursors, RCAs differ from incapacitating chemical agents (ICAs) in that they "can produce rapidly in humans sensory irritation or disabling physical effects which disappear within a short time following termination of exposure" (in line with the CWC definition of an RCA[64]). Experiments with mice have shown that an aerosol of fentanyl causes no apparent sensory irritation,[61] and experiences reported by survivors of the Moscow Theatre Siege chemical aerosol[22,65,66] tend to confirm that this lack of irritancy extends to humans. This insidious effect makes aerosols of fentanyls much more hazardous than those of RCAs. The solid RCA 'tear gases' CS or CR stimulate nerve endings *via* activation of transient receptor potential ankyrin 1 (TRPA1) receptors,[67–70] and respiratory frequency lowers in response to sensory irritation (protecting the lung).[70] One of the effects of lung irritation is a pause between respiratory cycles.[71] In mice exposed to aerosolised fentanyl, no pause or delay was observed in inspiration or expiration, suggesting that airborne fentanyl remained undetected by the sensory pathway (mouse and human TRPA1 receptors are functionally conserved,[72] and TRPA1 activation *via* electrophile sensing[72] and irritation[73–75] appear similar in both species). Unlike RCAs, the disabling physical effects of aerosolised fentanyl compounds do not disappear within a short time following termination of exposure (except in very rare situations where an exceedingly small dose has been absorbed), although the potentially life threatening effects of fentanyls can be reversed by timely administration of an opioid antagonist drug and assisted ventilation. These differences classify fentanyl compounds as toxic chemicals with physiologically distinct profiles to RCAs, whose confirmed high margins of safety for humans are tens of thousand times greater than those predicted for the least potent fentanyls.[76,77]

Opioid drugs including fentanyls are a socioeconomic burden and cause of morbidity and mortality.[78] Repetitive use of opioids can lead to tolerance and addiction through drug induced neuronal dysfunction and neurotoxicity.[79] The drugs imitate the endogenous opioid neuropeptides that activate the same receptors, causing release of dopamine,[80] which has been linked to reward mechanisms and the sensation of pleasure.[81] Complicating the defence and security against fentanyls is their production in illicit drug laboratories and availability as heroin substitutes on the black market. This aspect is discussed next.

8.5 Illegal Trade

Some fentanyl compounds are targeted for illegal trade because of their ease of synthesis and ability to cause euphoria, and appear in the United Nations Single Convention on Narcotic Drugs (of 1961).[82] Their chemical structures are shown in Figure 8.3. Street names for illicit fentanyl include Apache, China Girl, China White, Dance Fever, Friend, Goodfella, Jackpot, Murder

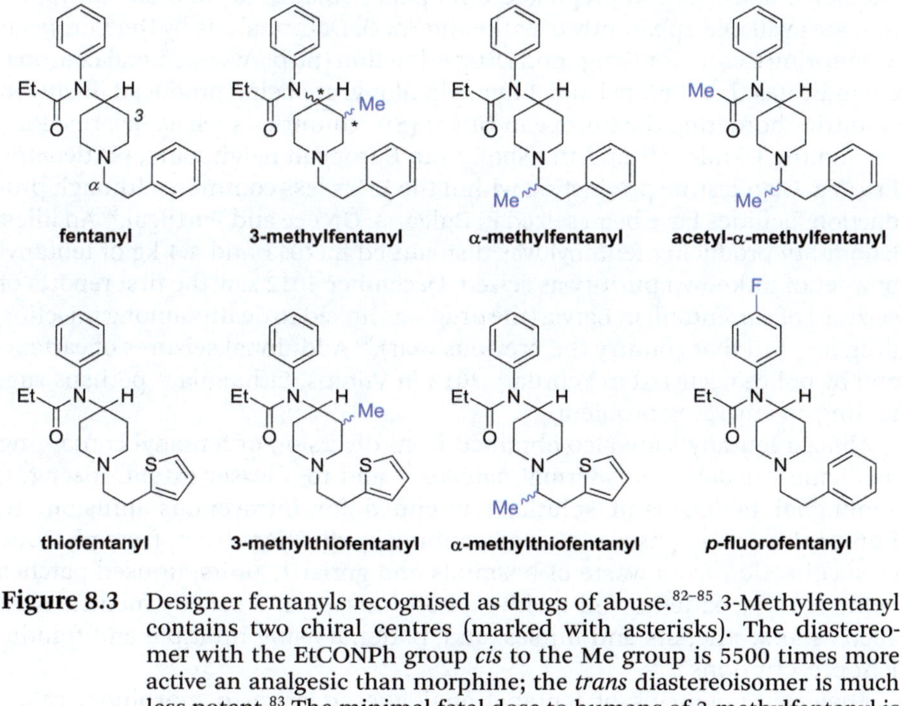

Figure 8.3 Designer fentanyls recognised as drugs of abuse.[82–85] 3-Methylfentanyl contains two chiral centres (marked with asterisks). The diastereomer with the EtCONPh group *cis* to the Me group is 5500 times more active an analgesic than morphine; the *trans* diastereoisomer is much less potent.[83] The minimal fatal dose to humans of 3-methylfentanyl is stated to be ~250 mg per 70 kg bodyweight.[83]

8, TNT, Perc-O-Pop, Lollipop, and Tango and Cash.[78] Since the mid-1970s, fentanyl has been abused by drug addicts as a substitute for heroin. The biological effects of fentanyls are indistinguishable from those of heroin.[37] However, fentanyls may be hundreds of times more potent analgesics and their misdosing leads to many accidental deaths.[78] Fentanyl patches are abused by extracting the liquid contents and injecting or ingesting them. Patches have also been frozen, sliced, and the strips placed in the cheek or under the tongue for oral fentanyl absorption.[78] Used patches are sought by abusers as a large percentage of fentanyl often remains in them. Fentanyl lozenges and injectable formulations are also misused by recreational drug takers and heroin addicts.[78]

Fentanyl abuse is a problem worldwide.[83,86] Estonia has an endemic pattern of fentanyl use and high associated mortality (1100 deaths during 2005–2013 alone).[86] Fentanyl abuse is rising in Europe due to a shortage of street heroin purportedly imposed by Taliban controls on opium production. (The Taliban is an Islamic fundamentalist political movement in Afghanistan.) Fentanyl and 3-methylfentanyl have been marketed as heroin replacements in countries affected by a heroin shortage (*e.g.* Bulgaria and Slovakia). Finland, Germany, and the UK have reported outbreaks of fentanyl related deaths in recent years.[86] The supply of contraband fentanyls into Europe's drug market stems from illicit production, the diversion of medicines from regulated supply chains, and the online sale of non-controlled new psychoactive substances (fentanyl and some analogues impregnated onto paper squares or 'blotters' for ingestion are available apparently over the Internet). Data analysis by the European Monitoring Centre for Drugs and Drug Addiction (http://www.emcdda.europa.eu) indicates that fentanyl and 3-methylfentanyl are being produced illicitly in countries bordering the European Union (EU; countries such as Belarus, Russia and the Ukraine),[86] and transported to European neighbours, particularly Estonia. Clandestine production within the EU is less common, although production facilities have been seized in Bulgaria, Greece and Portugal.[86] An illicit laboratory producing fentanyl was dismantled in 2011 and 4.4 kg of fentanyl powder of unknown purity was seized. December 2012 saw the first reports of seizures of carfentanil in Latvia (the drug was linked to deaths among injecting drug users in that country the previous year).[86] Additional seizures of carfentanil by police occurred in February 2013 in Vilnius, Lithuania,[86] perhaps suggesting an emerging problem.

Abused fentanyls are also obtained from diversion of fentanyl containing medicines, usually transdermal patches,[87] and to a lesser extent, lozenges, sublingual tablets, and solutions intended for intravenous infusion. In Europe this encompasses "over-prescribing by clinicians; theft from pharmacies; collection from waste of hospitals and geriatric units; unused patches being sold by patients and relatives; both misuse and sale by medical staff such as anaesthetists and nurses; and, patients using multiple and fraudulent prescriptions".[86]

Analgesic potencies of fentanyl analogues relative to morphine, calculated after oral administration to mice,[88] appear in Table 8.2. Oral overdose

Table 8.2 Data for some designer opioid agonist drugs, summarising their analgesic potencies compared with morphine and fentanyl, measured by oral administration to mice[88]

Drug	Oral ED_{50} (mg kg^{-1})	Oral LD_{50} (mg kg^{-1})	Potency ratio to morphine	Potency ratio to fentanyl
Morphine	0.33	470	1.0	0.02
Acetyl-α-methylfentanyl	0.106	125	3.1	0.06
p-Fluorofentanyl	0.021	9.3	15.7	0.29
α-Methylfentanyl	0.0058	8.6	56.9	1.10
Fentanyl	0.0061	62	54.1	1.00

presumably accounts for accidental deaths of drug addicts taking such compounds. Deaths from medicinal fentanyl formulations are common and accounts of police investigations are available.[89–97] These investigations prompted the development of analytical techniques for retrospective detection of fentanyls in environmental and biomedical samples robust enough to withstand scrutiny in court during criminal casework. (Note that environmental samples include material collected from soil, water, air, inanimate surfaces and objects present in the environment, or vegetation. Biomedical samples include material of biological origin from a human or animals; most commonly blood or urine. Any sample of biological tissue or fluid taken from a victim of a suspected chemical agent exposure would be considered a biomedical sample.) The next section recalls the first proven use of fentanyl compounds by military forces, during the Moscow Theatre Siege that took place 14 years ago, after analysis of environmental and biomedical samples obtained by the UK identified the chemical composition of the aerosol used.

8.6 Moscow Theatre Siege

On 23 October 2002, Chechen terrorists seized the Melnikov Street Theatre in Moscow during a sell-out performance of a musical, taking over 800 hostages and demanding withdrawal of Russian troops from Chechnya.[65,66] The siege ended in the early morning of 26 October after Russian Special Forces pumped a chemical aerosol, initially described by the authorities in Moscow as a 'sleeping gas', into the building and stormed it later.[98–106] At least 33 terrorists and 129 hostages died during or shortly after the raid. The terrorists were shot dead after falling unconscious due to the effects of the aerosol, and explosives strapped to them and a bomb in the auditorium were deactivated. Two hostages were shot by the terrorists, while 125 died through a combination of the aerosol and inadequate medical intervention after the rescue.[22] The official Russian Government figures are as follows:[65]

- Rescue services evacuated a total of 778 hostages from the theatre, including 101 dead bodies.
- 667 persons were dispatched to various hospitals.

- 21 arrived at hospital in a pre-agonal or agonal state, or were in a state of clinical death and could not be saved.
- Out of 656 persons who were eventually admitted to hospital, seven people died, including three who died of causes unrelated to the use of the aerosol.

Medical treatment of the 656 casualties who were admitted to hospitals was complicated because the Russian Government did not reveal the composition of the aerosol immediately. (Although the Russian health minister did however state several days after the event that an aerosolised opiate based on fentanyl had been used.[22,65,103]) Medics caring for the casualties nonetheless realised that their signs and symptoms matched those of opiate intoxication. They noted that the opiate antagonist naloxone (see Section 8.8.3), used routinely to treat cases of heroin overdose, alleviated the symptoms.[65,66,103] This confirmed initial suspicions that an opioid, or a mixture of opioids, had been employed, rather than an organophosphorus nerve agent, as initially suspected.[106] Atropine, a component of nerve agent therapy,[107] was found to be ineffective,[106] which discounted this possibility.

Clothing samples (Figure 8.4) from British survivors held in the theatre throughout the siege were received at the Defence Science and Technology Laboratory (Dstl), Porton Down, UK, on 28 October 2002 for analysis. A jumper and leather jacket from Casualty 1 (male) and a shirt from Casualty 2 (female) were provided. Analysis of solvent extracts of the leather jacket proved negative. Low concentrations of two fentanyl compounds—carfentanil and remifentanil—were detected by liquid chromatography-tandem mass spectrometry (LC-MS/MS) with multiple reaction monitoring (MRM) in aqueous extracts of the shirt (Figures 8.5 and 8.6). Analysis of a single urine specimen received from a man (Casualty 3) who had survived the siege, but

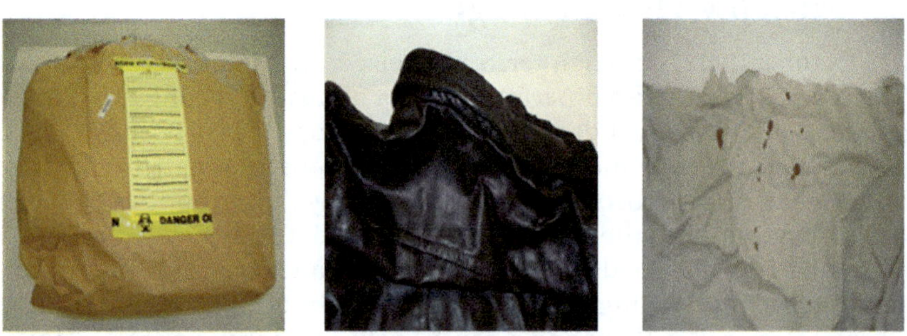

Figure 8.4 The parcel (left) containing separately packaged items of clothing from two British survivors of the chemical aerosol used to end the Moscow Theatre Siege. A black leather jacket (middle) was donated by Casualty 1 (male). A bloodstained white shirt was provided by Casualty 2 (female). The items were received for analysis at Dstl Porton Down 2 days after the use of the chemical aerosol. Concentrated aqueous extracts of the shirt of Casualty 2 proved positive for carfentanil and remifentanil, whose relative proportions the study was unable to identify.[22]

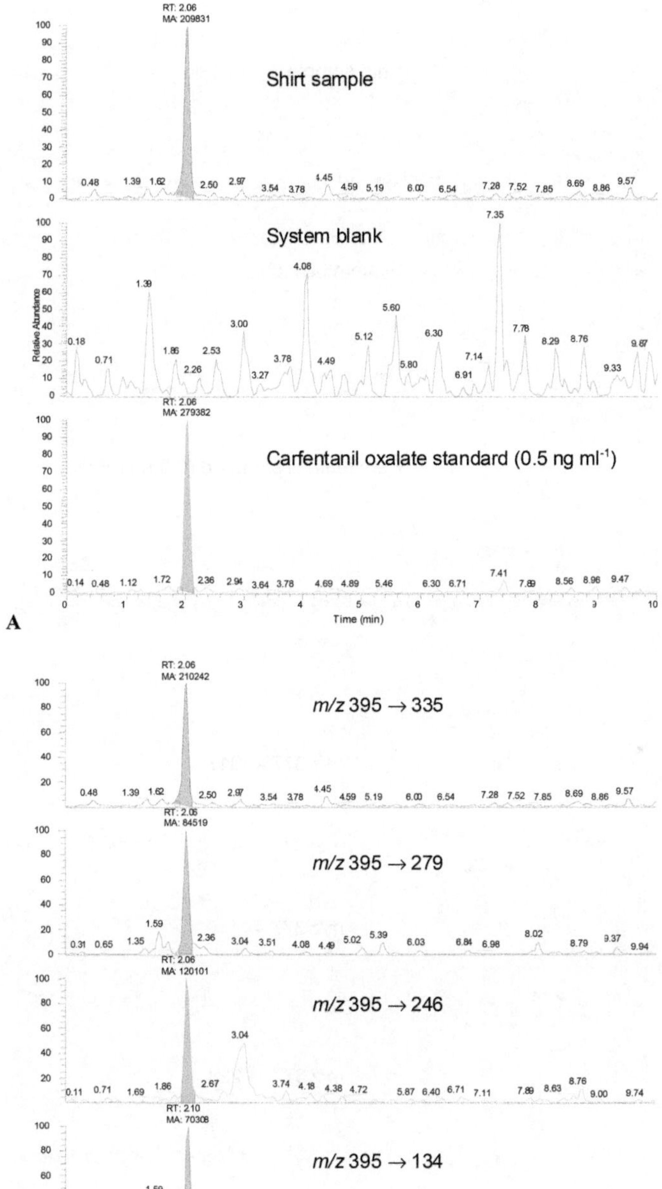

Figure 8.5 LC-MS/MS MRM detection of carfentanil on the shirt of Casualty 2. (A) Detection of carfentanil: monitoring fragmentation (upper, *m*/*z* 395.3 → 335.1), glassware control (middle, baseline magnified ~10 times), and a carfentanil standard (lower). (B) Detection of carfentanil in the shirt extract, monitoring four fragmentations of the protonated molecule (*m*/*z* 395.3). Figure reproduced from ref. 22.

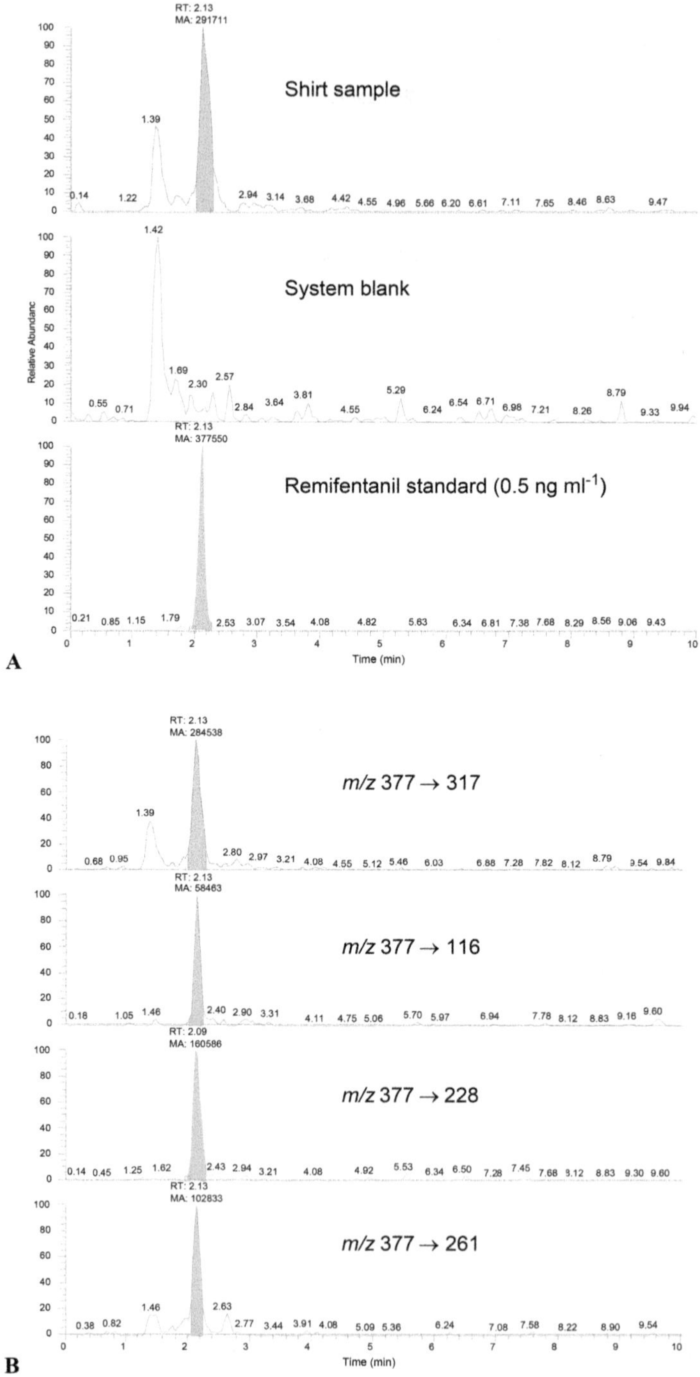

Figure 8.6 LC-MS/MS MRM detection of remifentanil on the shirt of Casualty 2. (A) Detection of remifentanil: monitoring fragmentation (upper, *m*/*z* 377.1 → 317.1), glassware control (middle), and a remifentanil standard (lower). (B) Detection of remifentanil in a shirt extract, monitoring four fragmentations of the protonated molecule (*m*/*z* 377.1). Figure reproduced from ref. 22.

felt unwell afterwards, identified norcarfentanil, a probable metabolite of carfentanil (this result is discussed in Section 8.10.2). The environmental and biomedical sample analyses suggest that the Russian Special Forces used a mixture of carfentanil and remifentanil to facilitate the end of the siege. This is consistent with the outcome arising from its use, because data discussed already suggest a very small margin of safety between the anaesthetic and lethal doses of the opioids in humans, and a high lethality in the absence of prompt and appropriate medical intervention.

8.7 Resurgence of Military Interest

The Moscow Theatre Siege focussed attention on how such episodes might be treated with respect to the provisions of the Chemical Weapons Convention[108] and the use of potent narcotic drugs in law enforcement (internal security) operations. International condemnation of the use of the aerosol, killing 15% of those exposed, was not forthcoming. Some observers may have viewed the outcome of the use of opioids in the siege as an operational success, considering that it may have played a role in preventing the explosives from being detonated, which could have resulted in a greater loss of life. A comparison of open literature publications before and after the siege from government scientists from around the world suggests an increased interest in fentanyl compounds and other potential incapacitating agents.[22,61,62,109–168] A lack of international or legal agreement of the definition of an 'incapacitating agent' complicates discussions on how to curb dual-use research of fentanyls that have legitimate medical uses. An appreciation of their biological effects is necessary to help direct such discussions to a satisfactory and peaceful conclusion in the future.

8.8 Biological Effects

Aspects of the biology of fentanyls are now described: inhalation toxicity, dermal toxicity, opioid antagonists, and opioid receptors.

8.8.1 Inhalation Toxicity

Fentanyl and analogues can be absorbed by the body through inhalation,[51–53,169] intranasal absorption,[59,60,169–171] intravenous or intramuscular injection,[172–174] oral administration,[175,176] or skin contact.[87,177,178] In a defence context, where such materials are most likely to be delivered in aerosol form, several of these routes may contribute to the toxicity. The principal route of exposure in the Moscow Theatre Siege was inhalation.[22] To consider human inhalation data for opioids it is necessary to rewind 25 years, to developments in analgesic drug delivery. At that time, it was realised that the large and highly permeable surface of the lung is accessible to analgesics during a single inhalation, and that this route might be useful for rapidly acting drugs.[50] It was discovered in the late 1980s that morphine could be absorbed by the human lung[179,180] and pain-relief could be achieved. However, bioavailability was low (17%).[179,181] This led to the idea that aerosolised opioids could be useful clinically if their bioavailability could be increased.

Human trials on nebulised fentanyl were performed from the 1990s onwards. These showed that pulmonary fentanyl was an effective means of pain relief.[50–53,182,183] Disappointingly, bioavailability in these studies was only 12% compared with intravenous fentanyl.[183] In a separate study,[51] healthy volunteers received 100–300 μg of aerosolised fentanyl free base generated from a 28:72 v/v mixture of $CFCl_3$ and CF_2Cl_2. This mixture was dispersed using a microprocessor controlled nebuliser. The mean respirable fraction (mass of fentanyl in aerosol droplets <5.8 μm) comprised 50% of the dose. The mass median aerodynamic diameter (MMAD) of the aerosol was 1.8 μm. Plasma concentration–time data were compared with those from the same doses given to the same subjects by intravenous injection. Fentanyl plasma concentrations of 0.4–3.0 ng ml^{-1} were obtained from 100–300 μg intravenous doses; the plasma fentanyl concentrations were proportional to dose. Pulmonary bioavailability was found to be high despite the well known propensity for sequestration of blood borne fentanyl in the lungs.[184,185]

Fentanyl and its analogues cross the blood–brain barrier rapidly.[186] Thermally generated aerosols, as fast onset medications[54] or from heating fentanyl patches,[187] are hazardous because of the risk of severe poisoning by inhalation.[187] How the Russian Special Forces generated the chemical aerosol that was introduced into the Moscow Theatre remains enigmatic. It is clear that an aerosol was produced that may have been absorbed through the upper airway, cornea, and skin. As the pharmacokinetics of fentanyl administered by inhalation and intravenous injection are similar,[51,53] data derived from intravenous clinical studies can be used to estimate the probable toxicity of fentanyl to humans by inhalation. The LD_{50} after intravenous injection in the rat[3] is 3 mg kg^{-1} and in the monkey (species not specified)[188] is 0.03 mg kg^{-1}. A 100 fold difference between the two animal species exists. The LD_{50} in humans is unknown, but since the monkey is considered a better model for aerosol inhalation exposure in humans than other species, one would estimate the human LD_{50} after inhalation of fentanyl to be 0.03 mg kg^{-1} or 2.1 mg for a 70 kg person[60] (but only with 100% pulmonary bioavailability). However, the lethal toxicity for inhaled agent is usually measured as the concentration (mg m^{-3}) multiplied by the time of exposure (t; min) that causes 50% lethality, *i.e.* LCt_{50}, in mg min m^{-3}. The calculation supports the earlier conclusion that fentanyl and its analogues, which can exceed the analgesic potency of fentanyl 10 000 fold, rank among the most toxic synthetic compounds known (alongside CW agents such as organophosphorus nerve agents[1,2]).

In humans, during the first half hour after a bolus intravenous injection of 3.5 μg kg^{-1} fentanyl, the probability of respiratory depression exceeds that of anaesthesia.[189] The duration and degree of respiratory depression are dose related[165] and the maximum effect occurs 5–10 min after injection of a single intravenous dose. Together with apnoea, bradycardia (resting heart rate below 60 beats per min), and muscular rigidity (especially respiratory muscles), respiratory depression constitutes a life threatening state that if untreated can rapidly cause death. Other documented toxic effects include blood pressure fluctuation, dizziness, blurred vision, nausea, and emesis.[8] Human volunteers receiving intravenous or inhaled fentanyl reported feelings of sedation, relaxation, difficulty concentrating, tiredness, light headedness, vagueness, mild disorientation, heaviness in the limbs, mental slowness, and pruritis.[51,190] There is an inherent and unavoidable variability in response by humans to fentanyl[172,174] and presumably its analogues.

Carfentanil is expected to be particularly hazardous to humans due to its high biological activity. Thirty times as potent as fentanyl, and about twice as potent as sufentanil (from comparison of the lowest ED_{50} values obtained from tail withdrawal tests on rats),[3] its sole approved use is by veterinarians to incapacitate wildlife for surgical procedures;[45] it is not approved for use in humans. Depending on dosage and weight of the animal, induction of immobilisation is very fast (from 5 to 15 min).[3] The first documented human exposure to carfentanil[47] became available in 2010. It described the accident of a 47 year old man splashing his eyes and mouth with the contents of a tranquilliser dart containing 1.5 mg carfentanil citrate. He washed his face immediately with water, but became drowsy 2 min later. His colleagues, understanding that he had been poisoned, administered 100 mg of the reversal agent naltrexone (whose antagonistic potency is approximately twice that of naloxone). Presumably this saved the man's life: he complained an hour later, while in hospital, of mild and transient chest discomfort, but this disappeared and he was discharged in a stable condition a day later. This case history, coupled with the high mortality from the chemical aerosol used in the Moscow Theatre,[22] confirms that carfentanil exposures may cause severe intoxication or fatality in the absence of prompt and appropriate medical treatment. The same conclusion can be drawn for remifentanil[191] and probably many other fentanyl compounds. Both carfentanil and remifentanil have narrow safety margins in humans, meaning that potentially fatal side effects, including respiratory depression, can occur at doses similar to those producing incapacitation.

8.8.2 Dermal Toxicity

Permeation of the skin by fentanyl[192] was reported in 1975. Clinical evaluation of transdermal fentanyl patches occurred in the 1980s, and they became available commercially in the 1990s. The first patches contained the drug in a reservoir with a membrane controlling the rate of delivery to the skin, and a separate adhesive to ensure skin contact. Advances in adhesive technology thereafter provided patches containing an adhesive matrix, where the adhesive served as the drug carrier. Misapplication of opioid containing patches by humans, or the use of multiple patches, has resulted in severe intoxication[87,193] and/or death.[96]

Fentanyl has a low molecular mass of 336.5 g mol^{-1} (≤500 g mol^{-1} is usually optimal for dermal penetration[194]). It has an octanol : water distribution ratio (D) of 860 (see Section 8.9.1), indicating high lipophilicity and sufficient water solubility to allow passage across the skin.[195] Drugs applied to unbroken skin must penetrate the lipophilic stratum corneum, and then the more hydrated lower epidermis and dermis to reach the blood vessels. A compound that is only lipophilic will cross the stratum corneum but the rate of penetration will decline as it encounters hydrophilic layers below, and its diffusion decreases (this is called the 'reservoir effect').[194] A chemical of low molecular mass soluble in the lipophilic layer, and additionally the more aqueous structures, generally has the greatest permeability through the skin.[196] Fentanyl has a bioavailability close to unity (0.92). On skin, it is not degraded by microflora or cutaneous enzymes,[197,198] and diffuses to blood vessels below the epidermis without significant loss.

The rate of fentanyl absorption 4–8 h after application of a transdermal patch has been recorded as 92 ± 26 μg h^{-1}.[198] Absorption continues at a declining rate after patch removal, indicating that a cutaneous depot of the drug accumulates. The permeability of aqueous fentanyl citrate (50 μg ml^{-1}) and fentanyl through patches (Duragesic®, delivering fentanyl at a rate of 25 μg h^{-1}) through human skin measured using a Franz diffusion cell was identical.[199] Dermal penetration between individuals can vary substantially in maximal flux, from 21 to 105 ng cm^{-2} h^{-1}, following application of an infinite dose of fentanyl to human skin in static diffusion cells.[199] The more potent analgesic sufentanil is also formulated in patches. The skin of younger people (aged 22–40 years) is generally more permeable to chemicals than that of older people aged >65 years.[200]

Accidental skin exposure of chemical production plant workers wearing air fed protective suits and three pairs of disposable gloves (worn over one another) has occurred.[201] The workers were engaged in the synthesis and isolation of five 30 kg batches of fentanyl (made using a 500 l reactor) and sufentanil, as dried powders. Thus, although the inhalation route for fentanyl compounds poses the gravest threat from a defence viewpoint, in terms of immediate health consequences, the dermal route of exposure after an aerosol challenge may also be important. Time weighted average occupational exposure limits for aerosols of sufentanil, fentanyl, and alfentanil have been established as 0.03, 0.1, and 1 μg m^{-3}, respectively.[201] These low concentrations serve as a reminder of the high biological activity of these chemicals.

8.8.3 Opioid Antagonists

To appreciate the evolution of opioid antagonists it is necessary to return to the constituents of opium, from which they are formally derived.[8] Morphine was first isolated from opium in 1804 by German pharmacist Friedrich Sertürner (1783–1841).[202] Codeine, like morphine, occurs naturally in opium (Figure 8.7). It is about one tenth as potent as morphine, but taken orally is absorbed more efficiently. It is often combined with aspirin (acetylsalicylic

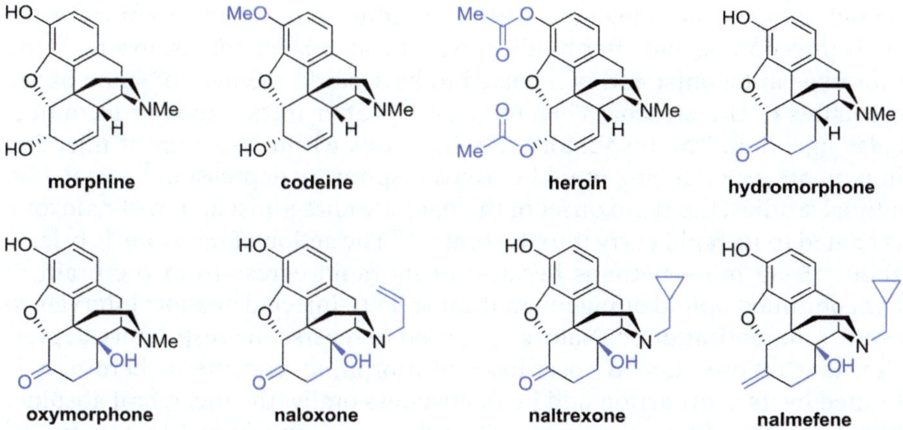

Figure 8.7 Chemical elaboration of morphine gives the painkilling drug codeine, the street drug heroin, and the lethal execution drug hydromorphone (top row). Modification of the μ-opioid receptor agonist oxymorphone yields the opioid receptor antagonists: naloxone, naltrexone, and nalmefene (bottom row). These are used clinically to reverse the pharmacological action of the μ-opioid receptor agonists. Naloxone was used to treat casualties of the Moscow Theatre Siege exposed to the carfentanil–remifentanil aerosol.[65,103]

acid) or acetaminophen (paracetamol) in pain relief tablets. The plasma half-life and duration of action of codeine is about 3–4 h. Heroin or diamorphine is synthetic diacetyl morphine. It was first marketed as a medicine by the German company Bayer in the 1890s before its addictive potential was realised. Heroin derives its name from the Greek word *heros*, in reference to its 'heroic' power. Its analgesic potency is about twice that of morphine by the intravenous route.[8] Its increased lipid solubility results in a faster onset of action; it causes an intense rush upon injection or inhalation (heroin free base can be smoked).

Heroin is metabolised in humans rapidly to 6-acetylmorphine, which has a greater analgesic potency than morphine.[203] The 6-acetylmorphine is then metabolised to morphine. Hydromorphone (Dilaudid®, Palladone®)[204] and oxymorphone (Numorphan®, Opana®)[205] are more potent analgesics than morphine. Executions by lethal injection for capital punishment have been conducted in the USA with a mixture of hydromorphone hydrochloride and midazolam hydrochloride[206] as recently as 2014. The main cause of death from this lethal injection is cessation of breathing due to the central action of the hydromorphone, a μ-opioid receptor agonist, with midazolam, a benzodiazepine, added to suppress convulsions (and presumably to augment the opioid effects).[38]

Three drugs related to oxymorphone are available clinically for treating opioid intoxication: naloxone hydrochloride (Narcan®, aqueous solution), naltrexone hydrochloride (Trexan®, tablets) and nalmefene hydrochloride (Revex®, aqueous solution) (Figure 8.7).[207,208] The three drugs are 'pure opioid antagonists'; they bind with high affinity to opioid receptors, especially μ-receptors, and after binding exert no agonist action. Naloxone is the prototype antagonist and is reported to have saved the lives of some of the casualties of the Moscow Theatre Siege[65,103] after intravenous or intramuscular injection. The respiratory rate increases within 1–2 min of injecting in patients experiencing opioid derived respiratory depression.[209] Based on animal studies, the rapid onset of the narcotic antagonist action of naloxone is related to its rapid entry into the brain.[210] The action of naloxone is brief—about 15–30 min—perhaps because of its rapid egress from the brain.[210] For continued opioid antagonism it must be re-injected at short intervals to avoid 'renarcotisation'.[211] Naloxone is used to reverse the respiratory depression that follows narcotic overdoses of morphine, codeine or heroin. It is limited by its short action and ineffectiveness orally (the mean oral absolute bioavailability of naloxone was ≤2% at doses ranging from 5 to 120 mg).[212] Intranasal naloxone is a viable alternative to intravenous naloxone for initial treatment of narcotic overdose.[213]

While naloxone was reportedly effective in reviving some casualties of the Moscow Theatre Siege,[65,103] the short elimination half-life and rapid reaction kinetics of naloxone might complicate the reversal of toxicity of high affinity opioids such as carfentanil. The duration of action of carfentanil might outlast that of naloxone, necessitating constant monitoring of naloxone treatment, with repeat dosing as required. (Naloxone is able to reverse alfentanil induced respiratory depression.[214]) Emergency planners have been encouraged "to consider sufficient stocking of naloxone to deal with a terrorist event such as that reported in the Russian theatre incident".[215]

Naltrexone emerged in 1985 as the first clinically available orally absorbed pure opioid antagonist. It resembles in action naloxone, but in contrast, is orally bioavailable and has a longer action (mean elimination half-life in humans of 4 h).[216] Naltrexone is used to treat heroin addicts[217] and self-harm patients.[218] Naltrexone reverses carfentanil mediated respiratory depression in large mammals.[45–47,219,220] Nevertheless, carfentanil 'recycling' can occur as it has a high affinity for fatty tissue and is sequestered there and slowly released; its biological half-life exceeds that of naltrexone.[220] Once the latter is metabolised and eliminated from the body, carfentanil can recirculate from the fatty tissue, causing renarcotisation. Hourly administration of naltrexone antagonises the behavioural and antinociceptive effects of a high dose of remifentanil in cats.[221]

Nalmefene, of similar structure and activity to naltrexone, has the advantage of greater oral bioavailability,[222] a longer mean elimination half-life in humans (11 h),[223] prolonged central μ-opioid receptor occupancy after single and repeat dosing in humans,[224] and no dose dependent liver toxicity after oral administration.[225] In rats, nalmefene hydrochloride counters the loss of righting reflex and respiratory depression induced by carfentanil more effectively than naloxone.[226] Nalmefene hydrochloride has been used to restore normal function to African elephants (*Loxodonta africana*) immobilised with single intramuscular injections of carfentanil citrate.[227]

8.8.4 Opioid Receptors

Opiates and opioids bind to opioid receptors, members of the superfamily of G-protein coupled receptors, in the brain and in the peripheral nervous system. Natural peptide ligands for the receptors occur in the body and many of these ligands have been identified in the brain. They belong to families classified according to their chemical structure: dynorphins, endomorphins, endorphins, enkephalins, morphiceptin, and nociceptin/orphanin FQ.

Several opioid receptor subtypes exist.[228] Each subtype is designated by a Greek letter: μ (mu), κ (kappa), or δ (delta), while the 'nociception/orphanin FQ peptide receptor' remains unabbreviated. These receptors are targets for antidepressants, anti-anxiety drugs, anti-addiction medications, and painkillers.[228] The μ-opioid receptors are binding sites linked to the mediation of pain relief.[229] The body produces opiate like peptides (endorphins) as part of a chemical messenger system; thus, the brain is "pre-tuned to receive the music of the poppy".[230] The traditional model of opioid receptor signalling proposes that the binding of an opioid to a receptor activates an associated G-protein, which then triggers the biological response. The first direct evidence for the mode of binding of opioids was published in 2012 for opioid antagonists docked into high resolution crystal structures of the receptors in ligand bound conformations.[231–234] The four opioid receptor structures reveal several evolutionarily conserved ligand–receptor interactions in the receptors' binding pockets, which are contained within the seven transmembrane helices. Transmembrane structures of the four opioid receptors are similar, and so are the structures of the non-homologous loop regions; a 'β-hairpin' system creates a wide opening that allows ligands unobstructed access to a primary binding pocket within the transmembrane area. Subsequent studies have provided structural insights into the mechanism of μ-opioid receptor activation.[235,236]

Fentanyl analogues bind to subclasses of opioid receptor with different affinities and efficacies. Each analogue elicits a different physiological response according to the sum of occupancies of the different receptor types and the associated binding kinetics.[237] From rat brain ligand binding studies, the ranking of fentanyl potency (carfentanil > sufentanil > fentanyl > alfentanil) and severity of respiratory depression, also determined in rats, followed the same order.[238] Affinities for μ-opioid receptors were between 1 and 600 fold greater than for the δ-opioid receptor. This implicates the μ-opioid receptor in respiratory depression caused by fentanyls. This association is supported by the finding that it may be possible to develop selective δ-opioid receptor agonists that do not produce respiratory depression.[239] Pharmacological profiles of lofentanil, carfentanil and fentanyl for μ, δ and κ receptors in guinea pig whole brain membranes have also been determined.[240] Affinities for the receptors decrease in the order μ- > δ- > κ-opioid receptor. Affinities for the μ-opioid receptor, specifically, decrease in the drug order: lofentanil ~ carfentanil > fentanyl > *N*-methylcarfentanil > *N*-methylfentanyl.[240] This study supported the high binding selectivity of carfentanil[48,241,242] and fentanyl[243] for the μ-opioid compared with the δ-opioid receptor. Receptor selectivity can vary between animal species making extrapolation of results to humans difficult.

The binding affinities of fentanyl analogues for the μ-opioid receptor were identical in rat and marmoset tissues.[244] Binding affinities for the δ-opioid receptor were dissimilar between the two species and support the hypothesis that the structure of the receptor shows phylogenetic differences.[244] In rat membranes, carfentanil was non-selective for μ- and δ-opioid receptors. In marmoset membranes, it had much greater affinity for the μ-opioid receptor. Anyone attempting to select a 'safe' fentanyl compound for law enforcement based on rodent toxicity and/or receptor binding data may underestimate the potential of the compound to cause lethality in humans through respiratory depression mediated by μ-opioid receptor agonism. Not only is the effect on humans a function of dose (which cannot be controlled precisely by aerosol delivery) and the age and health of those affected, it also depends on human opioid sensitivity, which is determined genetically[245,246] and is gender dependent.[247] Females are more sensitive than males to opioid receptor agonists; males are predicted to require 30–40% higher doses of opioid analgesics than females to achieve similar pain relief in the clinic.[248] Because of this, females may experience respiratory depression and other adverse effects more profoundly after receiving the same doses as males.

8.9 Chemistry

Aspects of the chemistry of fentanyls relevant to defence and security are discussed next, including: physicochemical properties, pyrolysis, hydrolysis, decontamination, and detection. Not much information on the last two topics is available publically.

8.9.1 Properties

The physicochemical properties of fentanyls determine their biological action. Fentanyl (*D* 860) is more lipophilic than morphine ($D < 1$) (Table 8.3) and its passage from the bloodstream into the CNS is consequently faster. The pK_a of the piperidine nitrogen atom in fentanyl (8.4) can be lowered by replacing the NCH_2CH_2Ph group by a more electronegative NCH_2CH_2 heterocyclic group (*e.g.* sufentanil, 8.0, or alfentanil, 6.5) in order to produce in physiological solution more of the unionised form of the drug. This traverses the blood–brain barrier quickly, causing a fast onset of action,[15] which may rationalise why sufentanil and alfentanil are faster acting than fentanyl. Remifentanil, with a $-NCH_2CH_2CO_2Me$ substituent, has a pK_a of 7.1 and is also fast acting. In the acidic environment of the stomach, fentanyls are highly ionised and therefore poorly absorbed. Drug compounds with basic amine groups and pK_a values >8 are generally absorbed by the lungs.[50]

Fentanyl is stable to light.[251] It is unchanged after exposure to white fluorescent light at ambient temperature,[251] or ultraviolet light of wavelength

Table 8.3 Selected physical data for some common fentanyl drugs[g,249]

Compound (free base)	Mw (g mol^{-1})	Density (g ml^{-1})	Mp (°C)	Solubility in water (g ml^{-1})	*D*	pK_a (ring nitrogen atom)	% unionised at physiological pH (pH 7.4)
Morphine	285.3	1.32	255	0.345	0.7	7.9	24
Fentanyl	336.5[a]	1.11	84	0.025	860	8.4[c]	9
Carfentanil	394.5	1.14	508[b]	0.026	—	8.1	17
Sufentanil	386.5[c]	1.12	97	0.076	2842	8.0	20
Alfentanil	416.5[d]	—	140[e]	Moderate	13.1[f]	6.5	89
Remifentanil	376.5	1.20	195[e]	Moderate	17.9[f]	7.1	67

[a]Citrate Mw: 528.6; Mp: 149–151 °C.
[b]Boiling point (°C) at 760 mmHg.
[c]Sufentanil citrate Mw: 578.7.
[d]Alfentanil hydrochloride Mw: 471.0 and Mp: 138 °C (from acetone).
[e]Melting point for the hydrochloride salts.
[f]Data taken from ref. 250.
[g]Abbreviations: D: distribution ratio, the ratio of concentrations of the compound in an immiscible 1-octanol/water mixture, at equilibrium, Mp: melting point, Mw: molecular weight.

Table 8.4 Physical parameters for fentanyl free base obtained by TGA[146]

Liquid phase vapour pressure (Pa)	Solid phase vapour pressure (Pa)	Enthalpy of sublimation at 25 °C (kJ mol^{-1})	Normal boiling point (°C)
$(4.6 \pm 2.7) \times 10^{-6}$	$(5.9 \pm 4.7) \times 10^{-7}$	144.6 ± 7.2	390.7 ± 49.5

365 nm (300 mW cm^{-2} at 6″) over the course of a week.[252] Thermogravimetric analysis (TGA) has been used to estimate the vapour pressure and properties of fentanyl free base.[146] Benzoic acid was used to calibrate a TGA instrument and the vapour pressure of fentanyl estimated at different temperatures ranging from 150 to 220 °C. Extrapolation of the measurements to 25 °C gave the vapour pressure of subcooled fentanyl and related physical constants (Table 8.4). These data confirm that fentanyl is stable at temperatures below 200 °C when heated for a short time. Further thermal stability data are discussed in the next section.

8.9.2 Pyrolysis

No decomposition is observed when fentanyl citrate is heated to 90 °C for 6 h.[251] Two major and three minor products were evident however when 99% pure fentanyl was heated to 300 °C for 5 min on a hotplate, whereupon 30% degradation occurred.[54] Placing fentanyl free base in a sealed glass tube in a furnace heated to 350 °C for 5 min, then analysing a solution of the residue in methanol using electrospray ionisation mass spectrometry (ESI-MS) and atmospheric pressure chemical ionisation-mass spectrometry (APCI-MS) revealed five main degradation products (Figure 8.8).[252]

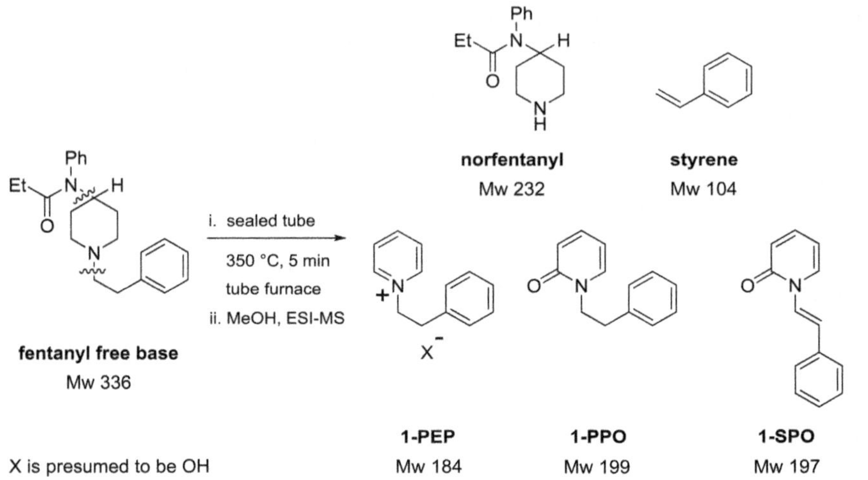

Figure 8.8 Pyrolysis of fentanyl free base in a sealed tube furnace at 350 °C for an average residence time of 5 min gives five products identifiable by ESI-MS.[252] Mw: molecular weight.

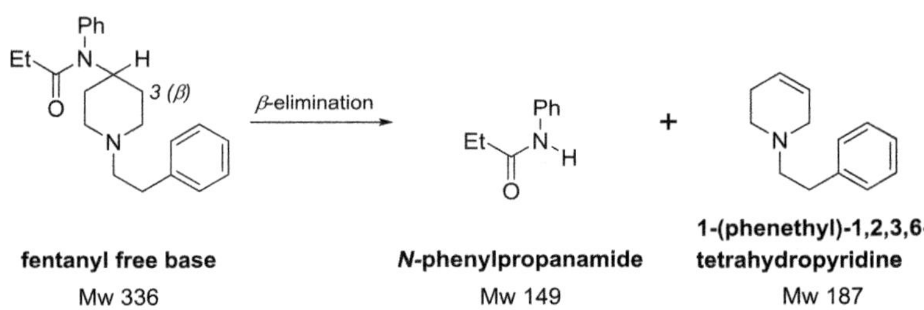

Figure 8.9 Pyrolysis of fentanyl free base results in β-elimination to provide *N*-phenylpropanamide and 1-(phenethyl)-1,2,3,6-tetrahydropyridine.[147,252] Mw: molecular weight.

Cleavage of the fentanyl free base occurred at the exocyclic C–N positions to generate norfentanyl, styrene, and 1-phenethylpyridinium salt (1-PEP), 1-phenethyl-1*H*-pyridin-2-one (1-PPO), and (*E*)-1-styryl-1*H*-pyridin-2-one (1-SPO).[252] The identity of the last three analytes was confirmed by comparison of mass and ^{1}H NMR spectra with those of synthesised standards. Mechanisms for the formation of 1-PEP, 1-PPO, and 1-SPO were proposed (not shown). The main point of interest is a postulated initial 3-*H* β-elimination to yield *N*-phenylpropanamide and 1-(phenylethyl)-1,2,3,6-tetrahydropyridine (Figure 8.9), which is speculated to transform through several steps to 1-PEP. The initial 3-*H* β-elimination also occurs when fentanyl free base is pyrolysed.[147] Flash pyrolysis of *N*-phenylpropanamide at 750 °C yields two major products: phenyl isocyanate and 3-methylindole.[147] An isomer of 1-(phenethyl)-1,2,3,6-tetrahydropyridine is formed upon ESI-MS of fentanyl.[253]

Analytical pyrolysis has been used for studying the thermal decomposition of drugs that addicts inhale after heating metal foils or transdermal delivery systems. Pyrolysis of a transdermal patch containing fentanyl citrate under aerobic conditions using a pyroprobe system (maximum temperature 750 °C, average residence time 10 s) coupled to a GC-MS instrument returned fentanyl (7%) and *N*-phenylpropanamide (93%).[254] Under anaerobic conditions, fentanyl (21%), *N*-phenylpropanamide (50%), styrene (20%), and pyridine (9%) were produced.

Pyrolysis of fentanyl hydrochloride generates HCl vapour, which reacts with the fentanyl species present to yield under aerobic conditions benzyl chloride and phenethyl chloride, and under anaerobic conditions phenethyl chloride (Figure 8.10).[254] Other products identified under both aerobic and anaerobic conditions included *N*-phenylpropanamide, and with less abundance, norfentanyl, styrene, benzaldehyde, despropionyl fentanyl, pyridine, and aniline. It is thus possible from the pattern of pyrolysis products to identify retrospectively the type of fentanyl salt pyrolysed: citrate or hydrochloride. This could assist any investigation of alleged use if weapons containing a fentanyl, or mixture of fentanyls, are suspected.

8.9.3 Hydrolysis

Titration of fentanyl salts with aqueous alkali or strong organic bases neutralises the salts and liberates fentanyl free base.[251] The free base cannot react further and sites of potential cleavage, the CO–NPh and N–CH_2 bonds, resist basic hydrolysis. The free base is practically insoluble in aqueous media at pH 9 and this insolubility retards hydrolysis. When heated in 5 M aqueous sodium hydroxide to 70 °C for 24 h, the free base remains unaltered.[252] It resists hydrolysis under neutral to strongly alkaline conditions. The story differs under acidic conditions. The amide bond is protonated in strong acids. However, only upon heating in 3 M hydrochloric acid to a temperature of 90 °C for 2 h does a proportion (21%) of the fentanyl hydrochloride decompose through amide bond cleavage (Figure 8.11).[251] Fentanyl heated in 5 M aqueous HCl to 70 °C for 24 h hydrolyses to propanoic acid and despropionyl fentanyl. Both products are expected to have low biological activities and acute toxicities. The reaction may therefore constitute a decontamination process. However, even under these harsh conditions, conversion is slow: the yield of despropionyl fentanyl is low (35%) and much of the fentanyl free base remains.

Remifentanil differs from other medicinal fentanyls in that it contains a hydrolytically labile methyl ester group.[17] A solution of remifentanil free base in water has a pH of 3 and hydrolyses spontaneously to remifentanil acid (Figure 8.12).[250] The acid is not significantly biologically active. It has a very low opioid agonist potency and is the principal metabolite of remifentanil in humans.[17,250]

Carfentanil and related analogues are likely to resist alkaline hydrolysis in the same way as fentanyl. However, data to confirm this are unavailable in the open literature at present. Some experiments are warranted to provide evidence of hydrolytic resilience. Treatment with acid is anticipated to promote exocyclic C–N peptide bond cleavage similar to the case described for fentanyl free base.

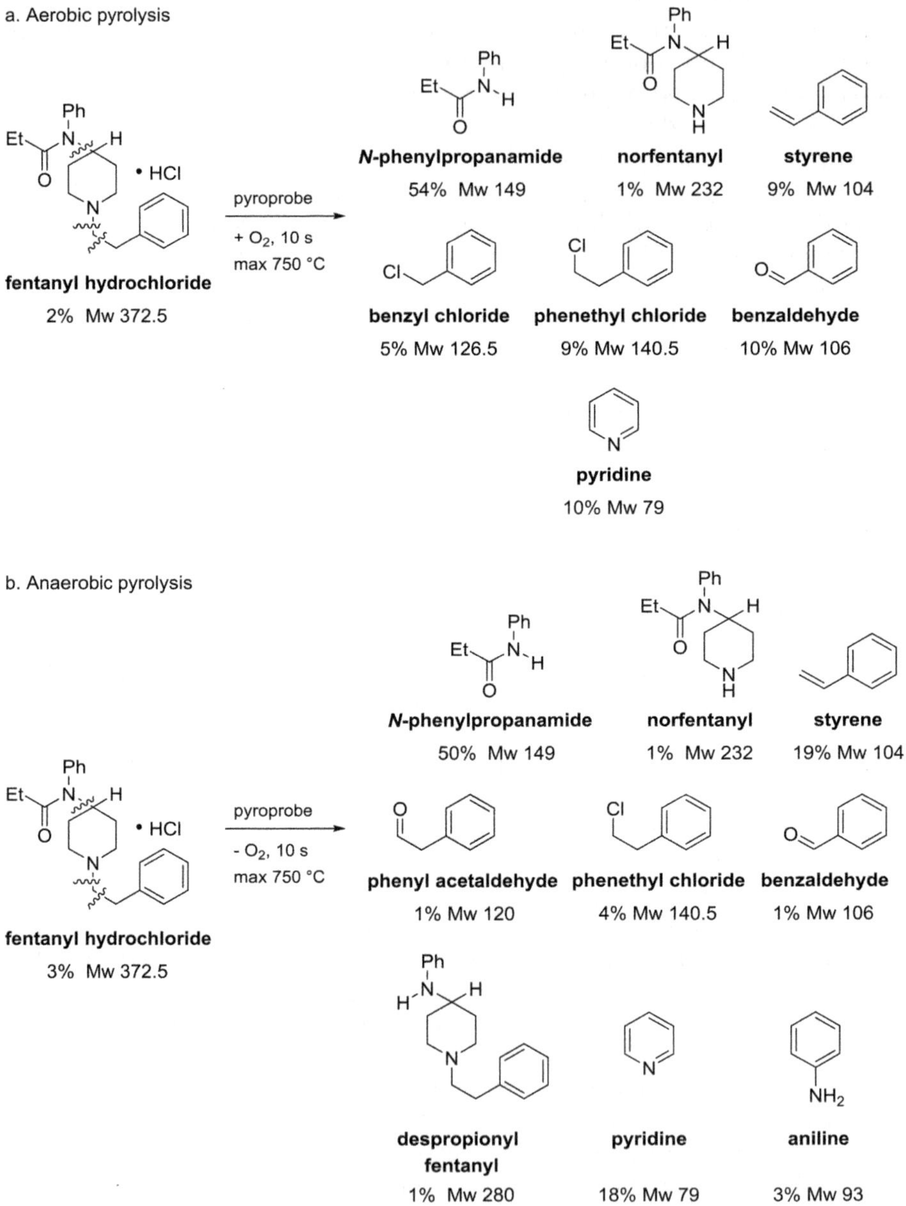

Figure 8.10 Pyrolysis of fentanyl hydrochloride under (a) aerobic or (b) anaerobic conditions in a pyroprobe apparatus (maximum temperature 750 °C, average residence time 10 s) gave different products identified by GC-MS (percentage proportions and Mw are shown for all products).[254] Mw: molecular weight.

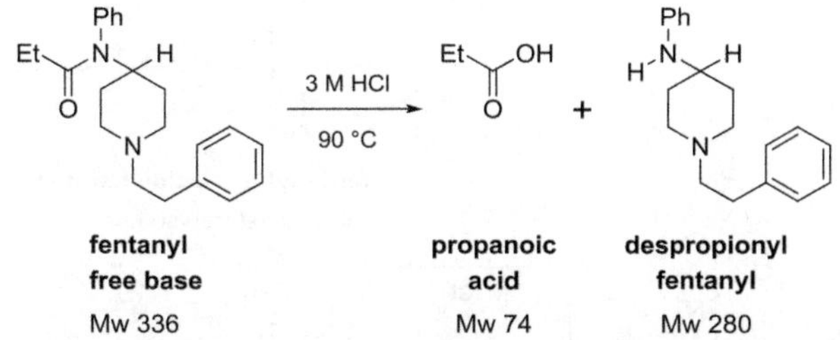

Figure 8.11 Fentanyl free base heated with 3 M hydrochloric acid at 90 °C for 2 h undergoes exocyclic C–N peptide bond cleavage to give propanoic acid and despropionyl fentanyl.[251] Mw: molecular weight.

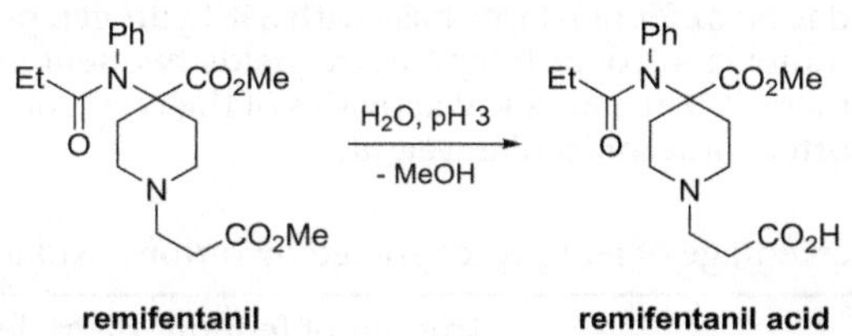

Figure 8.12 The least hindered methyl ester group in remifentanil in aqueous acidic solution hydrolyses to methanol and remifentanil acid,[17] a reaction that is catalysed in human blood by esterases, accounting for the short biological action of remifentanil.[250] Remifentanil acid has 1/300 to 1/2000 the analgesic potency of the parent compound in humans.[250]

8.9.4 Decontamination

Reviews of decontamination of traditional CW agents[255,256] do not include commentary on fentanyl compounds. The recommendation in US Army Field Manual No. 3–9 for removing fentanyls from contaminated surfaces is by scrubbing them with water acidified with acetic acid.[257] Under these mild conditions, cleavage of the amide bond is unlikely to occur. Therefore, this approach may not constitute an effective decontamination, but rather a method of shifting and diluting the toxic chemical. Public information on the decontamination of fentanyl compounds is scarce: the literature appears to contain only two papers describing various approaches by Chinese defence chemists.[159,160] The usual routes of decontamination of CW agents involve hydrolysis and/or oxidation typically by hypochlorites or peroxides.[255,256] Similar methods researched for the decontamination of fentanyl are now discussed.

Fentanyl free base is capable of transformation in the presence of oxidising agents. Exposure of fentanyl to 0.3% hydrogen peroxide in acetonitrile produces a 1 : 9 molar ratio of two *N*-oxides (Figure 8.13)[252] distinguishable by LC-MS and ^{1}H NMR spectroscopy. Nuclear Overhauser Effect spectroscopy (NOESY) failed to distinguish the dominant isomer. From steric considerations the β-*N*-oxide is expected to preponderate, with the *N*-phenylpropanamide and *N*′-phenylethyl groups in a 1,4-*trans*-diaxial arrangement

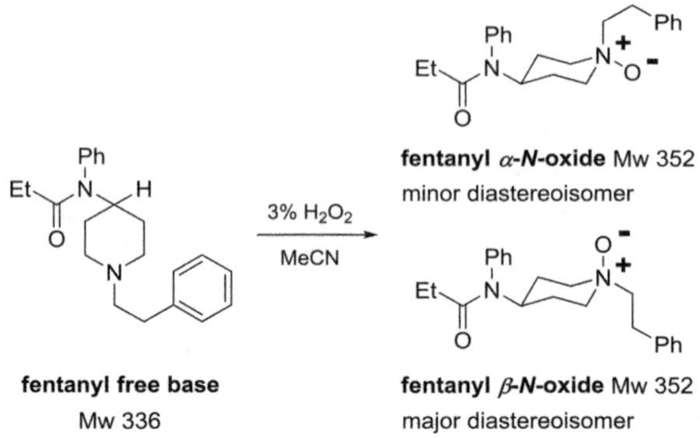

Figure 8.13 Oxidation of fentanyl free base with 3% hydrogen peroxide in aqueous acetonitrile at room temperature yields two fentanyl *N*-oxide diastereomers.[252] The biological activities of the two products have not been reported. Mw: molecular weight.

Table 8.5 The percentage of fentanyl degraded by various oxidants over time[a,b,159]

		Amount of fentanyl degraded (%)				
Oxidant	pH	2 min	5 min	10 min	30 min	60 min
$K_2S_2O_8$	6	—	4	6	33	46
H_2O_2	5	—	10	15	35	53
$KHSO_5$	5	—	24	28	45	44
MMPP	5	—	47	52	63	77
SPC	4	—	19	36	24	45
$MeCO_3H$	8	—	91	92	93	95
SPC-TAED	8	82	92	92	96	99
SPC-TAED	10	76	81	91	91	93
TCCA	5	97	99	99	100	ND
$Ca(OCl)_2$	12	86	59	42	39	37

[a]ND: not determined.
[b]

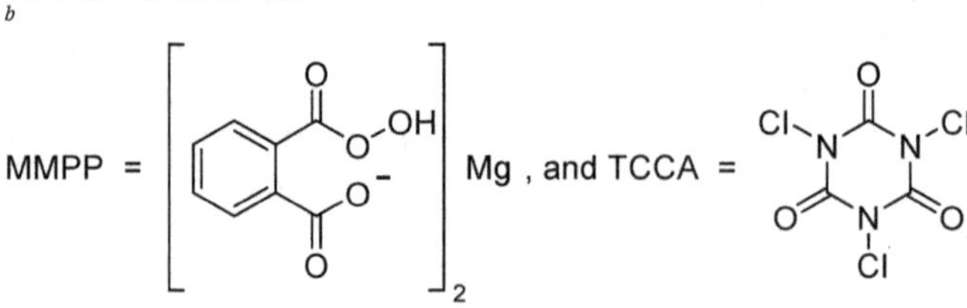

on opposite faces of the six membered ring, in presumably the lowest energy configuration.

The decontamination of fentanyl hydrochloride in stirred aqueous phosphate buffer by oxidants with active oxygen concentrations of 0.2 mol l^{-1} has been studied (Table 8.5).[159] The oxidants used included: potassium persulphate ($K_2S_2O_8$), hydrogen peroxide (H_2O_2), potassium peroxymonosulphate ($KHSO_5$), magnesium monoperoxyphthalate (MMPP; structure drawn in the footnote of Table 8.5), sodium percarbonate (SPC; $Na_2CO_3{\cdot}1.5H_2O_2$), peracetic acid ($MeCO_3H$), and aqueous sodium percarbonate and *N*,*N*,*N*′,*N*′-tetraacetylethylenediamine (SPC-TAED; effective in decontaminating some classical CW agents[258]). The amount of surviving fentanyl in the oxidant solution was monitored by adjusting the solution to pH 12 (to convert fentanyl hydrochloride to the free base) with 2 M aqueous NaOH and periodic analysis by GC with flame ionisation detection (GC-FID).

The results are summarised in Table 8.5. Analysis of the reaction mixture obtained using hydrogen peroxide, by GC- and LC-MS, suggested that the amide grouping of fentanyl was cleaved, the *N*-phenethyl group was removed, and the piperidinyl nitrogen atom oxidised (yielding norfentanyl, norfentanyl oxime, and styrene), and that a C–C cleavage also occurred, to give *N*-(1-formylpiperidinyl)-*N*-phenylpropanamide and benzaldehyde (Figure 8.14).

The decomposition pathways of fentanyl hydrochloride differed upon treatment with aqueous trichloroisocyanuric acid (TCCA) or calcium hypochlorite [$Ca(OCl)_2$] in aqueous phosphate buffer (both oxidants had 0.2 mol l^{-1} of available chlorine).[159] Addition of the aqueous fentanyl hydrochloride solution to the $Ca(OCl)_2$ solution caused solid fentanyl free base to precipitate due to its poor solubility in strongly basic aqueous solution, leading to erratic calculated

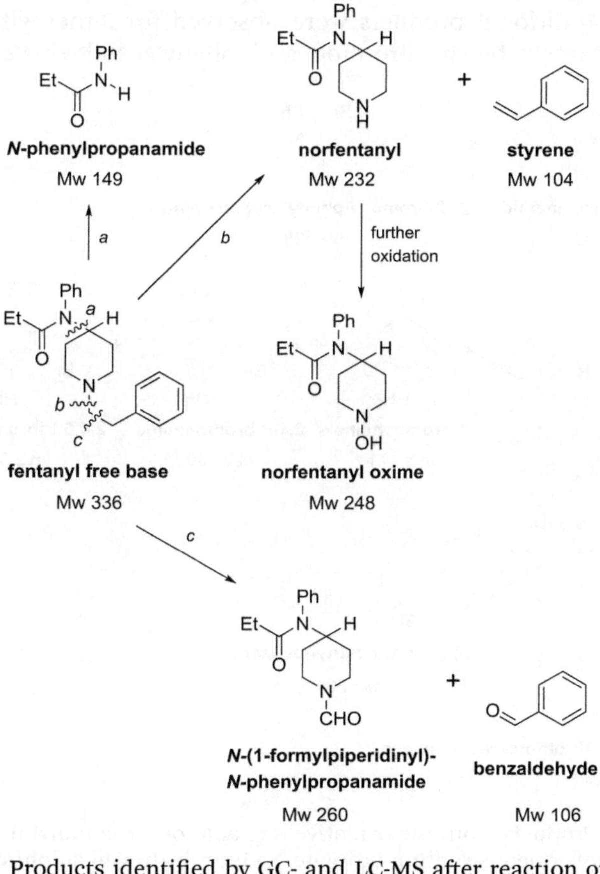

Figure 8.14 Products identified by GC- and LC-MS after reaction of fentanyl free base with hydrogen peroxide at pH 5.[159] Mw: molecular weight. *a*, *b* and *c* denote different cleavages of the fentanyl free base.

percentages of degraded fentanyl by GC-FID. Analysis of the TCCA solution by GC- and LC-MS revealed simultaneous fentanyl decomposition and *ortho*/*para*-chlorination reactions of the aromatic degradation products (to yield 2- and 4-chlorobenzaldehyde, 2-chlorobenzyl chloride, and 2,6-dichlorobenzyl chloride).[159] The presence of chlorine in some of the postulated products, not observed in peroxide based decontamination, suggests that if a fentanyl was disseminated and the exposed area subject to a decontamination attempt, it might be possible to identify retrospectively the type of decontaminant employed.

Under acidic conditions the reaction between sodium bromate, sodium hydrogen sulphite, and sodium sulphite produced active intermediates able to degrade fentanyl, 3-methylfentanyl, carfentanil, and sufentanil.[160] At pH 4 and a molar ratio of $NaBrO_3:NaHSO_3:Na_2SO_3$ equal to 20:3:7, degradation of fentanyl, 3-methylfentanyl, and carfentanil exceeded 99.9% in 30 min when the molar ratio of sodium bromate: fentanyl compounds surpassed 50:1. The molar ratio of sodium bromate: sufentanil needed to exceed 65:1 to ensure the complete destruction of the sufentanil in 30 min. Degradation products identified by GC-MS suggested C–C and C–N bond cleavages had occurred. The products identified after degradation of fentanyl are shown Figure 8.15. Additional products were observed for 3-methylfentanyl and carfentanil, namely benzyl bromide and phenylacetaldehyde. Sufentanil

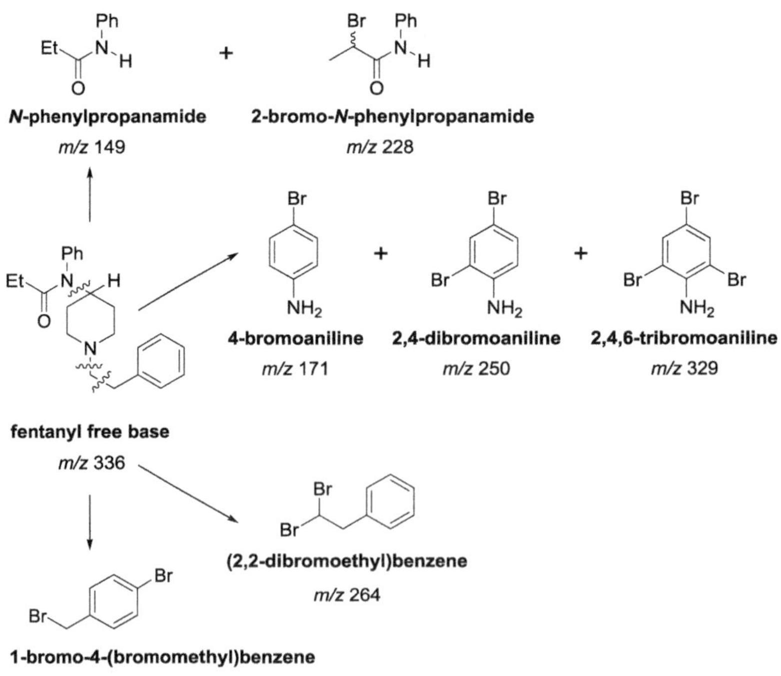

Figure 8.15 Products from the oxidative degradation of fentanyl using a mixture of aqueous sodium bromate, sodium hydrogen sulphite, and sodium sulphite, at pH 4.[160] Mw: molecular weight.

generated, in addition to the products depicted in Figure 8.15, benzyl bromide, α,α-dibromotoluene, and 2,3,4-tribromothiophene.

8.9.5 Detection

Detection of fentanyl, alfentanil, and remifentanil by forming ion pairs with azo dyes, mixing in citrate buffer, extraction into chloroform, and analysis of the ion pair *via* UV-visible spectrophotometry has been reported by Czech defence scientists.[153] The azo dyes used were Acid Orange 7, Acid Red 88, Crocein Orange G, and Ethyl Orange sodium salt (Figure 8.16). An electrochemical method for destroying fentanyl, developed by a scientist from the Russian State Institute of Organic Chemistry and Technology (GosNIIOKhT) in Moscow, has been noted, but not described in detail.[259]

Immunoassay test tickets for detecting fentanyls in urine, other biological fluids, or water are available, having been developed in the late 1980s for detecting drug doping in horses.[260,261] Enzyme immunoassays for fentanyl have been developed using horseradish peroxidase and 3,3′,5,5′-tetramethylbenzidine, and luminol as colorimetric and chemiluminescence substrates, respectively (detection limits for fentanyl: 0.045 and 0.005 ng ml^{-1}, respectively).[262] These commercially available systems offer the potential for detecting fentanyls in the field, and could allow preliminary identification prior to confirmatory analysis in the laboratory in the event of an allegation of military use.

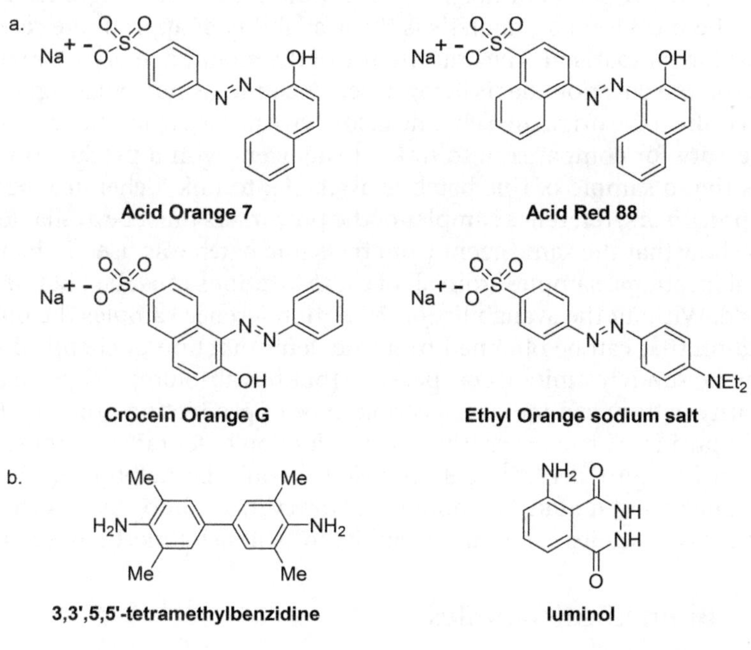

Figure 8.16 Chemicals for the detection of fentanyl compounds: (a) azo dyes,[153] and (b) reagents used for colorimetric and chemiluminescent detection.[262]

8.10 Identification

This section describes the identification of fentanyl compounds in environmental and biomedical samples. Transformations of fentanyls in the body are reviewed, as these impact the methods of analysis developed for their identification in biological fluids.

8.10.1 Environmental Samples

Sampling and analysis (S&A) delivers evidence for the presence or absence of chemicals relevant to the CWC. Methods for sample analysis, both on- and off-site, are essential for investigations of the alleged use of chemical weapons. Identification of chemical impurities in environmental samples containing CW agents is important because of the possibility of attributing the material to the perpetrator. Unique identifiers must be matched to the source for confident attribution, and this may not be possible if matching of sample chemical profiles cannot be achieved. However, the identification of impurities may allow the history of a CW agent[263–265]—whether it has been decontaminated[266] or treated by fire[267]—to be discerned.

The Director General of the OPCW, the implementing body of the CWC based in The Hague, has commented that it is due to the "strong deterrent value of advanced S&A that will make violations of the Convention increasingly difficult to hide".[268] Chemical forensics relevant to the CWC have been reviewed by the OPCW laboratory.[269] This review notes that "A significant challenge in chemical forensic analysis is the availability of appropriate reference materials for comparison. The exact nature of the required reference materials depends on the question that is being asked. If a unique molecular signature is used to confirm the origin of a chemical, known samples from the same origin are necessary for comparison; to link a toxic agent with a production batch requires that a sample of this batch is available; to link a chemical agent to certain precursors, reference samples of the precursors must be available; similarly to show that the same agent from the same batch was used in incidents at several locations, samples from all of these locations must be obtained and compared. Without the availability of the right reference samples the possible information that can be obtained from the determination of chemical signatures can be severely limited. One possible (but not absolute) exception is that an impurity pattern can indicate a certain type of production process." Examples of impurities carried over from the production of fentanyls commercially are shown in Figure 8.17.[252] Such knowledge could be helpful for chemical forensic analysis of fentanyl compounds. However, inhomogeneous chemical profiles across samples can limit the ability to establish links between them.

8.10.2 Biomedical Samples

In considering analytes that might be identified by analysis of biomedical samples, it is necessary to understand the transformations fentanyls undergo in humans. After intravenous injection, fentanyl enters the liver in a single pass and

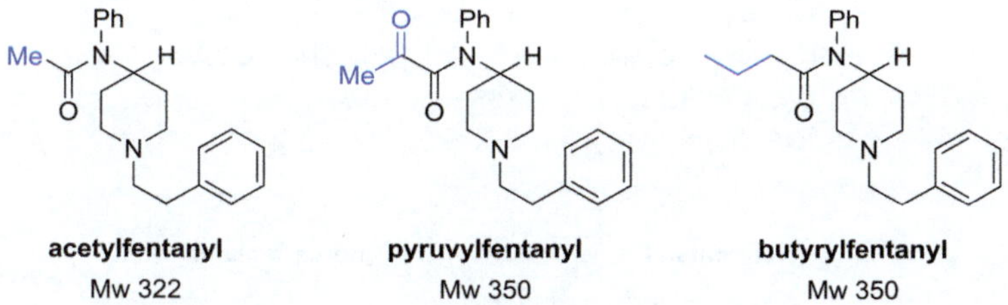

Figure 8.17 Impurities in some batches of fentanyls intended for pharmaceutical use.[252] Mw: molecular weight.

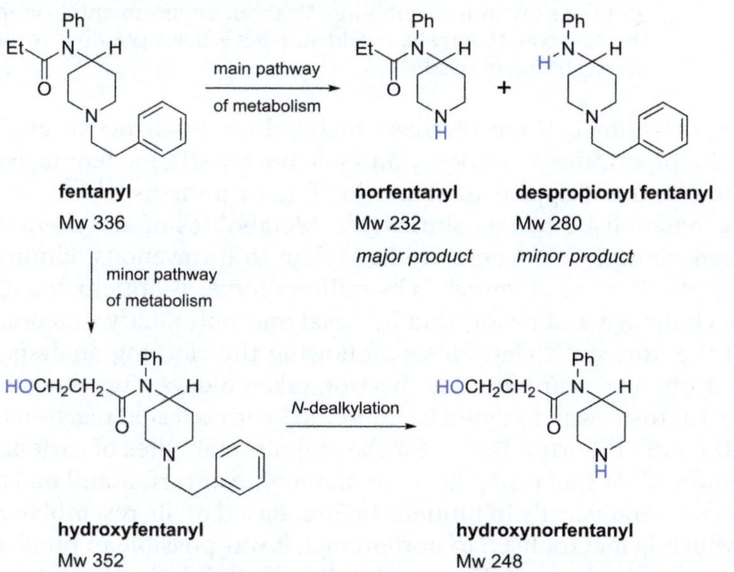

Figure 8.18 Metabolic transformations of fentanyl and the four main metabolites. Mw: molecular weight.

is metabolised there rapidly.[172,270] Concentrations of [^{3}H]-fentanyl fall quickly and 99% of the administered dose (3.2 or 6.4 μg kg^{-1}) is eliminated from plasma in 60 min; terminal elimination from the body is slow [half-life of elimination ($t_{1/2}\beta$) 219 min] due to the recycling of unaltered drug from a peripheral to a central compartment, where elimination occurs after biotransformation.[270] Some 85% of the dose appeared in the urine and faeces within 72 h, but less than 8% comprised unchanged fentanyl. Fluctuations were observed in plasma fentanyl concentrations during elimination. The long $t_{1/2}\beta$ and plasma level fluctuations may contribute to the prolonged and recurrent respiratory depression effects of the drug.[270] Liver metabolism of fentanyl is mediated by cytochrome P450 3A4, and metabolites detectable by GC-MS, quantifiable by using deuterated internal standards,[271] are shown in Figure 8.18.

The principal metabolic transformation of fentanyl is piperidine *N*-dealkylation to give norfentanyl (Figure 8.18). Minor metabolites are despropionyl fentanyl and hydroxyfentanyl. The latter is *N*-dealkylated to yield

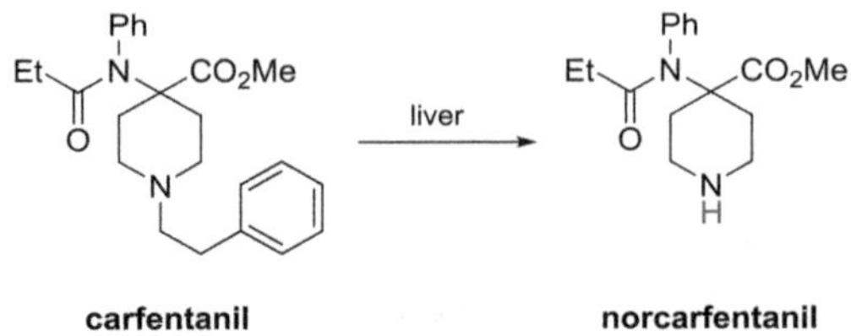

Figure 8.19 Proposed metabolic transformation of carfentanil in humans.[22] Note that the nor-metabolites do not permit unequivocal identification of the parent fentanyl compounds in many cases because of the close similarity of the parent structures (*e.g.* sufentanil and alfentanil would give the same nor-metabolite). Without environmental samples from the Moscow theatre it would not have been possible to be certain about the agent used.

hydroxynorfentanyl. None of these metabolites is an active analgesic.[271] Metabolic piperidine *N*-dealkylation is characteristic for fentanyls: sufentanil and alfentanil appear to share this fate in humans.[272,273] α-Methylfentanyl is metabolised by rats similarly.[274] Metabolites of acetylfentanyl have also been identified.[274] These studies relate to intravenous administration of fentanyls. The use of fentanyls by military forces is anticipated to involve aerosol challenge and absorption by nasal and pulmonary mucosae. In the case of the Moscow Theatre Siege, following the clothing analysis, a urine sample from a 56 year old male survivor, taken 5 days after exposure to the chemical aerosol, was analysed by LC-MS/MS with selected reaction monitoring (SRM) at Dstl Porton Down, for the major metabolites of carfentanil and remifentanil.[22] At that time, the main metabolite of carfentanil had not been identified unequivocally in humans before. Based on its resemblance to fentanyl, which is metabolised to norfentanyl, it was possible to predict a likely candidate: norcarfentanil (Figure 8.19). Remifentanil, characterised by a very short action and potency similar to fentanyl, is metabolised quickly in the blood by esterases,[17] with a mean half-life in humans of ~2 h, to remifentanil acid (refer to Figure 8.12).[250,275–277]

The analysis identified norcarfentanil in the man's urine (Figure 8.20), but no remifentanil. The identification of norcarfentanil confirmed the finding from the clothing analysis that carfentanil had been a component of the chemical aerosol used by the Russian Special Forces.[22] The detection of norcarfentanil so many days after the inhalation of the aerosol was presumably a consequence of the high fat solubility of carfentanil, which had limited its elimination from the body, and *N*-dealkylation by the liver of the proportion of the drug that had 'leached' into the hepatic system. The absence of remifentanil acid in the urine sample was unsurprising given the 5 day lapse between the man's exposure to the aerosol and the analysis.

In any future investigations of alleged use involving suspected exposure to fentanyl compounds it is probably worth screening urine samples for antagonist drugs such as naloxone. Morphine is metabolised by humans through conjugation to a glucuronide group by uridine diphosphate-glucuronosyltransferase-2B7

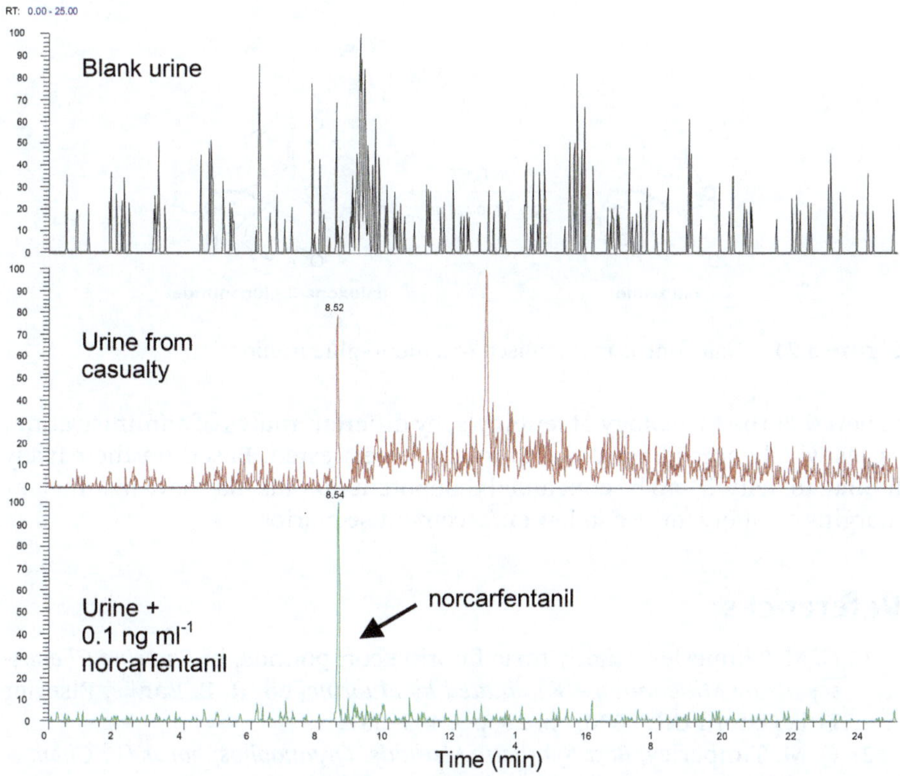

Figure 8.20 LC-MS/MS SRM chromatogram for the urine sample from Casualty 3. Transition *m*/*z* 291.0 → 259.0 from an extract of blank urine (top), urine from Casualty 3 (middle) and spiked urine (bottom) showing the presence of norcarfentanil. Figure reproduced from ref. 22.

(UGT2B7), a phase II metabolism isoenzyme present in the liver, to give morphine-3β-glucuronide (which is inactive as an analgesic and constitutes 75% of excreted morphine) and morphine-6β-glucuronide (which is a potent analgesic).[278–280] Morphine is also *N*-demethylated by cytochrome P450 3A4 (like fentanyl) and to a lesser extent cytochrome P450 2C8 to give normorphine (not shown).[281,282] Naloxone, like morphine, is glucuronidated by UGT2B7 to give naloxone-3-glucuronide[283] (Figure 8.21). Naltrexone is metabolised similarly.[283] LC-MS/MS analysis of opiates and opioids in urine has been reviewed.[284]

8.11 Conclusions

Our publication revealing the composition of the chemical aerosol used to end the Moscow Theatre Siege[22] has raised awareness of the hazards posed by the military application of fentanyls. The lack of an acceptable safety margin is probably universal for all fentanyls, when used for the purposes of inducing a state of mental/physical incapacitation. It is evident from this

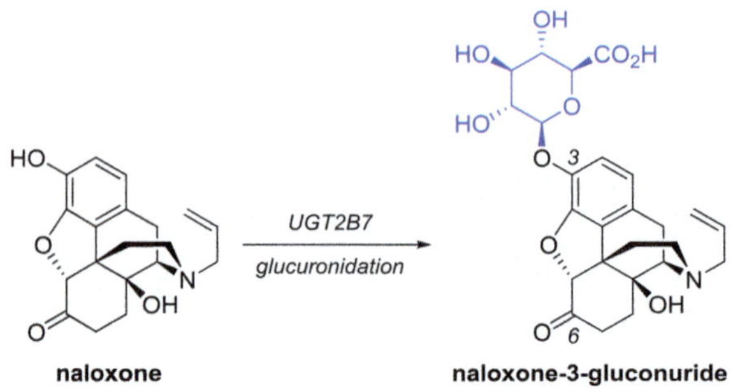

Figure 8.21 Naloxone is metabolised to a mono-glucuronide.[283]

review that the toxicology of fentanyls, by different routes of administration, varies widely according to the animal species tested. Based on their likely human toxicity, it can be concluded that potent opioids may have insufficient margins of safety for use in law enforcement scenarios.

References

1. C. M. Timperley, Highly-toxic fluorine compounds, in *Fluorine Chemistry at the Millennium - Fascinated by Fluorine*, ed. R. E. Banks, Elsevier Ltd., Oxford UK, 2000, ch. 29, pp. 499–537.
2. C. M. Timperley, *Best Synthetic Methods: Organophosphorus (V) Chemistry*, Elsevier Ltd., Oxford UK, 2015, pp. 1–89.
3. P. A. J. Janssen, The development of new synthetic narcotics, in *Opioids in Anesthesia*, ed. E. G. Estafenous, Butterworths Publishers, Boston MA, USA, 1984, ch. 7, pp. 37–44.
4. T. H. Stanley, T. D. Egan and H. Van Aken, A tribute to Dr. Paul A. J. Janssen: entrepreneur extraordinaire, innovative scientist, and significant contributor to anesthesiology, *Anesth. Analg.*, 2008, **106**, 451–462.
5. L. Iversen, *Drugs: A Very Short Introduction*, Oxford University Press, Oxford UK, 2001.
6. J. G. Cannon, *Analgesics. 1: General considerations and non-opioid analgesics, Pharmacology for Chemists*, Oxford University Press, Oxford UK, 2nd edn, 2007, ch. 11, pp. 191–207.
7. A. O'Donnell, *Anaesthesia: A Very Short Introduction*, Oxford University Press, Oxford UK, 2012.
8. A. F. Casy and R. T. Parfitt, *Opioid Analgesics: Chemistry and Receptors*, Plenum Press, London UK, 1986.
9. L. N. Chan, Opioid analgesics and the gastrointestinal tract, *Pract. Gastroenterol.*, 2008, 37–50.
10. P. W. Atkins, Morphine, in: *Molecules*, Scientific American Library, New York USA, 1987, pp. 165–166.
11. P. A. J. Janssen and J. F. Gardocki, *Method for producing analgesia*, US Patent 3,141,823, 1964.

12. K. W. Bentley and H. M. E. Cardwell, The morphine-thebaine group of alkaloids. Part V. The absolute stereochemistry of the morphine, benzylisoquinoline, aporphine, and tetrahydroberberine alkaloids,*J. Chem. Soc.*, 1955, 3252–3260.
13. P. G. H. Van Daele, M. F. L. De Bruyn, J. M. Boey, S. Sanczuk, J. T. M. Agten and P. A. J. Janssen, Synthetic analgesics: *N*-(1-[2-arylethyl])-4-substituted 4-piperidinyl) *N*-arylalkanamides, *Arzneim. Forsch.*, 1976, **26**, 1521–1531.
14. W. F. M. Van Bever, C. J. E. Niemegeers, K. H. L. Schellekens and P. A. J. Janssen, *N*-4-Substituted 1-(2-arylethyl)-4-piperidinyl-*N*-phenylpropanamides, a novel series of extremely potent analgesics with unusually high safety margin, *Arzneim. Forsch.*, 1976, **26**, 1548–1551.
15. J. R. Bagley, S. A. Thomas, F. G. Rudo, H. K. Spencer, B. M. Doorley, M. H. Ossipov, T. P. Jerussi, M. J. Benvenga and T. Spaulding, New 1-(heterocyclylalkyl)-4-(propionanilido)-4-piperidinyl methyl ester and methylene methyl ether analgesics,*J. Med. Chem.*, 1991, **34**, 827–841.
16. W. F. M. Van Bever, C. J. E. Niemegeers and P. A. J. Janssen, Synthetic analgesics. Synthesis and pharmacology of the diastereoisomers of *N*-[3-methyl-1-(2-phenylethyl)-4-piperidyl]-*N*-phenylpropanamide and *N*-[3-methyl-1-(1-methyl-2-phenylethyl)-4-piperidyl]-*N*-phenylpropanamide,*J. Med. Chem.*, 1974, **17**, 1047–1051.
17. P. L. Feldman, M. K. James, M. F. Brackeen, J. M. Bilotta, S. V. Schuster, A. P. Lahey, M. W. Lutz, M. R. Johnson and H. J. Leighton, Design, synthesis, and pharmacological evaluation of ultrashort- to long-acting opioid analgetics,*J. Med. Chem.*, 1991, **34**, 2202–2208.
18. P. A. J. Janssen and C. A. M. Van der Eycken, in *Drugs affecting the CNS*, ed. A. Burger, Dekker, New York USA, 1968, vol. 2, p. 25.
19. Z. Y. Lu, S. Y. Zhao, X. M. Yuan and Y. L. Yang, Studies and analgesic activity of 4-*N*-propionyl analogs of 4-methoxycarbonyl fentanyl, *Acta Pharm. Sin. (Yao Xue Xue Bao)*, 1990, **25**, 336–339(in Chinese).
20. Y. L. Yang, Z. Y. Lu, Z. J. Yang, S. Y. Zhao, J. B. Zhang and L. Y. Xiao, Synthesis and analgesic activity of analogs of 4-methoxymethyl fentanyl, *Acta Pharm. Sin. (Yao Xue Xue Bao)*, 1991, **26**, 493–498(in Chinese).
21. E. A. Antonov, A. A. Zhirov, A. T. Kirsanov, Yu. A. Krivolapov, A. A. Sorokin, Yu. D. Markovich and A. V. Panfilov, Synthesis of 5-(2-chloroethyl)-4-methylthiazole using the reaction of 5-(2-hydroxyethyl)-4-methylthiazole with phosphorus pentachloride, *Pharm. Chem. J.*, 1999, **33**, 658–660.
22. J. R. Riches, R. W. Read, R. M. Black, N. J. Cooper and C. M. Timperley, Analysis of clothing and urine from Moscow Theatre Siege casualties reveals carfentanil and remifentanil use,*J. Anal. Toxicol.*, 2012, **36**, 647–656.
23. R. B. Rothman, X. Hu, M. Seggel, A. E. Jacobson, K. C. Rice, G. A. Brine and F. I. Carroll, RTI-4614-4: an analog of (+)-cis-3-methylfentanyl with a 27,000-fold binding selectivity for mu *versus* delta opioid binding sites, *Life Sci.*, 1991, **48**, 111–116.

24. G. A. Brine, P. A. Stark, Y. Liu, F. I. Carroll, P. Singh, H. Xu and R. B. Rothman, Enantiomers of diastereomeric cis-N-[1-(2-hydroxy-2-phenylethyl)-3-methyl-4-piperidyl]-N-phenylpropanamides: synthesis, X-ray analysis, and biological activities, *J. Med. Chem.*, 1995, **38**, 1547–1557.
25. Z. X. Wang, Y. C. Zhu, W. Q. Jin, X. J. Chen, J. Chen, R. Y. Ji and Z. Q. Chi, Stereoisomers of N-[1-(2-hydroxy-2-phenylethyl)-3-methyl-4-piperidyl]-N-phenylpropanamide, *J. Med. Chem.*, 1995, **38**, 3652–3659.
26. Z. H. Liu, Y. He, W. Q. Jin, X. J. Chen, Q. X. Shen and Z. Q. Chi, Effect of chronic treatment of ohmefentanyl stereoisomers on cyclic AMP formation in Sf9 insect cells expressing human μ-opioid receptors, *Life Sci.*, 2004, **74**, 3001–3008.
27. W. Q. Jin, H. Xu, Y. C. Zhu, S. N. Fang, X. L. Xia, Z. M. Huang, B. L. Ge and Z. Q. Chi, Studies on the synthesis and relationship between analgesic activity and receptor affinity for 3-methylfentanyl derivatives, *Sci. Sin. B*, 1981, **24**, 710–720.
28. Z. M. Huang, J. Zhou, X. J. Chen, W. J. Zheng, H. P. Zhang, Z. Q. Chi, Z. G. Li and W. L. Chen, Analgesic activity and toxicity of potent analgesics ohmefentanyl, and mefentanyl, *Acta Pharmacol. Sin. (Zhongguo Yao Li Xue Bao)*, 1984, **5**, 153–158(in Chinese).
29. H. Xu, J. Chen and Z. Q. Chi, Ohmefentanyl – a new agonist for mu-opiate receptor, *Sci. Sin. B*, 1985, **28**, 504–511.
30. W. Q. Jin, X. J. Chen and Z. Q. Chi, The choice of opioid receptor subtype in isolated preparations by ohmefentanyl, *Sci. Sin., Ser. B*, 1987, **30**, 176–181.
31. W. Q. Jin, Z. X. Wang, J. Chen, X. J. Chen and Z. Q. Chi, Analgesic activity and selectivity for opioid receptors of enantiomers of ohmefentanyl, *Acta Pharmacol. Sin.*, 1996, **17**, 421–424.
32. G. W. Guo, Y. He, W. Q. Jin, Y. Zou, Y. C. Zhu and Z. Q. Chi, Comparison of physical dependence of ohmefentanyl stereoisomers in mice, *Life Sci.*, 2000, **67**, 113–120.
33. B. Y. Chen, W. Q. Jin, X. J. Chen, Y. C. Zhu and Z. Q. Chi, Analgesic activity and opioid receptor selectivity of stereoisomers of ohmefentanyl isothiocyanate, *Eur. J. Pharmacol.*, 2001, **424**, 195–198.
34. Z. Yong, W. Hao, Y. Weifang, D. Qiyuan, C. Xinjian, J. Wenqiao and Z. Youcheng, Synthesis and analgesic activity of stereoisomers of cis-fluoro-ohmefentanyl, *Pharmazie*, 2003, **58**, 300–302.
35. G. A. Brine, F. I. Carroll, T. M. Richardson-Leibert, H. Xu and R. B. Rothman, Ohmefentanyl and its stereoisomers: chemistry and pharmacology, *Curr. Med. Chem.*, 1997, **4**, 247–270.
36. R. S. Vardanyan and V. J. Hruby, Fentanyl-related compounds and derivatives: current status and future prospects for pharmaceutical applications, *Future Med. Chem.*, 2014, **6**, 385–412.
37. Fentanyl factsheet, Drug Enforcement Administration, Office of Diversion Control, Drug & Chemical Evaluation Section, Washington D.C. 20537, USA, December 2008.

38. Fentanyl datasheet, Medsafe, New Zealand Medicines and Medical Devices Safety Authority; http://www.medsafe.govt.nz/profs/datasheet/f/Fentanylinj.htm, accessed on 6 June 2014.
39. T. H. Stanley, Opiate anaesthesia, *Anaesth. Intens. Care*, 1987, **15**, 38–59.
40. G. M. Hall, Fentanyl and the metabolic response to surgery, *Br. J. Anaesth.*, 1980, **52**, 561–562.
41. M. R. Murphy and C. H. Hug, The anesthetic potency of fentanyl in terms of its reduction of enflurane MAC, *Anesthesiology*, 1982, **57**, 485–488.
42. C. E. Rosow, Sufentanil citrate: a new opioid analgesic for use in anaesthesia, *Pharmacotherapy*, 1984, **4**, 11–19.
43. D. R. Miller, M. Wellwood, S. J. Teasdale, D. Laidley, J. Ivanov, P. Young, M. Madonik, P. McLaughlin, D. A. G. Mickle and R. D. Weisel, Effects of anaesthetic induction on myocardial function and metabolism: a comparison of fentanyl, sufentanil and alfentanil, *Can. J. Anaesth.*, 1988, **35**, 219–233.
44. Sufenta® product label: http://www.hospira.com/en/images/EN-3604_tcm81-5428.pdf accessed on 1 November 2015.
45. Carfentanil citrate: sterile injection anesthetic for immobilization of Cervidae, ZooPharm™ Drugs Designed for Darts™, Application Note, Fort Collins, Colorado USA, http://www.wildpharm.com.
46. J. C. Haigh, L. J. Lee and R. E. Schweinsburg, Immobilisation of polar bears with carfentanil, *J. Wildl. Dis.*, 1983, **19**, 140–144.
47. A. V. George, J. J. Lu, M. V. Pisano, J. Metz and T. B. Erickson, Carfentanil – an ultra-potent opioid, *Am. J. Emerg. Med.*, 2010, **28**, 530–532.
48. N. Hagelberg, S. Aalto, L. Tuominen, U. Pesonen, K. Någren, J. Hietala, H. Scheinin, A. Pertovaara and I. K. Martikainen, Striatal μ-opioid receptor availability predicts cold pressor pain threshold in healthy human subjects, *Neurosci. Lett.*, 2012, **521**, 11–14.
49. I. Fleming, *Goldfinger* (first published in 1959 by Jonathan Cape Ltd.), Penguin Classics Ltd., London UK, 2004, p. 207.
50. F. Boer, Drug handling by the lungs, *Br. J. Anaesth.*, 2003, **91**, 50–60.
51. L. E. Mather, A. Woodhouse, M. E. Ward, S. J. Farr, R. A. Rubsamen and L. G. Eltherington, Pulmonary administration of aerosolized fentanyl: pharmacokinetic analysis of systemic delivery, *Br. J. Clin. Pharmacol.*, 1998, **46**, 37–43.
52. M. J. Higgins, A. J. Asbury and M. J. Brodie, Inhaled nebulised fentanyl for postoperative analgesia, *Anaesthesia*, 1991, **46**, 973–976.
53. D. B. MacLeod, A. S. Habib, K. Ikeda, D. A. Spyker, J. V. Cassella, K. Y. Ho and T. J. Gan, Inhaled fentanyl aerosol in healthy human volunteers: pharmacokinetics and pharmacodynamics, *Anesth. Analg.*, 2012, **115**, 1071–1077.
54. J. E. Rabinowitz, M. Wensley, P. Lloyd, D. Myers, W. Shen, A. Lu, C. Hodges, R. Hale, D. Mufson and A. Zaffaroni, Fast-onset medications through thermally generated aerosols, *JPET*, 2004, **309**, 769–775.

55. G. Edwards, Part two: opiates, *Matters of Substance – Drugs: Is Legalization the Right Answer – or the Wrong Question?*, Penguin Books, London UK, 2004, pp. 76–139.
56. H. Hobhouse, *Seeds of Change – Six Plants that Transformed Mankind*, Papermac: Macmillan Publishers Ltd., London UK, 1999, pp. 148–149.
57. M. J. Balick and P. A. Cox, *Plants, People, and Culture – The Science of Ethnobotany*, Scientific American Library, New York USA, 1996, pp. 172–173.
58. J. Mann, *Murder, Magic & Medicine*, Oxford University Press, Oxford UK, 2000, 2nd edn, pp. 190–202.
59. S. L. Banks, M. J. Paech, S. Lim, W. M. Rucklidge, M. J. Roberts and V. B. Sunderland, Pharmacokinetics of nasal fentanyl, *J. Pharm. Pract. Res.*, 2003, **33**, 59–63.
60. J. L. Corriveau and M. Feasel, Incapacitating agents, in *Inhalation Toxicology*, ed. H. Salem and S. A. Katz, CRC Press, London UK, 2015, ch. 12, 3rd edn, pp. 245–255.
61. L. Manral, N. Muniappan, P. K. Gupta, K. Ganesan, R. C. Malhotra and R. Vijayaraghavan, Effect of exposure to fentanyl aerosol in mice on breathing pattern and respiratory variables, *Drug Chem. Toxicol.*, 2009, **32**, 108–113.
62. S. K. Yadav, D. Swami, P. Kumar, M. K. Meena, C. K. Maurya, P. K. Gupta, K. Ganesan, A. K. Jain and R. Bhattacharya, Acute inhalation toxicity of smoke of fentanyl and its 1-substituted analogs in Swiss albino mice, *Cell Mol. Biol.*, 2014, **60**, 1–9.
63. Note by the Technical Secretariat, Declaration of Riot Control Agents: Advice from the Scientific Advisory Board, Organisation for the Prohibition of Chemical Weapons (OPCW) Office of Strategy and Policy, Document S/1177/2014, 1 May 2014, available at http://www.opcw.org.
64. Article II Definitions and Criteria, Section II(7) 'Riot Control Agent'; Convention on the Prohibition of the Development, Production, Stockpiling and Use of Chemical Weapons and on their Destruction, OPCW, The Hague, available at http://www.opcw.org.
65. Case of Finogenov and others v. Russia, Judgement of the European Court of Human Rights (First Section), Application No. 18299/03 and 27311/03, Strasbourg, France, 20 December 2011.
66. V. Vandova, The European Court of Human Rights' judgement in the case Finogenov and others v. Russia, in *Report of an Expert Meeting, "Incapacitating Chemical Agents": Law Enforcement, Human Rights Law and Policy Perspectives, Montreux, held on 24-26 April 2012*, International Committee of the Red Cross, Geneva, Switzerland, 2013, pp. 46–49.
67. B. Brône, P. J. Peeters, R. Marrannes, M. Mercken, R. Nuydens, T. Meert and H. J. M. Gijsen, Tear gasses CN, CR, and CS are potent activators of the human TRPA1 receptor, *Toxicol. Appl. Pharmacol.*, 2008, **231**, 150–156.

68. H. J. M. Gijsen, D. Berthelot, M. Zaja, B. Brône, I. Geuens and M. Mereken, Analogues of morphanthridine and the tear gas dibenz[b,f][1,4]oxazepine (CR) as extremely potent activators of the human transient receptor potential ankyrin 1 (TRPA1) channel, *J. Med. Chem.*, 2010, **53**, 7011–7020.
69. C. D. Lindsay, C. Green, M. Bird, J. T. A. Jones, J. R. Riches, K. K. McKee, M. S. Sandford, D. A. Wakefield and C. M. Timperley, Potency of irritation by benzylidenemalononitriles in humans correlates with TRPA1 ion channel activation, *R. Soc. Open Sci.*, 2015, **2**, 140160.
70. V. D. Hauschild, Risk management and public health considerations of riot control agents, in *Riot Control Agents – Issues in Toxicology, Safety and Health*, ed. E. J. Olojos and W. Stopford, CRC Press Ltd., London UK, 2004, ch. 15, p. 290.
71. A. Davies and M. Roumy, The effect of transient stimulation of lung irritant receptors on the pattern of breathing in rabbits, *J. Physiol.*, 1982, **324**, 389–401.
72. K. Kang, S. R. Pulver, Y. C. Panzano, E. C. Chang, L. C. Griffith, D. L. Theobald and P. A. Garrity, Analysis of Drosophila TRPA1 reveals an ancient origin for human chemical nociception, *Nature*, 2010, **464**, 597–601.
73. Y. Alarie, Irritating properties of airborne materials to the upper respiratory tract, *Arch. Environ. Health*, 1966, **13**, 433–449.
74. Y. Alairie, I. Wakisaka and S. Oka, Sensory irritation by sulfur dioxide and chlorobenzylidene malononitrile, *Environ. Physiol. Biochem.*, 1973, **3**, 53–64.
75. Y. Alairie, Dose-response analysis in animal studies: prediction of human responses, *Environ. Health Perspect.*, 1981, **42**, 9–13.
76. H. Salem, M. Feasel and B. Ballantyne, Inhalation toxicology of riot control agents, in *Inhalation Toxicology*, ed. H. Salem and S. A. Katz, CRC Press Ltd., London UK, 2015, 3rd edn, ch. 11, pp. 211–243.
77. P. Blain, Tear gases and irritant incapacitants. 1-Chloroacetophenone, 2-chlorobenzylidene malononitrile and dibenz[b,f]-1,4-oxazepine, *Toxicol. Rev.*, 2003, **22**, 103–110.
78. Fentanyl leaflet, Drug Enforcement Administration Office, Office of Diversion Control, Drug & Chemical Evaluation Section, Washington DC 20537, USA, March 2009.
79. T. R. Kosten and T. P. George, The neurobiology of opioid dependence: implications for treatment, *Sci. Pract. Perspect.*, 2002, pp. 13–21.
80. F. Weiss and G. F. Koob, Drug addiction: functional neurotoxicity of the brain reward systems, *Neurotoxicol. Res.*, 2001, **3**, 145–156.
81. T. Cunha-Oliveira, A. C. Rego and C. R. Oliveira, Cellular and molecular mechanisms involved in the neurotoxicity of opioid and psychostimulant drugs, *Brain Res. Rev.*, 2008, **58**, 192–208.
82. United Nations Single Convention on Narcotic Drugs, New York, USA, 1961 (also that amended by the 1972 protocol).

83. A. V. Godunov, A. V. Kireeva and S. V. Volchenko, Determination of 3-methylfentanyl by GC/MS in biological and non-biological objects, *Forensic Sci. Int.*, 2007, **169S**, S29–S35.
84. C. A. Valdez, R. N. Leif and B. P. Mayer, An efficient, optimized synthesis of fentanyl and related analogs, *PLoS One*, **9**(**9**), e108250.
85. W. H. Soine, Clandestine drug synthesis, *Med. Res. Rev.*, 1986, **6**, 41–74.
86. J. Mounteney, I. Giraudon, G. Denissov and P. Griffiths, Fentanyls: are we missing the signs? Highly potent and on the rise in Europe, *Int. J. Drug Policy*, 2015, **26**, 626–631.
87. C. Regnard and A. Pelham, Severe respiratory depression and sedation with transdermal fentanyl: four case studies, *Palliat. Med.*, 2003, **17**, 714–716.
88. Y. Higashikawa and S. Suzuki, Studies on 1-(2-phenethyl)-4-(*N*-propionylanilino)piperidine (fentanyl) and its related compounds. VI. Structure-analgesic activity relationship for fentanyl, methyl-substituted fentanyls and other analogues, *Forensic Toxicol.*, 2008, **26**, 1–5.
89. J. C. Garriott, R. Rodriguez and V. J. Di Maio, A death from fentanyl overdose, *J. Anal. Toxicol.*, 1984, **8**, 288–289.
90. E. M. Pare, J. R. Monforte, R. Gault and H. Mirchandani, A death involving fentanyl, *J. Anal. Toxicol.*, 1987, **11**, 272–275.
91. R. J. Matejczyk, Fentanyl related overdose, *J. Anal. Toxicol.*, 1988, **12**, 236–238.
92. B. Levine, J. C. Goodin and Y. H. Caplan, A fentanyl fatality involving midazolam, *Forensic Sci. Int.*, 1990, **45**, 247–251.
93. P. K. Lilleng, L. I. Mehlum, L. Bachs and I. Morild, Deaths after intravenous misuse of transdermal fentanyls, *J. Forensic Sci.*, 2004, **49**, 1364–1366.
94. R. E. Johnstone, R. L. Katz and T. H. Stanley, Homicides using muscle relaxants, opioids, and anesthetic drugs: anesthesiologist assistance in their investigation and prosecution, *Anesthesiology*, 2011, **114**, 713–716.
95. H. Andresen, A. Gullans, M. Veselinovic, S. Anders, A. Schmoldt, S. Iwersen-Bergmann and A. Mueller, Fentanyl: toxic or therapeutic? Postmortem and antemortem blood concentrations after transdermal fentanyl application, *J. Anal. Toxicol.*, 2012, **36**, 182–194.
96. V. Coopman, J. Cordonnier, K. Pien and D. Van Varenbergh, LC-MS/MS analysis of fentanyl and norfentanyl in a fatality due to application of multiple Durogesic® transdermal therapeutic systems, *Forensic Sci. Int.*, 2007, **169**, 223–227.
97. T. L. Martin, K. L. Woodall and B. A. McLellan, Fentanyl-related deaths in Ontario, Canada: toxicological findings and circumstances of death in 112 cases (2002-2004), *J. Anal. Toxicol.*, 2006, **30**, 603–610.
98. B. C. Garrett and J. Hart, *Historical Dictionary of Nuclear, Biological, and Chemical Warfare: Historical Dictionaries of War, Revolution, and Civil Unrest, No. 33*, The Scarecrow Press, Inc., Plymouth UK, 2007, p. 142.

99. J. S. Ketchum, *Chemical warfare secrets almost forgotten – a personal story of medical testing of army volunteers with incapacitating chemical agents during the Cold War (1955-1975)*, ChemBooks Inc., CA, USA, 2006, p. 16 and pp. 265–266.
100. Q. Schiermeier, Hostage deaths put gas weapons in spotlight, *Nature*, 2002, **420**, 7.
101. M. Enserink and R. Stone, Questions swirl over knockout gas used in hostage crisis, *Science*, 2002, **298**, 1150–1151.
102. B. Van Damme, Moscow Theatre Siege: a deadly gamble that nearly paid off, *Pharm. J.*, 2002, **269**, 723–724.
103. L. Ember, Opiate ends hostage crisis, *Chem. Eng. News*, 2002, **80**, 6.
104. J. Rieder, C. Keller, G. Hoffmann and P. Lirk, Moscow theatre siege and anaesthetic drugs, *Lancet*, 2003, **361**, 1131.
105. R. M. Coupland, Incapacitating chemical weapons: a year after the Moscow theatre siege, *Lancet*, 2003, **362**, 1346.
106. P. M. Wax, C. E. Becker and S. C. Curry, Unexpected "gas" casualties in Moscow: a medical toxicology perspective, *Ann. Emerg. Med.*, 2003, **41**, 700–705.
107. C. M. Timperley and J. E. H. Tattersall, Toxicology and medical treatment of organophosphorus compounds, in *Best Synthetic Methods: Organophosphorus (V) Chemistry*, Elsevier Ltd., Oxford UK, 2015, pp. 33–89.
108. Convention on the Prohibition of the Development, Production, Stockpiling and Use of Chemical Weapons and on their Destruction, Organisation for the Prohibition of Chemical Weapons (OPCW), The Hague, The Netherlands, available at http://www.opcw.org.
109. N. S. Antonov, *Chemical Weapons at the Turn of the Century, English translation LN72–96*, Progress Publisher, Moscow, Russia, 1994.
110. L. Ya Erman, V. F. Mindrul, N. Yu. Khromova and V. K. Kurochkin, Molecular structure of 1(phenethyl)-4(3-trimethyl germyl) propioanilidopiperidine hydrochloride, *J. Struct. Chem.*, 1995, **36**, 520–524.
111. A. V. Panfilov, Yu. D. Markovich, I. P. Ivashev, A. A. Zhirov, A. F. Eleev, V. K. Kurochkin, A. T. Kirsanov and G. V. Nazarov, Sodium borohydride in reductive amination reactions, *Pharm. Chem. J.*, 2000, **34**, 76–78.
112. A. V. Panfilov, Yu. D. Markovich, A. A. Zhirov, I. P. Ivashev, A. T. Kirsanov and V. B. Kondrat'ev, Reactions of sodium borohydride in acetic acid: reductive amination of carbonyl compounds, *Pharm. Chem. J.*, 2000, **34**, 371–373.
113. V. A. Zlobin, L. P. Bukreeva, P. E. Kuznetsov, A. V. Panfilov, G. V. Nazarov and A. T. Kirsanov, Analysis of opiates by HPLC with indirect spectrophotometric detection, *Pharm. Chem. J.*, 2000, **34**, 279–280.
114. F. S. Dukhovich, E. N. Gorbatova, M. B. Darkhovskii and V. K. Kurochkin, Relationship between the dissociation constant and the lifetime for complexes of biologically active substances with receptors and enzymes, *Pharm. Chem. J.*, 2002, **36**, 248–254.

115. A. V. Panfilov, A. M. Aparkin, A. A. Zhirov, P. E. Kuznetsov, S. P. Los, Yu. D. Markovich, G. V. Nazarov, L. V. Starodubtseva and E. P. Yashchenko, Use of the spin-relaxation method for the analysis of drugs in biological samples, *Pharm. Chem. J.*, 2002, **36**, 557–558.
116. P. E. Kuznetsov, A. M. Aparkin, V. A. Zlobin, G. V. Nazarov, P. V. Kosterin, E. V. Lyubun and A. A. Shcherbakov, Analysis of opiates by spin-lattice relaxation techniques, *Pharm. Chem. J.*, 2002, **36**, 331–332.
117. P. E. Kuznetsov, A. A. Gracheva, V. A. Zlobin, G. V. Nazarov, N. B. Kuznetsova, S. M. Rogacheva, Optical properties of aqueous morphine solutions, *Proc. SPIE 5068*, Saratov Fall Meeting 2002: Optical Technologies in Biophysics and Medicine IV, **396**, 14 October 2003, DOI: 10.1117/12.518858.
118. P. E. Kuznetsov, A. M. Aparkin, V. A. Zlobin, G. V. Nazarov, S. M. Rogacheva, A. A. Gracheva and Z. A. Simonova, On the possibility of using poly(*N*-vinylcaprolactam) for the determination of some drugs in aqueous media, *Pharm. Chem. J.*, 2003, **37**, 507–510.
119. U. A. Murashova, N. P. Sadchikova, L. V. Skalkina and S. K. Smirnov, Quality evaluation and standardization of fentanyl and the related injection preparation, *Pharm. Chem. J.*, 2004, **38**, 336–338.
120. U. A. Murashova, L. V. Skalkina, N. P. Sadchikova and S. K. Smirnov, Harmonization of quality indicators of the domestic parent substance fentanyl, *Pharm. Chem, J.*, 2008, **42**, 550–552.
121. U. A. Murashova, L. V. Skalkina, E. N. Glukhan and S. K. Smirnov, Kinetics of 1-(2-phenylethyl)-4-phenylaminopiperidine acylation by propionyl chloride in nonaqueous media, *Pharm. Chem. J.*, 2010, **44**, 261–264.
122. F. S. Dukhovich, E. N. Gorbatova, M. B. Darkhovskii and V. K. Kurochkin, Relationship between the dissociation constant and the lifetime for complexes of biologically active substances with receptors and enzymes, *Pharm. Chem. J.*, 2002, **36**, 248–254.
123. F. S. Dukhovich and M. B. Darkhovskii, Molecular electrostatic potential as a factor of drug-receptor recognition, *J. Mol. Recognit.*, 2003, **16**, 191–202.
124. F. S. Dukhovich, M. B. Darkhovskii, E. N. Gorbatova and V. S. Polyakov, The agonist paradox: agonists and antagonists of acetylcholine receptors and opioid receptors, *Chem. Biodiversity*, 2005, **2**, 354–366.
125. N. E. Kuz'mina, E. S. Osipova, V. S. Kuz'min and V. B. Sitnikov, Electron properties of aryl moieties in agonists and antagonists of opioid receptors, *Pharm. Chem. J.*, 2005, **39**, 644–649.
126. N. E. Kuz'mina, E. S. Osipova, V. S. Kuz'min and V. B. Sitnikov, Effect of the tyramine fragment of opioid receptor ligands on their agonist and antagonist properties, *Pharm. Chem. J.*, 2006, **40**, 254–260.
127. N. E. Kuz'mina, E. S. Osipova, V. S. Kuz'min and V. B. Sitnikov, Geometric parameters as a criterion for assessment of the bioactive conformations of opiate receptor ligands, *Russ. Chem. Bull., Int. Ed.*, 2006, **55**, 1516–1522.
128. N. E. Kuz'mina, E. S. Osipova, V. S. Kuz'min and V. B. Sitnikov, A general model of the opiate pharmacophore 1. Regions of the opiate pharmacophore responsible for nonselective affinity for the opiate receptor, *Russ. Chem. Bull., Int. Ed.*, 2006, **55**, 1523–1529.

129. N. E. Kuz'mina, E. S. Osipova, V. S. Kuz'min and V. B. Sitnikov, General model of the opiate pharmacophore 2. Regions of the opiate pharmacophore defining agonistic properties of the opiate receptor ligands, *Russ. Chem. Bull., Int. Ed.*, 2008, **57**, 1277–1284.
130. N. E. Kuz'mina, E. S. Osipova, V. S. Kuz'min and V. B. Sitnikov, General model of the opiate pharmacophore 3. Regions of the opiate pharmacophore determining antagonistic properties of the opiate receptor ligands, *Russ. Chem. Bull., Int. Ed.*, 2008, **57**, 1285–1298.
131. N. E. Kuz'mina and V. S. Kuz'min, Development of concepts on the interaction of drugs with opioid receptors, *Russ. Chem. Rev.*, 2011, **80**, 145–169.
132. N. E. Kuz'mina and I. N. Stankov, Role of saturability of noncovalent interactions in the analysis of the three-dimensional structure-opioid activity relationship, *Russ. Chem. Bull., Int. Ed.*, 2012, **61**, 1207–1214.
133. N. E. Kuz'mina, V. A. Yashkir, V. A. Merkulov and E. S. Osipova, Method for estimating a compound's opiate activity based on a versatile three-dimensional model of nonselective opiate pharmacophore, *Russian J. Bioorg. Chem.*, 2012, **38**, 507–519.
134. A. I. Golovko, Heterogeneity of mu-opioid receptors as one of the factors sensitive to narcotic analgesics, *Biology Bull. Rev.*, 2013, **3**, 139–151.
135. H. Fakhraian, T. Nezamoleslam, M. B. Panbehriseh and B. Javahery, Structural-activity relationship, atomic electron density and conformational investigation of fentanyl analogues, summary of oral presentation, *Fourth International Symposium Computational Methods in Toxicology and Pharmacology Integrating Internet Resources in 2007 Symposium Proceedings*, Moscow, 2007.
136. T. Nezamoleslam, B. Javahery, N. M. Shakiba and H. Fakhraian, Structure-activity relationship, atomic electron density and conformational investigation of fentanyl analogues, *J. Passive Def. Sci. Technol.*, 2010, **1**, 23–32 (in Farzi).
137. M. Ghaffarzadeh, S. Heidarifard, F. Feraji and S. S. Joghan, Synthesis of amides from imines using Et_3SiH/Zn system, *Appl. Organomet. Chem.*, 2012, **26**, 103–107.
138. H. Kamranpey, Aerosolization of medetomidine hydrochloride as an incapacitating agent, *J. Passive Def. Sci. Technol.*, 2011, **3**, 51–56.
139. H. Toulabi and H. Fakhraian, The synthesis of medetomidine and its naphtalenic derivative, *Org. Chem. J.*, 2014, **3**, 49–54.
140. H. Fakhraian, H. Toulabi, E. Choobdari, M. H. Peyrovi and H. H. Ghanbary, Synthesis and enantiomeric resolution of medetomidine, *Org. Prep. Proced. Int.*, 2015, **47**, 141–148.
141. E. Choobdari, H. Fakhraian and M. H. Peyrovi, Prediction and experimental determination of the binary and ternary phase diagrams of (±)medetomidine hydrochloride, *Tetrahedron: Asymmetry*, 2013, **24**, 801–806.
142. E. Choobdari, H. Fakhraian and M. H. Peyrovi, Anion effect on the binary and ternary phase diagrams of chiral medetomidine salts and conglomerate crystal formation, *Chirality*, 2014, **26**, 183–188.

143. P. K. Gupta, K. Ganesan, A. Pande and R. C. Malhotra, A convenient one-pot synthesis of fentanyl, *J. Chem. Res.*, 2005, **36**, 452–453.
144. P. K. Gupta, L. Manral, K. Ganesan and D. K. Dubey, Use of single-drop microextraction for determination of fentanyl in water samples, *Anal. Bioanal. Chem.*, 2007, **388**, 579–583.
145. L. Manral, P. K. Gupta, K. Ganesan and R. C. Malhotra, Gas chromatographic retention indices of fentanyl and analogues, *J. Chromatogr. Sci.*, 2008, **46**, 551–555.
146. P. K. Gupta, K. Ganesan, P. K. Gutch, L. Manral and D. K. Dubey, Vapor pressure and enthalpy of vaporization of fentanyl, *J. Chem. Eng. Data*, 2008, **53**, 841–845.
147. L. Manral, P. K. Gupta, M. V. S. Suryanarayana, K. Ganesan and R. C. Malhotra, Thermal behaviour of fentanyl and its analogues during flash pyrolysis, *J. Therm. Anal. Calorim.*, 2009, **96**, 531–534.
148. P. Yadov, J. S. Chauhan, K. Ganesan, P. K. Gupta, D. Chauhan and P. D. Gokulan, Synthetic methodology and structure activity relationship study of *N*-[1-(2-phenethyl)-piperidin-4-yl]propionamides, *Pelagia Research Library Der Pharm. Sin.*, 2010, **1**, 126–139.
149. P. K. Gupta, S. K. Yadov, Y. D. Bhutia, P. Singh, P. Rao, N. L. Gujar, K. Ganesan and R. Bhattacharya, Synthesis and comparative bioefficacy of *N*-(1-phenethyl-4-piperidinyl)propionanilide (fentanyl) and its 1-substituted analogues in Swiss albino mice, *Med. Chem. Res.*, 2013, **22**, 3888–3896.
150. S. K. Yadov, C. K. Maurya, P. K. Gupta, A. K. Jain, K. Ganesan and R. Bhattacharya, Synthesis and biological evaluation of some novel 1-substituted fentanyl analogues in Swiss albino mice, *Interdiscip. Toxicol.*, 2014, **7**, 93–102.
151. O. Navrátil, Z. Kobliha and E. Halámek, Solvent extraction of some incapacitating agents, *J. Radioanal. Nucl. Chem.*, 2004, **262**, 429–432.
152. L. Hess, J. Schreiberova and J. Fusek, Pharmacological non-lethal weapons, in *Third European Symposium on Non-Lethal Weapons*, Ettlingen, Germany, 10–12 May 2005, http://non-lethal-weapons.org.
153. R. Jelinkova, E. Halámek and Z. Kobliha, The possibility of identifying selected opioids by spectral analysis, *Mil. Med. Sci. Lett.*, 2013, **82**, 1–8.
154. E. Halámek and Z. Kobliha, Potential chemical warfare agents, *Chem. Listy*, 2011, **105**, 323–333.
155. V. Pitschmann, Overall view of chemical and biochemical weapons, *Toxins*, 2014, **6**, 1761–1784.
156. Z. Yang and J. Zhang, The synthesis of the potent analgesic sufentanil, *Yiyao Gongye*, 1985, **16**, 241–242.
157. J. Hu, Y. Li, J. Chen, F. Guo and Y. Liu, Crystal structure of the *N*-[4-acetyl-1-(2-cyclohexylethyl)-4-piperidinyl]-*N*-phenylpropionamide, *Jiegon Huaxue*, 1987, **6**, 53–57.
158. K. Lingce, Z. Guomin, L. Guangqiang, C. Zhenxing and C. Weiping, Surface-enhanced Raman spectroscopy for trace fentanyl detection in water, *Chin. J. Light Scattering*, 2010, **22**, 34–38.

159. L. Qi, Z. Cheng, G. Zao, S. Li and Q. Fan, Oxidative degradation of fentanyl in aqueous solutions of peroxides and hypochlorites, *Def. Sci. J.*, 2011, **61**, 29–34.
160. L. Xu, L. Ren, Z. Wang, X. Tian, L. Qi, Q. Fan and Y. Xiang, Oxidative treatment of fentanyl compounds in water by sodium bromate combined with sodium sulphite, *Water Sci. Technol.*, 2015, **72**(**1**), 38–44.
161. R. G. Thompson, D. Menking and J. J. Valdes, *Opiate receptor binding properties of carfentanil*, Chemical Research, Development & Engineering Center, Aberdeen Proving Ground, Maryland, USA; Technical Report CRDEC-TR-88029, November 1987 (unclassified).
162. H. D. Banks and C. P. Ferguson, *The metabolites offentanyl and its derivatives*, Chemical Research, Development & Engineering Center (CRDEC), Aberdeen Proving Ground, Maryland, USA, Technical Report 88139, September 1988 (unclassified).
163. R. Mioduszewski, S. Reutter and D. Berg, Pharmacological effects of opioid agonist and antagonist co-administered in ferrets, in *Proceedings of the 1989 U.S. Army Chemical Research, Development and Engineering Center Scientific Conference on Chemical Defense Research, Aberdeen MD, USA, held on 14-17 November 1989*, 1990, pp. 903–909, (unclassified).
164. L. P. Reiff and P. B. Sollman, *Process of making carfentanil and related analgesics*, US Patent 5,106,983, 1992.
165. R. J. Mioduszewski, *Opiate analgesic formulation with improved safety*, US Patent 5,834,477, 1998.
166. J. M. Lakoski, W. B. Murray and J. M. Kenny, *The Advantages and Limitations of Calmatives for Use as a Non-Lethal Technique*, College of Medicine Applied Research Laboratory, Pennsylvania State University, USA, 30 October 2000.
167. H. Shankaran, F. Adeshina and J. C. Teeguarden, Physiologically-based pharmacokinetic model for fentanyl in support of the development of provisional advisory levels, *Toxicol. Appl. Pharmacol.*, 2013, **273**, 464–476.
168. A. J. Walz and F. L. Hsu, *Synthesis of intermediate anilino methyl esters used in the production of synthetic opioid analgesics*, US Patent 8,742,111 B1, 2014.
169. A. Dahan, A. Yassan, H. Bijl, R. Romberg, E. Sarton, L. Teppema, E. Olofsen and M. Danhof, Comparison of the respiratory effects of intravenous buprenorphine and fentanyl in humans and rats, *Br. J. Anaesth.*, 2005, **94**, 825–834.
170. S. Mercadante, G. Prestia, C. Adile and A. Casuccio, Intranasal fentanyl *versus* pectin nasal spray for the management of breakthrough cancer pain in doses proportional to basal opioid regimen, *J. Pain*, 2014, **15**, 602–607.
171. D. Taylor, L. Radbruch, J. Revnic, L. M. Torres, J. E. Ellershaw and M. Perelman, A report on the long-term use of fentanyl pectin nasal spray in patients with recurrent breakthrough pain, *J. Pain Symptom Manage.*, 2014, **47**, 1001–1007.

172. L. E. Mather, Clinical pharmacokinetics of fentanyl and its newer derivatives, *Clin. Pharmacokinet.*, 1983, **8**, 422–446.
173. L. E. Mather and G. K. Gourlay, Pharmacokinetics of fentanyl, in *Transdermal Fentanyl: A New Approach to Prolonged Pain Control*, ed. K. A. Lehmann and D. Zech, Springer-Verlag, Heidelberg, Germany, 1991, pp. 73–97.
174. C. S. Reilly, A. J. J. Wood and M. Wood, Variability of fentanyl pharmacokinetics in man. Computer predicted plasma concentrations for three intravenous dosage regimens, *Anaesthesia*, 1985, **40**, 837–843.
175. T. Kosugi, S. Hamada, C. Takigawa, K. Shinozaki, H. Kunikane, F. Goto, S. Tanda, Y. Shima, K. Yomiya, M. Matoba, I. Adachi, T. Yoshimoto and K. Eguchi, A randomized, double-blind, placebo-controlled study of fentanyl buccal tablets for breakthrough pain: efficacy and safety in Japanese cancer patients, *J. Pain Symptom Manage.*, 2014, **47**, 950–1000.
176. G. Zeppetella, A. Davies, I. Eijgelshoven and J. P. Jansen, A network meta-analysis of the efficacy of opioid analgesics for the management of breakthrough cancer pain episodes, *J. Pain Symptom Manage.*, 2014, **47**, 772–785.
177. M. L. Arvanitis and R. C. Satonik, Transdermal fentanyl abuse and misuse, *Am. J. Emerg. Med.*, 2002, **20**, 58–59.
178. T. P. Coon, M. Miller, D. Kaylor and K. Jones-Spangle, Rectal insertion of fentanyl patches: a new route of toxicity, *Ann. Emerg. Med.*, 2005, **46**, 473.
179. S. Chrubasik, J. Chrubasik, G. Friedrich, D. Niv, E. Geller, J. Meynadier and J. Schulte-Mönting, Postoperative pain treatment by means of a morphine aerosol: a multicenter study, in *Advances in Pain Therapy II*, ed. J. Chrubasik, E. Martin and M. J. Cousins, Springer-Verlag, Heidelberg, Germany, 1993, pp. 151–167.
180. N. Masters, G. Heap, J. Wedly and A. Moore, Inhaled nebulised morphine and diamorphine: useful in general practice?, *Practitioner*, 1988, **232**, 910–914.
181. J. Chrubasik, H. Wüst, G. Friedrich and E. Geller, Absorption and bioavailability of nebulized morphine, *Br. J. Anaesth.*, 1988, **61**, 228–230.
182. M. H. Worsley, A. D. MacLeod, M. J. Brodie, A. J. Astbury and C. Clark, Inhaled fentanyl as a method of analgesia, *Anaesthesia*, 1990, **45**, 449–451.
183. O. R. Hung, S. C. Whynot, J. R. Varvel, S. L. Shafer and M. Mezei, Pharmacokinetics of inhaled liposome-encapsulated fentanyl, *Anesthesiology*, 1995, **83**, 277–284.
184. D. L. Roerig, K. J. Kotrly, E. J. Vucins, S. B. Ahlf, C. A. Dawson and J. P. Kampine, First pass uptake of fentanyl, meperidine, and morphine in the human lung, *Anesthesiology*, 1987, **67**, 466–472.
185. D. L. Roerig, K. J. Kotrly, S. B. Ahlf, C. A. Dawson and J. P. Kampine, Effect of propranolol on the first pass uptake of fentanyl in the human and rat lung, *Anesthesiology*, 1989, **71**, 62–68.
186. T. K. Henthorn, Y. Liu, M. Mahapatro and K. Y. Ng, Active transport of fentanyl by the blood-brain barrier, *JPET*, 1999, **289**, 1084–1089.

187. K. A. Marquardt and R. S. Tharratt, Inhalation abuse of fentanyl patch, *J. Toxicol. Clin. Toxicol.*, 1994, **32**, 75–78.
188. D. Sutlović and M. Definis-Gojanović, Suicide by fentanyl, *Arh. Hig. Rada Toksikol.*, 2007, **58**, 317–321.
189. M. Boom, E. Olofsen, M. Neukirchen, R. Fussen, J. Hay, G. J. Groeneveld, L. Aarts, E. Sarton and A. Dahan, Fentanyl utility function: a risk-benefit composite of pain relief and breathing responses, *Anesthesiology*, 2013, **119**, 663–674.
190. A. Hindle, Intrathecal opioids in the management of acute postoperative pain, Continuing Education in Anaesthesia, *Crit. Care Pain*, 2008, **8**, 81–85.
191. T. D. Egan, S. E. Kern, K. T. Muir and J. White, Remifentanil by bolas injection: a safety, pharmacokinetic, pharmacodynamic, and age effect investigation in human volunteers, *Br. J. Anaesth.*, 2004, **92**, 335–343.
192. A. S. Michaels, S. K. Chandrasekaran and J. E. Shaw, Drug permeation through human skin: theory and in vitro experimental measurement, *AIChE J.*, 1975, **21**, 985–996.
193. H. Lövborg, M. Holmlund and S. Hägg, Medication errors related to transdermal opioid patches: lessons from a regional incident reporting system, *BMC Pharmacol. Toxicol.*, 2014, **15**, 31.
194. N. M. Zadymova, Colloidochemical aspects of transdermal drug delivery (a review), *Colloid J.*, 2013, **75**, 491–503.
195. G. Oliveira, J. Hadgraft and M. E. Lane, Toxicological implications of the delivery of fentanyl from gel extracted from a commercial transdermal reservoir patch, *Toxicol. In Vitro*, 2012, **26**, 645–648.
196. R. H. Guy, J. Hadgraft and D. A. Bucks, Transdermal drug delivery and cutaneous metabolism, *Xenobiotica*, 1987, **17**, 325–343.
197. S. D. Roy, S. Y. E. Hou, S. L. Witham and G. L. Flynn, Transdermal delivery of narcotic analgesics: comparative metabolism and permeability of human cadaver skin and hairless mouse skin, *J. Pharm. Sci.*, 1994, **83**, 1723–1728.
198. J. R. Varvel, S. L. Shafer, S. S. Hwang, P. A. Coen and D. R. Stanski, Absorption characteristics of transdermally administered fentanyl, *Anaesthesiology*, 1989, **70**, 928–934.
199. R. H. Larsen, F. Nielsen, J. A. Sørensen and J. B. Nielsen, Dermal penetration of fentanyl: inter- and intraindividual variations, *Pharmacol. Toxicol.*, 2003, **93**, 244–248.
200. K. V. Roskos and H. I. Maibach, Percutaneous absorption and age implications for therapy, *Drugs Aging*, 1992, **2**, 432–449.
201. N. F. J. Van Nimmen, K. L. C. Poels and H. A. F. Veulemans, Identification of exposure pathways for opioid narcotic analgesics in pharmaceutical production workers, *Ann. Occup. Hyg.*, 2006, **50**, 665–677.
202. A. P. Klockgether-Radke, F. W. Sertürner und die Entdeckung des Morphins, *Anästhesiol. Intensivmed. Notfallmed. Schmerzther*, 2002, **37**, 244–249.

203. C. J. Weitz, L. I. Lowney, K. F. Faull, G. Feistner and A. Goldstein, 6-Acetylmorphine: a natural product present in mammalian brain, *Proc. Natl. Acad. Sci. U. S. A.*, 1988, **85**, 5335–5338.
204. J. J. Vallner, J. T. Stewart, J. A. Kotzan, E. B. Kirsten and I. L. Honigberg, Pharmacokinetics and bioavailability of hydromorphone following intravenous and oral administration to human subjects, *J. Clin. Pharmacol.*, 1981, **21**, 152–156.
205. E. Prommer, Oxymorphone: a review, *Supportive Care Cancer*, 2006, **14**, 109–115.
206. J. Kemsley, Lethal injections under new scrutiny, *Chem. Eng. News*, 2014, 46–48.
207. J. H. Jaffe and W. R. Martin, Opioid analgesics and antagonists, in *Goodman and Gilman's The Pharmacological Basis of Therapeutics*, ed. A. G. Gilman, T. W. Rall, A. S. Nics and P. Taylor, Pergamon Press, Oxford UK, 1990, 8th edn, ch. 21, pp. 485–521.
208. R. M. Julien, *A Primer of Drug Action: A Concise, Nontechnical Guide to the Actions, Uses, and Side Effects of Psychoactive Drugs*, W. H. Freeman & Company, New York USA, ch. 10, pp. 282–318.
209. A. Dahan, L. Aarts and T. W. Smith, Incidence, reversal, and prevention of opioid-induced respiratory depression, *Anesthesiology*, 2010, **112**, 226–238.
210. B. A. Berkowitz, The relationship of pharmacokinetics to pharmacological activity: morphine, methadone and naloxone, *Clin. Pharmacokinet.*, 1973, **1**, 219–230.
211. S. F. J. Clarke, P. I. Dargan and A. L. Jones, Naloxone in opioid poisoning: walking the tightrope, *Emerg. Med. J.*, 2005, **22**, 612–616.
212. K. Smith, M. Hopp, G. Mundin, S. Bond, P. Bailey, J. Woodward and D. Bell, Low absolute bioavailability of oral naloxone in healthy subjects, *Int. J. Clin. Pharmacol. Ther.*, 2012, **50**, 360–367.
213. T. M. Robertson, G. W. Hendey, G. Stroh and M. Shalit, Intranasal naloxone is a viable alternative to intravenous naloxone for prehospital narcotic overdose, *Prehospital Emerg. Care*, 2009, **13**, 512–515.
214. E. Sarton, L. Teppema and A. Dahan, Naloxone reversal of opioid-induced respiratory depression with special emphasis on the partial agonist/antagonist buprenorphine, *Adv. Exp. Med. Biol.*, 2008, **605**, 486–491.
215. S. W. Borron and V. S. Bebarta, Asphyxiants, *Emerg. Med. Clin. North Am.*, 2015, **33**, 89–115.
216. M. C. Meyer, A. B. Straughn, M. W. Lo, W. L. Schary and C. C. Whitney, Bioequivalence, dose-proportionality, and pharmacokinetics of naltrexone after oral administration, *J. Clin. Psychiatry*, 1984, **45**, 15–19.
217. G. Gerra, A. Marcato and R. Caccavari, Clonidine and opiate receptor antagonists in the treatment of heroin addiction, *J. Subst. Abuse Treat.*, 1995, **12**, 35–41.
218. A. S. Roth, R. B. Ostroff and R. E. Hoffman, Naltrexone as a treatment for repetitive self-injurious behaviour: an open-label trial, *J. Clin. Psychiatry*, 1996, **57**, 233–237.

219. M. W. Miller, M. A. Wild and W. R. Lance, Efficacy and safety of naltrexone hydrochloride for antagonizing carfentanil citrate immobilization in captive Rocky Mountain elk (*Cervus elaphus nelsoni*), *J. Wildl. Dis.*, 1996, **32**, 234–239.
220. J. C. Haigh and C. C. Gates, Capture of wood bison (*Bison bison athabascae*) using carfentanil-based mixtures, *J. Wildl. Dis.*, 1995, **31**, 37–42.
221. B. H. Pypendop, R. J. Brosnan and J. E. Llkiw, Use of naltrexone to antagonize high doses of remifentanil in cats: a dose-finding study, *Vet Anaesth. Analg.*, 2011, **38**, 594–597.
222. R. Dixon, J. Gentile, H. B. Hsu, J. Hsiao, J. Howes, D. Garg and D. Weidler, Nalmefene: safety and kinetics after single and multiple oral doses of a new opioid antagonist, *J. Clin. Pharmacol.*, 1987, **27**, 233–239.
223. R. Dixon, J. Howes, J. Gentile, H. B. Hsu, J. Hsiao, D. Garg, D. Weidler, M. Meyer and R. Tuttle, Nalmefene: intravenous safety and kinetics of a new opioid antagonist, *Clin. Pharmacol. Ther.*, 1986, **39**, 49–53.
224. K. Ingman, N. Hagelberg, S. Aalto, K. Någren, A. Juhakoski, S. Karhuvaara, A. Kallio, V. Oikonen, J. Hietala and H. Scheinin, Prolonged central mu-opioid receptor occupancy after single and repeated nalmefene dosing, *Neuropsychopharmacology*, 2005, **30**, 2245–2253.
225. G. M. Keating, Nalmefene: a review of its use in the treatment of alcohol dependence, *CNS Drugs*, 2013, **27**, 761–772.
226. Z. Yong, X. Gao, W. Ma, H. Dong, Z. Gong and R. Su, Nalmefene reverses carfentanil-induced loss of righting reflex and respiratory depression in rats, *Eur. J. Pharmacol.*, 2014, **738**, 153–157.
227. E. R. Jacobson, G. V. Kollias, D. J. Heard and R. Caligiuri, Immobilization of African elephants with carfentanil and antagonism with nalmefene and diprenorphine, *J. Zoo Animal Med.*, 1988, **19**, 1–7.
228. M. Filizola and L. A. Devi, How opioid drugs bind to receptors, *Nature*, 2012, **485**, 314–317.
229. R. Al-Hasani and M. R. Bruchas, Molecular mechanisms of opioid receptor-dependent signalling and behaviour, *Anesthesiology*, 2011, **115**, 1363–1381.
230. G. Edwards, *Matters of Substance*, Penguin Ltd., London UK, 2004, p. 80.
231. A. Manglik, A. C. Kruse, T. S. Kobilka, F. S. Thian, J. M. Mathiesen, R. K. Sunahara, L. Pardo, W. I. Weis, B. K. Kobilka and S. Granier, Crystal structure of the μ-opioid receptor bound to a morphinan antagonist, *Nature*, 2012, **485**, 321–326.
232. H. Wu, D. Wacker, M. Mileni, V. Katritch, G. W. Han, E. Vardy, W. Liu, A. A. Thompson, X. P. Huang, F. I. Carroll, S. W. Mascarella, R. B. Westkaemper, P. D. Mosier, B. L. Roth, V. Cherezov and R. C. Stevens, Structure of the human κ-opioid receptor in complex with JDTic, *Nature*, 2012, **485**, 327–332.
233. S. Granier, A. Manglik, A. C. Kruse, T. S. Kobilka, F. S. Thian, W. I. Weis and B. K. Kobilka, Structure of the δ-opioid receptor bound to naltrindole, *Nature*, 2012, **485**, 400–404.

234. A. A. Thompson, W. Liu, E. Chun, V. Katritch, H. Wu, E. Vardy, X. P. Huang, C. Trapella, R. Gueurrini, G. Calo, B. L. Roth, V. Cherezov and R. C. Stevens, Structure of nociception/orphanin FQ receptor in complex with a peptide mimetic, *Nature*, 2012, **485**, 395–399.
235. W. Huang, A. Manglik, A. J. Venkatakrishnan, T. Lacremans, E. N. Feinberg, A. L. Sanborn, H. E. Kato, K. E. Livingston, T. S. Thorsen, R. C. Kling, S. Granier, P. Gmeiner, S. M. Husbands, J. R. Traynor, W. I. Weis, J. Steyaert, R. O. Dror and B. K. Kobilka, Structural insights into μ-opioid receptor activation, *Nature*, 2015, **524**, 315–321.
236. R. Sounier, C. Mas, J. Steyaert, T. Lacremans, A. Manglik, W. Huang, B. K. Kobilka, H. Déméné and S. Granier, Propagation of conformational changes during μ-opioid receptor activation, *Nature*, 2015, **524**, 375–378.
237. T. A. Bowdle, Adverse effects of opioid agonists and agonist-antagonists in anaesthesia, *Drug Safety*, 1998, **19**, 173–189.
238. M. Yeadon and I. Kitchen, Binding characteristics of [D-Ala^2-MePhe^4-Glyol^5] enkephalin and [D-Pen^2,D-Pen^5] enkephalin in rat brain: inhibition studies with fentanyl-like drugs, *NIDA Res. Monogr.*, 1986, **75**, 64–66.
239. H. H. Szeto, Y. Soong, D. Wu, N. Olariu, A. Kett, H. Kim and J. F. Clapp, Respiratory depression after intravenous administration of *δ*-selective opioid peptide analogues, *Peptides*, 1999, **20**, 101–105.
240. P. Maguire, N. Tsai, J. Kamal, C. Cometta-Morini, C. Upton and G. Loew, Pharmacological profiles of fentanyl analogs at μ, δ and κ opiate receptors, *Eur. J. Pharm.*, 1992, **213**, 219–225.
241. C. J. Endres, B. Bencherif, J. Hilton, I. Madar and J. J. Frost, Quantification of brain μ-opioid receptors with [^{11}C]carfentanil: reference-tissue methods, *Nucl. Med. Biol.*, 2003, **30**, 177–186.
242. L. Dosen-Micovic, M. Ivanovic and V. Micovic, Steric interactions and the activity of fentanyl analogs at the μ-opioid receptor, *Bioorg. Med. Chem.*, 2006, **14**, 2887–2895.
243. Y. S. Lee, J. Nyberg, S. Moye, R. S. Agnes, P. Davis, S. W. Ma, J. Lai, F. Porreca, R. Vardanyan and V. J. Hruby, Understanding the structural requirements of 4-anilidopiperidine analogues for biological activities at μ and δ opioid receptors, *Bioorg. Med. Chem. Lett.*, 2007, **17**, 2161–2165.
244. M. Yeadon and I. Kitchen, Differences in the characteristics of opioid receptor binding in the rat and marmoset, *J. Pharm. Pharmacol.*, 1988, **40**, 736–739.
245. A. Arias, R. Feinn and H. R. Kranzler, Association of an Asn40Asp (A118G) polymorphism in the μ-opioid receptor gene with substance dependence: a meta-analysis, *Drug Alcohol Depend.*, 2006, **83**, 262–268.
246. D. Nishizawa, K. Fukuda, S. Kasai, J. Hasegawa, Y. Aoki, A. Nishi, N. Saita, Y. Koukita, M. Nagashima, R. Katoh, Y. Satoh, M. Tagami, S. Higuchi, H. Ujike, N. Ozaki, T. Inada, N. Iwata, I. Sora, M. Iyo, N. Kondo,

M. J. Won, N. Naruse, K. Uehara-Aoyama, M. Itokawa, M. Koga, T. Arinami, Y. Kaneko, M. Hayashida and K. Ikeda, Genome-wide association study identifies a potent locus associated with human opioid sensitivity, *Mol. Psychiatry*, 2014, **19**, 55–62.

247. Y. Feng, X. He, Y. Yang, D. Chao, L. H. Lazarus and Y. Xia, Current research on opioid receptor function, *Curr. Drug Targets*, 2012, **13**, 230–246.
248. H. Pleym, O. Spigset, E. D. Kharasch and O. Dale, Gender differences in drug effects: implications for anesthesiologists, *Acta Anaesth. Scand.*, 2003, **47**, 241–259.
249. *The Merck Index: An Encyclopedia of Chemicals, Drugs, and Biologicals*, ed. M. J. O'Neil, Merck & Co. Inc., Whitehouse Station NY, USA, 14th edn, 2006.
250. P. S. A. Glass, Remifentanil: a new opioid, *J. Clin. Anesth.*, 1995, **7**, 558–563.
251. J. Lambropoulos, G. A. Spanos, N. V. Lazaridis, T. S. Ingallinera and V. K. Rodriguez, Development and validation of an HPLC assay for fentanyl and related substances in fentanyl citrate injection, USP, *J. Pharm. Biomed. Anal.*, 1999, **20**, 705–716.
252. A. Garg, D. W. Solas, L. H. Takahashi and J. V. Cassella, Forced degradation of fentanyl: identification and analysis of impurities and degradants, *J. Pharm. Biomed. Anal.*, 2010, **53**, 325–334.
253. W. Wichitnithad, T. J. McManus and P. S. Callery, Identification of isobaric product ions in electrospray ionization mass spectra of fentanyl using multistage mass spectrometry and deuterium labeling, *Rapid Commun. Mass Spectrom.*, 2010, **24**, 2547–2553.
254. R. K. Nishikawa, S. C. Bell, J. C. Kraner and P. S. Callery, Potential biomarkers of smoked fentanyl utilizing pyrolysis gas chromatography-mass spectrometry, *J. Anal. Toxicol.*, 2009, **33**, 418–422.
255. B. Singh, G. K. Prasad, K. S. Pandey, R. K. Danikhel and R. Vijayaraghavan, Decontamination of chemical warfare agents, *Def. Sci. J.*, 2010, **60**, 428–441.
256. K. Kim, O. G. Tsay, D. A. Atwood and D. G. Churchill, Destruction and detection of chemical warfare agents, *Chem. Rev.*, 2011, **111**, 5345–5403.
257. Potential Military Chemical/Biological Agents and Compounds, US Army Field Manual No 3-9 (FM 3-9), Department of the Army, Washington, DC, 12 December 1990, p. 50.
258. L. Qi, G. Zao, Z. Cheng, L. Wang and C. Zhou, Treatment of chemical warfare agents by combined sodium percarbonate with tetraacetylethylenediamine solution, *Chem. Eng. J.*, 2013, **229**, 197–205.
259. Presentation by V. V. Turygin of the Russian State Institute of Organic Chemistry and Technology (GosNIIOKhT), Moscow, at the 17th Conference on Electrochemistry of Organic Compounds, held on 27-30 September 2010 at the Tambov State Technical University, mentioned in: A. G. Krivenko, V. A. Kurmaz and V. P. Gul'tyai, *Russ. J. Electrochem.*, 2011, **47**, 968–971.

260. T. Tobin, S. Kwiatkowski, D. S. Watt, H. H. Tai, C. L. Tai, W. E. Woods, J. P. Goodman, D. G. Taylor, T. J. Weckman, J. M. Yang, J. D. Tai, S. D. Stanley, T. Wood, S. L. Chang, J. W. Blake, J. McDonald, S. Wie, C. A. Prange and C. E. Uboh, Immunoassay detection of drugs in racing horses. XI. ELISA and RIA detection of fentanyl, alfentanil, sufentanil and carfentanil in equine blood and urine, *Res. Commun. Chem. Pathol. Pharmacol.*, 1989, **63**, 129–152.
261. T. Tobin, H. H. Tai, C. L. Tai, P. K. Houtz, M. R. Dai, W. E. Woods, J. M. Yang, T. J. Weckman, S. L. Chang, J. W. Blake, J. McDonald, R. Gall, P. Wiedenbach, V. D. Bass, B. Deleon, F. J. Ozog, M. Green, C. Brockus, D. Stobert, S. Wie and C. A. Prange, Immunoassay detection of drugs in racing horses. IV. Detection of fentanyl and its congeners in equine blood and urine by a one step ELISA assay, *Res. Commun. Chem. Pathol. Pharmacol.*, 1988, **60**, 97–115.
262. Y. Dotsikas, Y. L. Loukas and I. Siafaka, Determination of umbilical cord and maternal plasma concentrations of fentanyl using novel spectrophotometric and chemiluminescence enzyme immunoassays, *Anal. Chim. Acta*, 2002, **459**, 177–185.
263. M. R. Gravett, F. B. Hopkins, M. J. Main, A. J. Self, C. M. Timperley, A. J. Webb and M. J. Baker, Detection of organophosphorus nerve agent VX and its hydrolysis products in white mustard plants grown in contaminated soil, *Anal. Methods*, 2013, **5**, 50–53.
264. M. R. Gravett, F. B. Hopkins, A. J. Self, A. J. Webb, C. M. Timperley and M. J. Baker, Evidence of VX nerve agent use from contaminated white mustard plants, *Proc. R. Soc. A*, 2014, **470**, 20140076.
265. M. J. Baker, M. R. Gravett, F. B. Hopkins, D. G. C. Rees, J. R. Riches, A. J. Self, A. J. Webb and C. M. Timperley, Plants as nerve agent detectors, *OPCW Today*, 2014, **3**(**1**), 27–36.
266. F. B. Hopkins, M. R. Gravett, A. J. Self, M. Wang, H. C. Chua, H. S. Nancy Lee, J. T. A. Jones, C. M. Timperley and J. R. Riches, Chemical analysis of bleach and hydroxide-based solutions after decontamination of the chemical warfare agent *O*-ethyl *S*-2-diisopropylaminoethyl methylphosphonothiolate (VX), *Anal. Bioanal. Chem.*, 2014, **406**, 5111–5119.
267. M. R. Gravett, F. B. Hopkins, A. J. Self, A. J. Webb, C. M. Timperley and J. R. Riches, Fate of the chemical warfare agent *O*-ethyl *S*-2-diisopropylaminoethyl methylphosphonothiolate (VX) on soil following accelerant-based fire and liquid decontamination, *Anal. Bioanal. Chem.*, 2014, **406**, 5121–5135.
268. A. Üzümcü, The Chemical Weapons Convention – disarmament, science and technology, *Anal. Bioanal. Chem.*, 2014, **406**, 5071–5073.
269. The OPCW Science & Technology Monitor – A sampling of Science and Technology Relevant to the Chemical Weapons Convention, vol. 2, Number 7, 1 June 2015, pp. 4–6 (http://www.opcw.org).
270. D. A. McClain and C. C. Hug, Intravenous fentanyl kinetics, *Clin. Pharmacol. Ther.*, 1980, **28**, 106–114.
271. R. B. Labroo, M. F. Paine, K. E. Thummel and E. D. Kharasch, Fentanyl metabolism by human hepatic and intestinal cytochrome P450 3A4:

implications for interindividual variability in disposition, efficacy, and drug interactions, *Drug Metab. Dispos.*, 1997, **25**, 1072–1080.

272. T. Tateishi, Y. Krivoruk, Y. F. Ueng, A. J. Wood, F. P. Guengerich and M. Wood, Identification of human liver cytochrome P-450 3A4 as the enzyme responsible for fentanyl and sufentanil N-dealkylation, *Anesth. Analg.*, 1996, **82**, 167–172.
273. W. Meuldermans, A. Van Peer, J. Hendrickx, R. Woestenborghs, W. Lauwers, J. Heykants, G. Vanden Bussche, H. Van Craeyvelt and P. Van der Aa, Alfentanil pharmacokinetics and metabolism in humans, *Anesthesiology*, 1988, **69**, 527–534.
274. Y. Higashikawa and S. Suzuki, Studies on 1-(2-phenethyl)-4-(*N*-proprionylanilino)piperidine (fentanyl) and its related compounds: novel metabolites in rat urine following injection of α-methylfentanyl, one of the most abused typical designer drugs, *J. Health Sci.*, 2008, **54**, 629–637.
275. J. F. Hoke, F. Cunningham, M. K. James, K. T. Muir and W. E. Hoffman, Comparative pharmacokinetics and pharmacodynamics of remifentanil, its principal metabolite (GR90291) and alfentanil, *JPET*, 1997, **281**, 226–232.
276. L. G. Michelsen and C. C. Hug, The pharmacokinetics of remifentanil, *J. Clin. Anesth.*, 1996, **8**, 679–682.
277. V. U. Navapurkar, S. Archer, S. K. Gupta, K. T. Muir, N. Frazer and G. R. Park, Metabolism of remifentanil during liver transplantation, *Br. J. Anaesth.*, 1998, **81**, 881–886.
278. R. W. Milne, R. L. Nation and A. A. Somogyi, The disposition of morphine and its 3- and 6-glucuronide metabolites in humans and animals, and the importance of the metabolites to the pharmacological effects of morphine, *Drug Metab. Rev.*, 1996, **28**, 345–472.
279. B. L. Coffmann, G. R. Rios, C. D. King and T. R. Telphy, Human UGT2B7 catalyzes morphine glucuronidation, *Drug Metab. Dispos.*, 1997, **25**, 1–4.
280. D. Paul, K. M. Standifer, C. E. Inturrisi and G. W. Pasternak, Pharmacological characterization of morphine-6 beta-glucuronide, a very potent morphine metabolite, *J. Pharmacol. Exp. Ther.*, 1989, **251**, 477–483.
281. S. Y. Yeh, C. W. Gorodetzky and H. A. Krebs, Isolation and identification of morphine 3- and 6-glucuronides, morphine-3,6-diglucuronide, morphine 3-ethereal sulfate, normorphine, and normorphine 6-glucuronide as morphine metabolites in humans, *J. Pharm. Sci.*, 1977, **66**, 1288–1293.
282. D. Projean, P. E. Morin, T. M. Tu and J. Ducharme, Identification of CYP3A4 and CYP2C8 as the major cytochrome P450s responsible for morphine *N*-demethylation in human liver microsomes, *Xenobiotica*, 2003, **33**, 841–854.
283. B. L. Coffman, C. D. King, G. R. Rios and T. R. Tephly, The glucuronidation of opioids, other xenobiotics, and androgens by human UGT2B7Y(268) and UGT2B7H(268), *Drug Metab. Dispos.*, 1998, **26**, 73–77.
284. D. French, The challenges of LC-MS/MS analysis of opiates and opioids in urine, *Bioanalysis*, 2013, **5**, 2803–2820.

Subject Index